Language Disabilities in Cultural and Linguistic Diversity

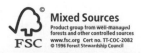

BILINGUAL EDUCATION & BILINGUALISM
Series Editors: Nancy H. Hornberger, *University of Pennsylvania, USA* and
Colin Baker, *Bangor University, Wales, UK*

Bilingual Education and Bilingualism is an international, multidisciplinary series
publishing research on the philosophy, politics, policy, provision and practice of
language planning, global English, indigenous and minority language education,
multilingualism, multiculturalism, biliteracy, bilingualism and bilingual education.
The series aims to mirror current debates and discussions.

**Full details of all the books in this series and of all our other publications can
be found on http://www.multilingual-matters.com, or by writing to Multilingual
Matters, St Nicholas House, 31-34 High Street, Bristol BS1 2AW, UK.**

BILINGUAL EDUCATION & BILINGUALISM
Series Editors: Nancy H. Hornberger, *University of Pennsylvania,*
USA and Colin Baker, *Bangor University, Wales, UK*

Language Disabilities in Cultural and Linguistic Diversity

Deirdre Martin

MULTILINGUAL MATTERS
Bristol • Buffalo • Toronto

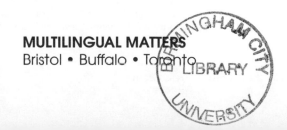

To my mother and father

Library of Congress Cataloging in Publication Data
A catalog record for this book is available from the Library of Congress.
Martin, Deirdre.
Language Disabilities in Cultural and Linguistic Diversity/Deirdre Martin.
Bilingual Education & Bilingualism
Includes bibliographical references and index.
1. Learning disabled children–United States–Language. 2. Language disorders in children–United States. 3. Communicative disorders in children–United States. 4. English language–Study and teaching–United States–Foreign speakers. 5. Linguistic minorities–Education–United States. 6. Multiculturalism–United States.
I. Title.
LC4704.85.M36 2009
371.91′4–dc22 2009009449

British Library Cataloguing in Publication Data
A catalogue entry for this book is available from the British Library.

ISBN-13: 978-1-84769-160-6 (hbk)
ISBN-13: 978-1-84769-159-0 (pbk)

Multilingual Matters
UK: St Nicholas House, 31-34 High Street, Bristol BS1 2AW, UK.
USA: UTP, 2250 Military Road, Tonawanda, NY 14150, USA.
Canada: UTP, 5201 Dufferin Street, North York, Ontario M3H 5T8, Canada.

The policy of Multilingual Matters/Channel View Publications is to use papers that are natural, renewable and recyclable products, made from wood grown in sustainable forests. In the manufacturing process of our books, and to further support our policy, preference is given to printers that have FSC and PEFC Chain of Custody certification. The FSC and/or PEFC logos will appear on those books where full certification has been granted to the printer concerned.

Typeset by Datapage International Ltd.
Printed and bound in Great Britain by the Cromwell Press Group.

Contents

Acknowledgements

Many people have supported me in writing this book and I would like to acknowledge my debt of gratitude to them. In particular I thank Colin Baker who has been the most supportive and encouraging of editors. I am also grateful to Tommi Grover and Multilingual Matters who have been steadfast publishers.

I am grateful to my colleagues in the School of Education at the University of Birmingham who awarded me sabbatical leave to begin writing this text. I am also indebted to my colleagues in the Centre of Socio-Cultural and Activity Theory in the School of Education which offered a forum for enquiry, discussion and empirical research in socio-cultural and Vygotskian thinking. Together with my colleagues on the ESRC TLRP funded research project, Learning in and for Interagency Work, they enabled me to develop my understanding of language and learning, although they may not recognise their contribution here.

This book would not have been written without the inspiration, confidence and support of my friends and family. I am most grateful.

Introduction

Rethinking Traditional Perspectives

The study of language disability is in a period of change. For some time, the psycho-bio-medical approach has orientated our understanding of language-related disabilities, such as specific speech and language impairment, dyslexia and deafness. The focus of research has been the nature (phenotypes) and core characteristics of language disabilities. Findings have been applied to practices concerned with identification, assessment and intervention of core features of disabilities. More recently, this approach has been extended to contexts of cultural and linguistic diversity (CLD) and sociolinguistic concerns (e.g. Genesee *et al.*, 2004; Centeno *et al.*, 2007). We are in a position now to consider the extent to which the traditional paradigm is a sufficient tool to explore and explain how language-related disabilities work in complex dimensions of social, cultural and linguistic diversity.

This book critiques the traditional approach to language-related disabilities through a sociocultural lens. The critique draws on Vygotskian and sociocultural perspectives to (re)interpret psychological and socio-linguistic research, and present a theoretically coherent view of language disabilities in culturally and linguistically diverse contexts. From a Vygotskian and sociocultural perspective, learning is both social and cognitive, and enabled by language. It is a particularly appropriate and powerful perspective for the purposes of this book. A reconceptualisation of language disabilities in contexts of diversity emphasises the central role of language(s) and communication for learning and transformation. A sociocultural approach has implications not only for research and practice with bilingual children with language disabilities, but also for interprofessional learning for work with families and colleagues who are culturally and linguistically diverse.

The Context

Changing demographics among school student populations, from homogenous to diverse, presents particular challenges for research and practice in the field of special education and language disabilities.

Although the number of bilingual children in many countries has increased dramatically in the last few decades, most research continues to be focused on monolingual children (for review see Leonard, 1998) and comparatively few studies deal with speech and language-related disabilities in bilingual children.

The capability of practitioners to meet the needs of diverse student populations remains a controversial professional education issue. Educators of practitioners have continued to question whether practitioners – both trained and preservice – have the requisite skills and the necessary sensitivity toward diversity to meet the challenges associated with effectively teaching culturally and linguistically diverse students (Marbley *et al.*, 2007). This book engages with the challenge of preparing practitioners and researchers, where the majority are likely to be monolingual English, monocultural and white, but not limited to that group, who work with an increasingly culturally and linguistically diverse student and client population.

A specific example of the need to develop practitioners' knowledge is revealed in findings from research studies concerning professional confusion about 'disentangling' *learning* needs from *language-learning* needs for schooling (e.g. Troyna & Siraj-Blatchford, 1993; Gillborn & Youdell, 2000; Cline & Shamsi, 2000; Lindsay *et al.*, 2006). That is, professional practices continue to confuse the educational needs embedded in learning English as an additional language (EAL) with cognitive learning needs and specific speech, language and communication needs. Professional confusion highlights an important theoretical and empirical site for further research and is a focus for discussions in this book.

Children who appear to learn language differently or with difficulty are a resource for understanding how we perform language learning. They may be situated in diverse sociolinguistic contexts, or they may be differently equipped biologically for language learning. These children afford opportunities for us to tease apart the cultural assumptions made about language development and practices within and across distinct language communities. They also provide a site for us to interrogate theoretical, empirical and professional assumptions about language development, difference and disability.

Terminology

Some terms that are used frequently in the text are introduced here and discussed more fully in subsequent chapters.

Bilingualism is understood in a variety of ways. Monolinguals in monolingual cultures may believe that being bilingual is for a few 'special' people. In fact, one in three of the world's population routinely uses two or more languages for work, family life and leisure. If we include those who use two or more languages occasionally, then monolinguals are the minority (Li Wei, 2000: 5). Bilingualism is not only a feature of individual capability, but also of a society's identity. As a social practice in communities and in schools, bilingualism is a site of social and political tension in many countries that traditionally see themselves as monolingual, such as the UK, USA and Australia. In the USA, the bilingual education movement has grown into a political movement. It is driven partly by the English For All/English Only legislation, which was passed in States, such as California, that have substantial bilingual and non-English-speaking populations. In the UK, there is no similar political movement for bilingual education. Nevertheless, discourses at national level about bilingualism in citizenship, and the need for language testing among minority linguistic communities, shape the everyday lives of bilingual learners and the practitioners who work with them. These discourses are recognised as important influences on research and practice, and they are the backdrop for discussions in this book.

Being bilingual primarily describes someone with possession of two or more languages and often refers to multilingual people as well. The terms *multilingual* and *bilingual* are often used interchangeably in the literature and they are in this book. These terms include speakers with varying degrees of proficiency across languages, from understanding only, to include speaking and literacy skills in both languages. While bilingualism may include school-taught foreign languages, particularly English as a foreign language (EFL), it usually refers to learning and using language on a regular basis for everyday use. Communicating through two or more languages is both an individual's skill, and also a collective practice in families and societies. Using a language is usually domain-specific, related to people, places or topic. Language is also linked closely with identity and allegiance; bilingual people's preference for using only one language may reflect their changes in self-identity and community allegiances (Baker, 1992; Myers-Scotton, 2006).

Second language learning. In addition to the terms bilingual and multilingual, there are many terms describing speakers of two or more languages. Some terms indicate the sequence of language acquisition while others index importance of one of the learners' languages. Among the most commonly used terms are *Second Language Acquisition* (SLA),

Second Language (L2) *learners,* learners of *English as an Additional Language* (EAL), *English as a Second Language* (ESL), and a term used mainly in the USA, *Limited English Proficiency* (LEP).

    Cultural and linguistic diversity (CLD) is a generic term that is increasingly used by researchers and practitioners. CLD indexes the range of sociocultural contexts and practices, including race, cultural heritage, religious beliefs, social class and socioeconomic status, which inform the social processes that shape the social and educational experiences of communities, families and individual learners. Through-out the book, I mainly use the terms: bilinguals, EAL learners and CLD. In citing studies, the terms of the authors are used.

    Diversity is a term often used to describe and to emphasise the heterogeneity and complexity of differences across disability, culture and language. Diversity offers an alternative to simplistic bipolar constructs. For example, the notion of disability is often understood as a homo-geneous 'other' that contrasts with the notion of able-ness (Norwich, 1990; Wedell, 2005). In this book, the main driver for discourses of diversity is the protection of minority groups from discriminatory descriptions. Discussions about diversity here, seek to make visible and conscious assumed (nonconscious) beliefs and to (re)present more fairly and inclusively groups in society that are vulnerable to majority exclusionary forces.

    Culture is often thought of in normative ways, as neatly bound traditions that help to differentiate groups of people, as when we say: 'Irish do this; English do that'. In this way, the concept of culture is presented as well-integrated, cohesive entities whose values are shared by all members of a group, each with its own predictable folk theory, values, socialisation patterns and academic outcomes (Moll, 2000: 257). Sociology has abandoned this structural construct and moved to a more process-based, dynamic understanding, where culture is multivoiced with unity and discords. This discourse of culture emphasises that *culture is in human practices* (Moll, 2000: 258). The term 'cultural and linguistic diversity' is informed by this concept, which enables us to recognise and conceptualise shared and diverse human practices both within and across apparent cultural structures. For example, understanding dis-ability through values of human dignity is shared across diverse culture groups and underpins similar social practices.

    The term *special education* specifically refers to specialist education provision for particular learners with disabilities and special educational needs (SEN). In the UK and many countries, it has been replaced by inclusive education. Most learners with additional learning needs are included in mainstream education supported by additional resources where necessary. In the USA, bilingual education is a part of 'special education' provision. Bilingual education in the UK refers to a small amount of provision for bilingual learners learning in two languages, namely in Wales and Scotland. Minority community languages, which in many countries are the first languages of bilingual children, are generally taught in supplementary schools outside mainstream provision in the UK (see Creese *et al.*, 2006). Bilingual learners of EAL are included in mainstream education in the UK.

Terms for disability vary within the field of disability studies and they emerge from different traditions. There are terms such as handicap, impairment, SEN and disability, as well as the descriptor terms for cognitive, sensory and physical categories of disability. Category terms can be used differently across countries. The term 'learning difficulties' in the UK is synonymous with 'mental retardation' in the USA, and 'dyslexia' or 'specific learning difficulties' in the UK is known as 'learning difficulties' in the USA. The terms 'disorder' and 'impairment' are from a medical discourse traditionally used in research and practice around language: specific language impairment, children's communication disorders. The terms 'difficulties' and 'needs' are from a discourse of social models of disability and are used in this book to describe language disabilities. Discourses of disability are discussed more fully in Chapter 3.

In this book I have chosen to examine what is traditionally known as 'categories of impairment', which concern language-related disabilities, specifically, speech and language difficulties, dyslexia and deafness. I have chosen them because they present a particularly sensitive site, around language and communication, where the axes for the construction of disability and diversity may be most easily confused. This site affords insightful exploration of how we conceptualise and perform practice in contexts of disability and diversity.

Blaming Diversity, Disabling Diversity

There are discourses that construct diversity as a problem. They present diversity and difference as interfering with the smooth running of aspects of mainstream society and services. Disruptions caused to mainstream life are the fault of individuals who are diverse or different. One analogy is that society is like a clock and when the clock breaks down it is not the *system* that is faulty, but rather individual elements within it (Paulston, 1992, in Baker, 2001: 399). Similar analogies are offered by Valencia (1997) concerning poorly made/broken spectacles, and escalators that damage people who use them, where customers, and not the manufacturers, are blamed for damaged goods. He uses these analogies to illustrate the ways that barriers to education and other services are constructed for culturally and linguistically diverse communities. The more powerful manufacturers/providers of goods blame the less powerful users for the resulting damage and harm, rather than accept responsibility for faulty and inadequate goods. From this perspective, when problems are perceived by the dominant majority group, such as perceived threats to health, wellbeing and educational achievement, advocates assert that it is not the mainstream provision that needs to be corrected, but rather specific culturally and linguistically diverse consumers.

Social practices of exclusion and inclusion around language diversity are under-researched and not widely recognised by well-intentioned practitioners. An important focus of this book is to examine the social processes that 'blame diversity' for challenging mainstream provision of services, and which construct diversity itself as disabling.

Disability, SEN and Diversity

There are substantial challenges – barriers even – to doing a literature review in the area of disability, SEN and diversity. Research and professional practices have kept these areas separated by their own traditions (Daniels *et al.*, 2001a). Research and practice in this area has yet to become a recognised discipline or field of study. The area of 'disability and cultural and linguistic diversity' remains a space for the creation of new knowledge. It is a space shaped and informed by a range of boundaried, compartmentalised disciplinary knowledges: biological, medical, health, education, disability, SEN, ethnicity, race, bilingualism, SLA, multiculturalism, equal opportunities, underachievement. It is a zone of potential reconceptualisation in future research.

A review of Canadian literature on the intersections of disability and race/ethnicity, heritage language and religion concludes that

> So much research is needed that it is impossible to prioritize, except to return to the need for research to recognise the full participation of ethno-racial people with disabilities and their communities in the research process, from their vantage point, recognizing and valuing their expertise and addressing their benefit. (Steinstra, 2002: 22)

Steinstra (2002) analyses the literature during the 1990s along strands of the Canadian context, looking in turn at the intersections of race, ethnicity, heritage languages and religion. She uses a social model of disability and identity frameworks to evaluate the studies. She concludes that there seem to be mainly two views of disability from a multicultural and multilingual perspective. Firstly, in the literature there is the 'either/or' construct, where disabled people from CLD heritages have a primary identity. People are constructed as having 'either' a primary identity as a disabled person who is also a member of a minority bilingual or cultural community, **or** conversely, they are primarily constructed as minority ethnic/linguistic with a disability. A second construct, 'both–and' posits dual or multiple identities for people with disability and diverse languages and cultures. For example, studies of minority ethnic people with deafness have explored both these notions of identity. They have examined the extent to which individuals construct themselves primarily *either* as Deaf and members of the Deaf community albeit from minority families *or* as being members of a minority ethnic/linguistic community who are also deaf. Alternatively, do they construct themselves as being *both* deaf *and* Deaf *and* a member of the minority ethnic community? In other words, identity is fluid and constructed *in situ* with the resources available. Research also needs to explore the extent to which service providers facilitate development of flexible multiple identities. How would a fluid identity of disability develop?

There are practices of exclusion in research on disability and diversity. Reflecting on one aspect of disability and diversity, Cline and Reason (1993: 30–34) observe about dyslexia and ethnicity:

> it seems strange that the research traditions on specific learning difficulties (dyslexia) and social and cultural differences have remained in different compartments.

Many researchers of bilingualism, SLA and CLD explicitly note that they exclude discussion of children and learners who have biologically based educational difficulties, such as deafness, severe learning difficulties. Researchers may focus on sociocultural, including racist, practices that marginalise diversity, which perform 'disabling diversity'. On the other hand, approaches to studying disability that are embedded in biomedical-based difficulties often demonstrate either a lack of curiosity and inertia/resistance to exploring the contribution that CLD could offer to understanding disability, or they exclude children and adults who are culturally, ethnically and linguistically diverse because these social factors 'contaminate' and complicate the research study (Diniz, 1999).

Nevertheless, there are important indicators that researching disability and diversity is emerging as a discipline of study, evidenced in handbooks on special education and diversity and working with speech and language disability in bilingualism (Baca & Cervantes, 1998, 2003; Battle, 2002; Centeno *et al.*, 2007; Duncan, 1989; Frederickson & Cline, 2002; Genesee *et al.*, 2004; Harry, 1992; Isaac, 2002; Kayser, 1995; Kohnert, 2007; Miller, 1984).

This text attempts to mark out a field of study on bilingualism and disability, and where its core and boundaries might be. It draws together two fields of research and practice in bilingualism studies and disability studies, and reveals parallels and relationships between them. An inevitable consequence of the multidisciplinary nature of the area of disability, ethnicity and CLD is the 'underlap' in studies, and the consequent 'underlap' in conceptualisation. This book contributes to the enterprise of developing conceptualisations of language-related disabilities in contexts of cultural and linguistic diversity.

Chapter Themes

In this book, I develop a coherent and cohesive understanding of disability, specifically, language-related disabilities, in contexts of diversity by drawing on a sociocultural lens to bring into focus other approaches, which are prevalent in this area. The book opens with some broad perspectives on disability in contexts of cultural and multilingual diversity and introduces more specialist ideas in later chapters.

The sociocultural orientation for this book is set out in Chapter 1 to inform subsequent chapters. The following chapters open with a case study vignette that illustrates issues being discussed. The second chapter examines sociocultural contexts and practices around CLD and the discourses that construct CLD as 'barriers' to access and take up of provision. The third chapter explores inclusive and exclusive practices of health and education provision to culturally and linguistically diverse families and children with language disabilities. The fourth chapter examines the dominant cognitive discourse of the nature of speech, language and communication difficulties in children developing two languages. The fifth chapter examines discourses around dyslexia and explores the inter-relatedness of psychological and sociocultural research for educational practice. The sixth chapter explores deafness and Deafness in children with bilingual minority linguistic families and issues of multiple identities being deaf in diverse cultures, religions and ethnicities. Chapter 7 critiques formal assessment methods of language disabilities in bilingual children and explores the advantages of using dynamic assessment approaches. Chapter 8 draws on learning theories to examine practices of intervention and teaching with bilingual children with language disabilities. Chapter 9 examines multidisciplinary collaboration among practitioners working to meet the needs of bilingual children with language difficulties. Chapter 10 explores practice and provision for bilingual parents and families with children with language disabilities.

The book works to achieve:

(1) a (re)conceptualisation of language disabilities within a socio-cultural perspective;
(2) a contribution to a community of research and practice around language-related disabilities in cultural and linguistic diversity;
(3) a resource for students and researchers in this emerging field;
(4) a resource for interprofessional development for mainstream and special needs teachers, psychologists, speech and language therapists and assistants involved in the field of language-related disabilities in culturally and linguistically contexts.

This book contributes to the small yet growing body of research, emergent conceptualisations and discourses in the field of language disability in linguistic diversity. It presents a critical reflection on, and (re)conceptualisation of, existing literature across pertinent areas of research and practice. The book is written for researchers and professionals from backgrounds in health and education who work with language-related disabilities in culturally and linguistic diversity. Its main focus and purpose is not so much on developing 'craft' and skills for practitioners' work, but rather on informing the assumptions that underpin policies and practice that frame practitioners and clients' daily routines. This approach supports professional development of masters and doctoral students, managers and policymakers in the fields of health, social work and education who work with each other as well as with and for those with language disabilities in culturally and linguistically diverse contexts. The next chapter presents key ideas about language and learning, context and diversity that orientate discussion throughout the book.

Chapter 1

A Sociocultural Activity Approach: Key Concepts

Introduction

This chapter presents the theoretical approach and key concepts used in further chapters to interpret research and practice with language-related disabilities and cultural and linguistic diversity (CLD). The dominant approach to understanding language disabilities is through linguistic, cognitive and psycholinguistic avenues of research and practice. While sociocultural and historical issues are always considered in practice with children and families with language disabilities, the importance of conceptualising this dimension is underscored in contexts of CLD. This chapter sets out a Vygotskian approach to understanding language difficulties in CLD contexts, and draws together linguistic, cognitive and psycholinguistic perspectives with sociocultural constructs. The chapter weaves these approaches across three sections. The first section examines relationships between reality and knowledge, in order to draw attention to the importance of self-consciousness and reflexion in contexts of diversity and difference between researcher/researched and practitioner/client. The second section looks specifically at models used to represent language development and disability, and the third section presents key concepts of a Vygotskian perspective concerning language and learning.

Knowledge and Representations

In this section, I discuss representations of language, language disability and diversity in the research literature. Relationships between reality and the representation of reality underpin our understanding of the world and the assumptions we bring to considering language learning, language disabilities and diversity. The conceptual power of theories and models informs different discourses and practices for language-related learning needs, and examining discourse and practice gives a window onto our construction of knowledge. With reference to language disability and diversity, models recruited to inform research and practice are constructions of understanding built up from social, cultural and historical traditions.

Wartofsky's (1979: xv) thoughts offer an important perspective:

> we create cognitive artifacts which not only go beyond the biological evolved and genetically inherited modes of perceptual and cognitive activity but which radically alter the very nature of learning... The cognitive artifacts we create are models: representations to ourselves of what we do, of what we want, and of what we hope for. The model is, therefore, not simply a reflection or a copy of some state of affairs, but beyond this, a putative mode of action, a representation of prospective practice, or of acquired modes of action... The model is taken to be a construction in which we organize symbols of our experience or of our thought in such a way that we effect a systematic representation of this experience or thought as a means of understanding it, or of explaining it to others.

Wartofsky argues here that we use our cognitive capacities to create new tools for thinking. These cognitive tools, models, do not reflect back to us our lived reality. Rather, they act on our experiences by abstracting them into symbolic signs and organising them into systems so that they re-present our lived reality for us and are a way of making sense of it to ourselves and to others. In this way, a distinction is maintained between the model and what it is a model of. I draw on this approach as a conceptual tool to discuss some of the powerful conceptual models that shape construction and use of knowledge by researchers and practitioners and by learners with language-related disabilities and their bilingual parents and families.

A powerful tool for organising our experiences is language. We use it internally to organise lived experiences in order to *make sense* of them alongside the other knowledge we have. We use language to organise what is external and social, in order to *make meaning* and create shared cognitions with others of what we perceive. Collective language practices are referred to as discourses, which transform issues, experiences and our reality into discursive objects that contribute to our conceptualisation of them. Talk and discourses are tools to organise problems and conceptualise knowledge. We distinguish lived reality from the representation by using cognitive tools for organising experience. Models of experience are built from nonlinguistic symbols, such as gestures, mathematics, pictures, as well as linguistic artefacts of discourse. Wartofsky argues that representing and making representations is something we *do*, rather than being in the nature of the represented/ representation. Furthermore, it is a reflexive activity:

> the active role which representation and the use of models plays in shaping our perception and cognition, and in serving as a heuristic guide to our theoretical or practical activity .. it is suggested that ... our perceptual and cognitive understanding of the world is in large part shaped and changed by the representational artifacts we ourselves create. We are in effect the products of our own activity, in this way: we transform our own perceptual and cognitive modes, our ways of seeing and of understanding, by means of the representations we make. (Wartofsky, 1979: xxiii)

This quote is important because it emphasises the reflexive relationship between reality and the constructs we use to interpret and enact reality. The representations and metaphors we use to talk about reality become our perceived reality. Thus, shared ways of talking and discourses of texts and policies about CLD and disability, particularly language-related disabilities, are the artefacts we use to shape practices with people who are culturally and linguistically diverse with language disabilities. A salient example is the different representations of knowledge held by researchers, professional groups and parents concerning two groups of bilingual children: those with language-learning difficulties in both their languages and those with difficulties learning a second language having successfully learnt their first. The cognitions that we have about each group of children take professionals, parents and researchers on different trajectories of thinking and behaving with these children in their practices and in research. The relationship between practice traditions and learning is revisited later in the chapter.

Metaphors of Language Development and Disability

Theories, models and metaphors are important cognitive devices to support human thinking as well as being shared conceptual tools to support communal thinking (Mercer, 2000: 173). I present three metaphors of learning language in contexts of disability and diversity with an emphasis on learning, and argue that sociocultural metaphors offer a best fit for the realities of language disabilities and diversity. Two metaphors are frequently used to describe learning and particularly language learning: *acquisition* and *participation*, and a more recent third metaphor is co-construction (Sfard, 1998; Donato, 2000; Hager, 2004).

Metaphors are used as tools for conceptual development by describing a subject in terms of another subject, so that our understanding is enhanced. Characteristics of the first subject are transposed to the second; often a concrete object or experience is used to relate to something abstract or conceptual. While conceptual understanding is enhanced in one way, it is also limited by the concrete dimensions and orientations of the metaphor. Hence, there is a dynamic in (re)searches for further metaphors that are a better fit for the characteristics of the abstract or conceptual reality. For example, the 'bucket theory' (Crystal, 1987) was recruited to explain language development and disability, and drew on the familiar metaphor of mind: a container with hierarchic levels and input. While this metaphor captured some salient characteristics of language development and disability, it could not capture the complexity of dynamic disability across language levels.

> A model of limited linguistic processing which is based on a notion of hierarchy is premature. Rather, a simpler model, referred to here as the "bucket" model, in which the different levels exercise mutual influence without priorities, is more appropriate in our present state of knowledge. (Crystal, 1987: 7)

For similar reasons, the container metaphor of language for bilingual development was abandoned. While it could represent the characteristic of two developing language codes, it could not represent the socio-linguistic complexities of bilingualism evident in reality, such as codeswitching. Crystal notes that the usefulness of metaphors is intimately related to our current understanding of reality. Metaphors for conceptual understanding are evident in research paradigms as well as in professional practices and policies. I discuss three metaphors for learning, specifically applied to language.

The *acquisition* metaphor is often used to explain the maturation of a biological predisposition of language. This nativist position is put by Pinker (1994: 8):

> I prefer the admittedly quaint term "instinct". It conveys the idea that people know how to talk in more or less the sense that spiders know how to spin webs. Web-spinning was not invented... spiders spin webs because they have spider brains which give them the urge to spin and the competence to succeed.

The acquisition metaphor foregrounds language, the assumption of a given source of language knowledge, often Universal Grammar, rather than learning. The acquisition metaphor represents language such that 'heads come fully loaded' and only need minimal triggering from the environment to grow to their full functionality (van Lier, 2000: 259). Metaphors of acquisition and language instinct capture nonconscious, tacit learning characteristics of first language development. It is a highly influential model of language development that shapes research paradigms in the field, with its emphasis on down-playing the impact of environment, and using (quasi) experimental paradigms, comparing 'real' talk with 'ideal' targets. It is most frequently associated with development as 'product', demonstrated in practices such as measuring language development by acquired items of language, in decontextualised scenarios. The acquisition metaphor is used to explain developmental difficulties in speech, language and communication due to a genetic predisposition. It supports a large body of empirical research focused on specific difficulties with language structure (see Chapter 4).

The acquisition metaphor also represents the *language information-processing* model. This model emphasises the powerful cognitive strategies involved in language development, and is highly influential in the field of speech and language development and disabilities. Metaphors for information processing are closely linked to historical developments in related areas of knowledge. The model emerged in the 1970s when widespread use of computers for problem solving and storing information led some psychologists to use computer processing as a representation of processing in the human mind. Cognitive processing models have provided powerful cognitive artefacts and heuristic devices for under standing processing and the breakdown in processing of speech and language information (e.g. Fodor, 1983; Dockrell & McShane, 1993; Stackhouse & Wells, 1997). Models have been developed to offer insights on structural hierarchic development, which embrace bilingual and additional language development (Pienemann, 2005, see Chapter 4). The metaphors in this perspective conceptualise speech and language knowledge in terms of internal representations stored in memory to be accessed, retrieved and manipulated. It, too, constructs learning as 'product' and draws on the container metaphor of mind-as-filing-cabinet, where new learning of content can be added, in an atomised, sequential way (Middleton & Brown, 2005). These conceptual tools have shaped research and practice by informing diagnostic practices, programmes of intervention and decisions about educational provision.

However, the acquisition metaphor of language development offers little insight for the purposes of culturally and linguistically diverse children with language disability. It is limited in its representation both of development through explicit teaching/learning and intervention, and of the effect of cultural practices and diverse language environments on language development and disability. The language instinct metaphor relies on an underspecified source of language knowledge for first language development and is unable to offer a source for additional language development. Cognitive approaches explain language learning and additional language learning through strategies. Cognitive models often use the mechanistic metaphor of 'input'/'output' to describe language development and teaching learning. Yet, this metaphor is unable to capture the complexity of dialogic and negotiated practice that is common in developmental and teaching-learning scenarios, either formally in class, or informally between parent and child or between peers. Nor does it capture concepts of language learning in contexts of CLD.

A consequence of the dominance and limitations of the acquisition metaphor in research on speech and language difficulties is that intervention is a relatively undertheorised and under-researched area. A similar pattern was evident in early second language acquisition (SLA) research, but teaching-learning in SLA and bilingual language development has become more researched in studies that draw on sociocultural approaches to language learning. Researchers (see Lantolf, 2000) working in a sociocultural approach, explore, in particular, multilingual learning in culturally diverse contexts around the activity of collective meaning making and sense making in children.

There are implications of the acquisition metaphor for policy and practice with language learning and language-related disability for children from culturally and linguistically diverse homes. The nativist model of the acquisition metaphor dominates research, which emphasises speed and ease of language acquisition and places little emphasis on language environments for language learning. While the cognitive model represents becoming bilingual as making increased demands on language knowledge and processing knowledge and thus more complex within-the-head processing. This approach may inform (mis)advice about simplifying 'input' to one language. Yet, it is evident that children across the gamut of ability can and do become bilingual. This real-life situation is a strong driver to consider other metaphors that represent more accurately language learning in disability and diversity.

The *participation* metaphor is frequently used to represent language learning as participating in practice, discourse and activity. Language development and learning is a process of change for the learner and their environment. Learning is situated, contextualised and influenced by cultural, historical and social factors. A metaphor for this understanding of learning is 'the gradually clearing of a fog in a landscape', indicating the gradual growth of understanding, rather than an all-or-nothing 'across-the-board' learning event represented in the acquisition metaphor (Hager, 2004: 8). To construct a rounded understanding of language growth, it may be unwise to adopt one metaphor over the other. The social is not absent in the acquisition metaphor and acquisition in the form of internalised social practices and conversation is not absent from the participation metaphor (Donato, 2000: 40). The participation metaphor has informed research and practice with bilingual language development and second/additional language learning, while its implications for informing conceptualising research and assessment practices, intervention and pedagogy with language disability are only beginning to be explored.

A more recent third metaphor is also used for learning and language learning: construction (Hager, 2004) and specifically *transformative through co-construction* (Wells, 1999). It contrasts with the acquisition metaphor by refuting assumptions that abilities and learning emerge independently from their historical and cultural settings. Co-construction captures the individual's engagement with the social context as well as the gradual building of knowledge and understanding, and is discussed next, through a Vygotskian perspective. All three metaphors are referred to in discussion of literature in subsequent chapters.

A Vygotskian Approach

Practitioners and researchers have drawn on theories for understanding disability and diversity, which straddle different traditions. Biomedical and psycholinguistic approaches are most often used to represent knowledge about language development and disability. On the other hand, knowledge about historical, cultural and social practices of marginalisation and 'disabling diversity' are usually drawn from sociocultural approaches. This analysis presents the familiar dualism of cognitive, inside-the-head, rationalist approaches and social, cultural, romanticist approaches. Yet, both approaches to representing knowledge are needed to inform ways of investigating and supporting language difficulties shown by bilingual children.

A Vygotskian perspective addresses this dualism and offers a way forward to understanding language disabilities in bilingualism. Researchers with this perspective assert that learning, including language learning, is understood as a cognitive endeavour (intrapsychological, intramental) at the same time as it is a social and cultural enterprise (interpsychological, intermental). Rather than giving primacy to either the individual or the social, sociocultural processes and individual functioning exist in an 'irreducible dynamic tension' (Wertsch, 2000). Language knowledge is created through individual sense making and collective meaning making. Individuals reconstruct and co-construct new language knowledge with each other and within themselves (John-Steiner & Meehan, 2000).

One interpretation of a sociocultural approach to language is offered by Thorne (2000: 223) as:

> a term applied to the efforts of Vygotsky and his students to formulate "a psychology grounded in Marxism" (Wertsch, 1985: 7) with an emphasis on locating the individual within collective, material and historical conditions. A sociocultural approach empha-sizes language as socially constructed rather than internally intrinsic, language as both referential and constructive of social reality and notions of distributed and assisted activity in contrast to individual accomplishment. Central to this approach is that human activity is mediated by material artifacts and by symbolic sign systems, the most important of which is language.

So, here we have a theory that has as its central focus mediation between CLD and individual bilingual language development. In line with the *co-construction* metaphor of language in learning, this book approaches understanding language disabilities in culturally and linguistically diverse populations based on the notion of mediation between that which is sociocultural (external and social) and that which is cognitive/psycholinguistic (internal and individual).

Key Concepts

Concepts that are central to understanding Vygotskian perspectives on social learning and language are presented here, and revisited and expanded in subsequent chapters. The relevance of this perspective to language-related disabilities and CLD is highlighted. Central notions of tools, particularly language, and context used to (co)construct social, cultural and historical shared meanings are discussed. First, I discuss four key ideas which inform Vygotsky's concept of learning: learning as social and individual, learning as a transformational process, the zone of proximal development (ZPD) and language as a tool for learning. Central to these ideas is the notion of mediation.

Mediation

When the individual acts upon the world and is acted upon by social, cultural and historical factors the activity is called mediation (Daniels, 2001: 14). In mediation, we use tools to act directly or indirectly on the object of learning. Language is one of the most powerful tools for mediating learning and language learning. As children develop language, they make things happen without having to do the thing themselves. Similarly, they can be influenced by others directly and indirectly through the mediating power of words and the culturally organised knowledge that words embody (Vygotsky, 1978). Vygotsky developed the insight that through the use of language, people alter and transform themselves. The importance of this notion for bilingual children is captured by Luria (1981: 35):

> With the help of language, children can deal with things that they have not perceived even indirectly and with things which were part of the experience of earlier generations. Thus, the word adds another dimension to the world of humans... Humans have a double world.

Historically, CLD extends Luria's idea of 'a double world'. Children, families and professionals with several languages and cultures will have 'multiple worlds'.

Figure 1.1 represents Vygotsky's basic learning relationship of mediation between people (actors, subjects) and the tools they use for mediating to accomplish the learning or 'activity' (object). A unified account of Vygotsky's original proposals on the nature and development of human learning and behaviour is presented by Leont'ev in Activity Theory (1978, 1981). Activity Theory is taken up in Chapter 9, in discussion of collaboration and interprofessional learning.

Mediation is the making of mind, that is, it concerns the relationship between the biological brain and the social, cultural and historical world.

> Luria (1973, 1979) refers to the system that results from the integration of artifacts into human activity, whether the activity be psychological or social as a functional system. Mind, according to Luria, is not, properly speaking, the activity of the biologically given brain, but it is a *functional system* formed when the brain's electro-chemical processes come under control of our cultural artifacts: foremost among these is language. (Lantolf, 2000: 8)

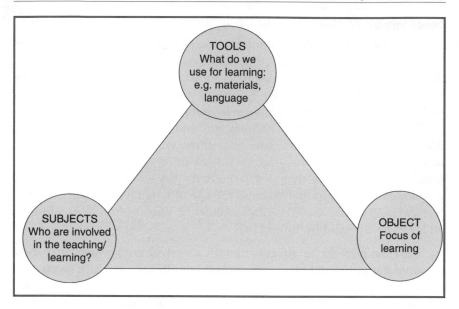

Figure 1.1 Learning 'Activity' system

Lantolf here clarifies that when cultural tools, such as language, mediate biological processes, then the human mind becomes a functional system. A functional system is one that *mediates* (can respond to and make sense of) external concerns in the world about us with our internal constructs of that world. We use cultural tools to make internal sense as well as external shared collective meaning among ourselves about the world around us. Children's minds emerge in joint mediated activity with the people around them. Their minds and language are co-constructed through tools from knowledge and expertise distributed around them. Artefacts can include physical tools, such as computers, books, food; symbolic tools, such as rituals, customs, dress; cultural tools such as communicative practices, language and literacy practices; as well as lived experiences, concepts and ideas.

In instances of language learning for first and additional languages and language disabilities, language is both the focus of learning as well as the tool for learning. In these cases, mediation relies on other psychological and cultural artefacts to develop language, such as developing an awareness of language, both as metacognitive and metalinguistic knowledge, as well as social and cultural communicative practices.

Learning as social and individual

Vygotsky is credited with understanding development, intelligence and learning as a readiness to use culturally transmitted knowledge and procedures as prostheses of the mind (Bruner, 1986: 141–142). That is, shared learning precedes and enables individual learning. Social, cultural, historical, *intermental* learning enables cognitive, inside-the-head *intramental* learning (Mercer, 2000). Learning is about developing cognitive capacities via social, collective learning capacities, and is as much about developing content knowledge as it is about learning self-awareness about how to learn, and creating new knowledge through social practices. The two planes are mediated by cultural tools, such as language, so that what were originally aspects of the interpersonal, social domain become internalised on the intramental cognitive plane. This understanding of internalisation reinterprets the cognitive approach, such that knowledge structures, like schemata, memory and language are defined as meaning-making tools that make sense of actions. For children in bilingual contexts this means that diverse sociocultural practices in the family are not extraneous to children's development, but core to developing their meaning-making capacities for making cognitive sense of their actions and interactions.

There are two important implications for children with language disabilities in culturally and linguistically diverse families. First, each language is a tool for learning intellectual and social cognitions as well as being the focus for learning. Second, for culturally and linguistically diverse families, when and which language is used for communication, learning and language learning is a situated choice. Selection of, or abandoning, a language has social, cultural, communicative and cognitive implications.

Learning as a transformational process

There are two main approaches to understanding the drivers of development, particularly language development, in children: developmental and determinist. Strong determinist interpretations of biological and social development do not hold out possibilities for changing the course of development. Biological endowment determines pace and extent of development of children. For example, for Piaget, growth happened 'naturally', that is, the child's mind developed through biological maturation and self-sufficiency within its own logic. Development did not consist in comparing its present status with what it would be later or might become under some special curricular dispensation (Bruner, 1986: 141). Piaget and others who represent development as being biologically bounded are determinists. From a Vygotskian perspective, biological and social determinism is eschewed, as Bruner (1986: 135) notes:

> Human culture is one of the ways by which "instructions" about how humans should grow are carried from one generation to the next – the other being the human genome... [hence] to say that a theory of development is "culture free" is to make not a wrong claim, but an absurd one.

Many sociological studies offer detailed and insightful accounts of cognitive and social stasis. From determinist perspectives, being born into poverty has largely unchangeable biological and cultural constraints on development. Similarly, social and religious class/caste is also presented as 'naturally' determined. More notoriously, determinist interpretations of racial differences argue that cognitive, emotional and social development is genetically determined (for review, see Valencia, 1999). The implications for culturally and linguistically diverse communities, many of which are often among the poorest in developed countries, are that determinist theories offer no means for change.

By contrast, 'Vygotsky is a growth theorist' (Bruner, 1986: 141). A Vygotskian approach does not interpret development as determined by biological, social or racial endowment. Vygotskian approaches to understanding development are primarily interested in how stasis in the individual and in society can be transformed. Researchers are concerned with social, cultural and historical formative events that bring about learning and development individually and collectively. They construct language as a key tool that bridges individual development with social culture. An approach that is focused on the knowledge of change, learning and the process of transformation could be highly useful for the study of and work with disability and social and racial disadvantage. An approach which places language as central to learning and transformation could offer a great deal for study and work with language-related disability in contexts of CLD.

Vygotsky posited that 'mediation' between the external and the internal brought about internalisation of new knowledge, meaning making and learning. The fundamental notion of learning is being able to think or do something that was previously beyond one's capability and do this learning in a social context with another or others. Vygotsky called the set of interactions in this space for learning, the zone of proximal development.

The zone of proximal development

Vygotsky observed that children respond in different ways to similar teaching, guidance and opportunities for learning, depending not only on their capabilities and potential to learn, but also on the engagement with teaching and guided joint practice. The difference between a child's original independent capability and eventual achievement with teaching, he called the child's zone of proximal development. To be effective, teaching and guided joint practice should work within the child's ZPD, at the boundaries of a child's or person's development to maximise their potential for learning, rather than work on what they can already do. It is future orientated: as Vygotsky said, what a child can do with help today she/he can do alone tomorrow (Vygotsky, 1978: 86). The notion of ZPD engages a new approach to assessing children's intellectual capabilities. Rather than measuring intellectual abilities as static, decontextualised skills, ZPD offered a way of looking at the dynamic process of learning, which was developing capacity.

From a critical perspective, changes in the child's ZPD have traditionally been characterised as individual changes that imply that the learner may do today what she/he could do yesterday with help. This led to an understanding that cognitive learning (internalisation) also included the transfer of social factors to the individual, and constituted the learner as a passive receiver of social material. However, a more accurate interpretation is that the main aspect of change in the ZPD is centred on the appropriation and acquisition of new forms of mediation. This appropriation does not just refer to individual learning after guided joint practice, but rather to the capacity of the learner to participate in new collaborative activities. The focus is not on the transfer of skills from those who know more to those who know less, but instead on the shared use of new forms of communication for creating and communicating meaning (de la Mata & Santamaria, 2001: 261). For children in bilingual families, this is evidenced in continuous learning and language learning in social and language routines across both (all) languages.

Opportunities for children to learn on their own and in community are framed culturally. Some cultures and individuals privilege the ideal of personal autonomy and independence and play down interdependence, while other cultures and individuals place great value on social and functional interdependencies, at the risk of being judged inferior. Most approaches to learning are mediated through negotiation with others and other tools in Vygotsky's notion of the ZPD. These tools and artefacts may be fit for purpose or have to be transformed by new understandings from their original purpose to a new one. Language is a key tool.

To be able to work in a learner's ZPD, the adult must judge carefully what the child understands at the time and base their communications with the child on this judgment. Adults need to modify the intellectual and language support they give the learner, to take account of developing knowledge and understanding. Bruner (1986, Wood *et al.*, 1976) use the metaphor of *'scaffolding'* for the temporary support that the adult, or other, gives a child as they co-construct learning. Scaffolding can be any guidance – nonverbal support, advice, simplifying the task – which helps the learner to accomplish a task which she/ he would not have been able to do on their own. Scaffolding for learning is

> the steps taken to reduce the degrees of freedom in carrying out some tasks so that the child can concentrate on the difficult skill she is in the process of acquiring. (Bruner, 1978: 19)

Scaffolding is a special kind of help. It is the important Other's, such as the teacher's, temporary, graduated assistance which helps a learner know how to do something so that they can complete a similar task alone.

For language development, even though the child has a biological predisposition to develop/learn language, the language of others is needed to mediate and support the development of language. For children with language disability there are implications for the kind of scaffolding in language intervention. There are implications for scaffolding language and content demands when teaching curriculum content to learners who have language disability and who are second language learners. For practitioners evaluating learners with language disability, dynamic assessment may be one way of making this judgment.

Language for learning

Language has been studied as a subject in its own right for a long time. Here, though, language is constructed in its relationship with learning, for communicative, social, cultural, emotional and academic purposes. Language is always closely associated with thinking, although primacy is contested. For Piaget, thought comes first. The maturational constraints of internal logic determine thinking, so that language reflects thought and does not determine it. Within his paradigm, there seems to be no avenue for socially and culturally developed ideas generated by language to disrupt the child's development. By contrast, one of Vygotsky's central metaphors is the notion of two separate streams of development that flow together: a stream of thinking and a stream of language. His view is that conceptual learning is a collaborative enterprise involving an adult or an important other who enters into dialogue with the child in a fashion that provides the child with hints and props that allow him/her to begin a new climb, guiding the child in graduated next steps before the child is capable of appreciating the significance on her/his own (Bruner, 1986: 132; Vygotsky, 1978).

Sociocultural theory, inspired by Vygotsky, has as its central claim that children's minds develop as a result of constant interactions with the social world. These interactions and experiences are shaped by 'cultural tools', such as social routines like meal times, parenting practices. The most important of these shared cultural tools is language – in terms of meaning, speech sounds, word strings and rules of communication. Language has a central role in Vygotsky's notion of learning in the zone of development. Language is a meaning-making tool that is used to negotiate and mediate actions.

Mercer (2000: 141) puts the emphasis on teaching-learning rather than assessment and refers to a learner's potential learning as the 'interthinking' process or the intermental zone of development (IZD). Learning potential is constructed by communication and negotiation and is particularly sensitive to dialogue. So, for practitioners to work with learners and for learners to learn with them, they must both use talk and joint activity to create a shared communicative space on the foundations of a shared context of common knowledge and aims. Thus, language is a tool kit that enables the negotiation and mediation of meaning making in teaching-learning activity (Wells, 1996). In culturally and linguistically diverse contexts, there are implications for using language for mediating learning and language learning. Language need not always be spoken by the child; watching language in use is a form of apprenticeship in becoming a language user. Children in bilingual environments develop receptive language knowledge by being present in communicative contexts without necessarily speaking the language (Romaine, 1995) and this seems to hold for those with language disabilities.

Next, I develop the sociocultural historical aspect of learning through two notions: learning as instrumental in terms of tools and artefacts involved in learning, the most important of which is language, and, second, the concept of context.

Sociocultural and historical meaning

Learning is the process of transformation in a child's, parent's or practitioner's relationship to her/his historical and social world. Learning is acquiring competence in situated practices with tools and artefacts. A tool for learning is more than just an implement to complete an activity, such as a pen for writing. The pen is imbued with cultural and historical meaning about its purpose. It is *'already* invested with cognitive and affective content... Tools and languages [are taken] to be objectifications of human needs and intentions' (Wartofsky, 1979: 204). The importance of understanding language as a tool in this sense, is that it contrasts with the structuralist (intramental) conceptualisation (Saussurre's notion of 'parole') of functional grammars that underpin much of the work in language disability and second language teaching. Languages in linguistically diverse societies are instruments imbued with cultural and historical meaning for the purpose of learning.

There are important implications of sociocultural and historical perspectives for children with language disabilities in culturally and linguistically diverse families. First, a linguistic analysis alone is insufficient to understand language and communication. The sociocultural and historical communicative practices in which children in families participate also need to be analysed, taking account of routines and the physical artefacts that are drawn on to perform them, such as toys, books and participation repertoires (Guttierrez & Rogoff, 2003). The emotional and motivational valiance of the home and other languages plays an important part in learning and maintaining communication (see Chapter 2 for further discussion).

Distributed cognition

The term 'distributed cognitions' has been used to describe

> how human knowledge is embodied as a collective resource in the tools, machines, and social routines we build and use together. (Mercer, 2000: 190)

From a Vygotskian perspective, knowledge learnt from shared collective activity (interpersonal) precedes individual cognitive learning (intrapersonal); so that individual capacities, such as language and social development, are developed through shared family activities around language and socialising. Thus, distributed cognition entails the notion that learning and communication are situated. Children with language learning difficulties are likely to perform optimally in situations where they are supported by shared resources of language and communication routines. Requiring children with language difficulties to perform in situations where they can rely only on their individual cognitive and linguistic resources is likely to elicit a less than optimal performance. There are implications for assessment practices and learning situations for bilingual children.

Affordance

Opportunities for learning are shaped by material and social *affordances* (van Lier, 2000). For example, a piece of lined writing paper can afford writing opportunities. If the lined paper is placed so that the lines run horizontally, the paper affords opportunities for writing in most alphabetic orthographies, but the paper would need to be turned so the lines ran vertically to afford writing opportunities for logographies, such as Japanese and Chinese. This example illustrates the implications for using materials and sociocultural knowledge to afford learning across cultures, languages and literacies. In a situation where a child does not engage with an activity offered by the practitioner, the child's reluctance may be interpreted as child deficit: lack of knowledge due to social and cultural disadvantage or to social or cognitive difficulties. An alternative explanation that does not negatively construct the child would be that the activity or materials did not offer affordances to the child to engage with. Scenarios such as looking at picture books, playing with particular toys in a particular way, parenting practices around child play, are often examples of (un)successful cultural affordances. Affordances are necessarily culturally and linguistically embedded to support language and learning.

Context

Much of the previous discussion about shared cultural knowledge and language use and development rests on the notion of context. Context is usually understood as 'that which surrounds' (Cole, 1996). The essential feature of context is that it is shared by the participants in the communication. There is a primary importance for creating context in interactions involving CLD. A shared language helps create a context for communication, and conversely where there is no shared language, it is difficult to create context and communication. Here are three examples that illustrate the importance of language, time and space in creating context in CLD.

Context can mean 'common knowledge' shared by speakers (readers/ writers). Families have shared memories, and members from the same community or heritage will have shared histories and experiences that they draw on to interpret the present. Where there is little shared prior knowledge, communication needs to make meanings more explicit and explanatory. There are implications for practitioners, researchers and linguistic minority families creating contexts to work together, and for minority families to access services and education. At a different level, professionals in the same discipline share technical knowledge through jargon and specialist language. There are implications for creating contexts to facilitate multidisciplinary work.

Context may be the physical or virtual surroundings shared by the speakers that construct *situated meaning*, where the situation surrounding the spoken or written text shapes the meaning. For example, how do you respond to the statement: *'The coffee's spilled'*? Do you bring a mop or a brush? (Gee, 2005). This illustration shows the intimate relationship between language, context, action or practice, and artefact for the individuals in communication. Learning and language learning is always situated practice and context dependent (Lave & Wenger, 1991; Lantolf, 2000), where context may be physical place, such as home, neighbour-hood, school, work, or an historical or imagined context, such as reading a book, or watching TV. Through situated practice, that is by living and interacting in these physical and virtual surroundings, individuals learn self-identity and about their position in their family, school, community and professional group.

The metaphor 'context as container' particularly as a container for learning is being eschewed by educational researchers (Ivanič, 2006). Context is understood as

> a relational phenomenon in which the "text" – what is going on – cannot be separated from the "con" what accompanies it. The "texture" of an event changes moment by moment as the elements which constitute it co-emerge: identities, relationships, actions, semiotic resources, the significance and use of space and time, all of which have historical trajectories, are networked to others, and are culturally shaped. (Ivanič, 2006: 8)

Context is created by activity, 'practice'. Practice traditions within institutions and communities constitute the social and cultural context and tools for learning. For example, each school has its own language practices, literacy practices as well as practices in the way curriculum subjects are taught, or homework practices. Children must learn the artefact (that is, the content of the practice), according to conditions of use, that is situated practice in context. For example, it is not enough to know the skills of reading, children need to be able to know how to enact the literacy practices of the school. There are implications for children with language disability learning sociocultural practices of school, and implications for language choice in bilingual families for children with language disability. For example, when children are asked to tell narratives (stories) as part of assessment, do they tell stories which come from school and curriculum culture or from home culture? There is likely to be a difference in these tasks which children themselves perceive and report. The language and cultural content of story telling are intimately interwoven (Blackledge, 1994).

Hedegaard *et al.* (2001) interpret Cole's (1996) definition of context 'that which surrounds' through Bourdieu's notion of 'field'. Each person is surrounded by different social fields, such as home, school, community and country. Families from ethnic and linguistic minority communities are usually surrounded by a complex set of fields constructed across minority and majority domains. Bourdieu's ideas are discussed further in later chapters as an important notion of context for understanding CLD when working with parents and families.

Before concluding the chapter, it is important to note that there are two groups of learners who are involved in developing knowledge about disability and diversity. One group is researchers, practitioners and their parents who have representations of knowledges of language disability and diversity which underpin their work with bilingual children with language disabilities. The other group is bilingual children and young people with language disabilities who need to develop and learn languages, literacies and other communication knowledges. Communication and language use is a sociocultural practice, and while individual children may have substantial difficulties learning their first and additional languages, the role of those who communicate with them plays a crucial part in their success learning language and communication practices.

Conclusions

This chapter has framed the discussion of language disabilities in linguistically and culturally diverse contexts within a Vygotskian orientation. Key concepts about learning and language have been introduced for reference and development in subsequent chapters.

I have argued that we draw on theoretical tools – concepts and metaphors – as representations of reality to understand language diversity and language-related disabilities. The constraints of acquisition and mentalist models are largely around their inability to specify the importance of CLD for developing language for bilingual children with language disabilities. These ideas may be familiar currency in practice for many practitioners and it is important to theorise practice. Abstracting the salient features of practices and contexts across space and time transforms practices into concepts which can 'travel', that is they can become tools to interpret and to inform past and future practices.

One of the purposes of this book is to address the question: to what extent can a Vygotskian approach offer a coherent and cohesive theoretical conceptualisation for language disabilities in linguistically and culturally diverse contexts? A Vygotskian perspective, that is a sociocultural historical and activity approach, focuses on language-for-learning, and identifies language as a key tool for learning and language learning. Learning is understood as the activity of mediating social and cultural participation with individual cognitive sense making. The phenomenon of social, cultural and linguistic diversity is positioned as primary for the development and growth of bilingual children and their families.

The book uses a Vygotskian lens to examine the notions of CLD, disability particularly language disabilities, assessment, intervention and working collaboratively with bilingual colleagues and families. In so doing, the book attempts to present a framework which elucidates the intimate relationship between social and cultural meaning making and individual sense making through the tool of language for individuals who have language-related disabilities growing up in families, schools, neighbourhoods and societies that are culturally and linguistically diverse.

Chapter 2

Provision for Communication Disabilities in Cultural and Linguistic Diversity

Case Study

A family, originally from Kosovo, are presently faced with removal from the UK to Germany from where they will be removed, by the German authorities, to Kosovo. The family has a son who has been 'diagnosed' as having 'significant language delay'. A year ago when he was 3 years 2 months, the local Speech and Language Therapy Department in the UK described him as having the understanding and expressive language of an 18 month old child and considered him in need of speech and language therapy in English. It was proposed that this therapy should be integrated into his pre-school nursery programme. The child speaks Albanian at home. The family currently live in south east England.

Could the speech and language therapist assess and report on the following:

(a) The child's present level of development and any speech and language therapeutic needs; and
(b) The consequences of removal to Germany and to Kosovo on his language development both in respect of
  (i) no longer being taught/treated in English
  (ii) the effect of the disruption/termination on a therapeutic programme and
  (iii) the consequent deterioration in his mother's (and main carer) mental state, having been diagnosed with post-traumatic stress disorder (PTSD).

(Taken from an email circulated to speech and language therapists in the UK, 2004)

Introduction

Language diversity is a characteristic of most countries in the 21st century, due to autochthonous (indigenous) language diversity, established transplanted culturally and linguistically diverse (CLD) communities, or due to movement of people driven by a variety of reasons. Economic reasons for migration explain most linguistic diversity in the UK, USA, Australia and Europe. Li Wei (2000) sums up the complex reasons: the growth of international travel; economically poor countries benefit from migration that generates foreign currency returning to the country; rich economies benefit from new labour, both open and hidden (ironically 'black markets'). Nonvolitional migration of refugees and asylum seekers is due to political reasons, such as security and war, as in the above case study example, as well as natural disasters. Furthermore, language diversity in non-English-speaking countries may be due to education requirements to access knowledge and learning through English as a foreign language (EFL).

Increasingly, countries that traditionally saw themselves as monolingual are becoming multilingual and multicultural because of migration and movement of peoples. This transformation due to cultural, linguistic and racial diversity is often a site of social processes of exclusion more than inclusion. The case study that introduces this chapter reflects a familiar scenario for culturally and linguistically diverse families and service providers in many countries. At the start of 2007, 9.9 million people were classified as refugees by the UN High Commissioner for Refugees (UNHCR), the multilateral body charged with their protection (UNHCR, 2007: 8). This marked a 14% increase on 2006, when the number of refugees (8.7 million) was the lowest since 1980, following a peak of 18.2 million in 1993 after the end of the Cold War (UNHCR, 2007). By the end of 2006, Europe, North America and Oceania hosted a quarter of the world's refugees and less than 14% of populations of concern to UNHCR, while Asia hosted nearly half of both (UNHCR, 2007). War is an important cause of population mobility, and increasingly, forcing people to leave their homes has become a direct aim in war. Where claims to political power have been framed in terms of ethnic, racial or religious identity, a group mobilises itself on the basis of that identity, and then tries to assert its right to power by excluding 'others' from the territory. An example is the conflict in Yugoslavia, with Serbs, Bosnians and Croats and its impact on the people of Kosova. Repatriation of refugees is one of the 'durable solutions' by the UNHCR.

The case study illustrates important characteristics of the relationship between provision and clients: families' transitory situation, the disjuncture between family language and that of the country of residence and service providers, monolingual practices of service providers that do not include the family's language, difficulties in communication and continuity across services and countries, the acute and pervasive nature of the child's and parents' needs and the range of interconnected services required to support them. These characteristics are formed by social processes of inclusion and exclusion, which operate in the interstices between culturally and linguistically diverse families and monolingual and monocultural service provision.

This chapter concerns practices of health and education provision in contexts of CLD for children with language-related disabilities and their families. The purpose of the chapter is to examine conceptualisations of CLD, which shape the practices of health and education provision for culturally and linguistically diverse children with communication disabilities and their families. I argue from a sociocultural perspective that the context for practitioners and clients is constituted by our collective actions and practices, which become institutionalised by traditions in service provisions.

First, I discuss Bourdieu's ideas that unequal valuing of people's social, cultural and linguistic capital contributes to the marginalisation and 'social disabling' of culturally and linguistically diverse disabled people for provision and research. In the next two sections, I use Bourdieu's ideas to interpret common practices by providers towards culturally and linguistically diverse families with children with language-related disabilities. I evaluate demographic profiling of ethnicity and language as a social practice of exclusion and inclusion in health and education provisions and which is orientated by service needs rather than by culturally and linguistically diverse client needs. In the third section, I discuss the social processes influencing service providers' choice of language for intervention with language-related disability in contexts of linguistic diversity. Finally, I draw some conclusions.

Social Theory and Provision

I draw on social theory and Bourdieu's (1977) ideas of *field*, *capital* and *habitus* to interpret social processes of inequality in health and education provision in CLD contexts. An important shared relationship between Bourdieu's ideas and Vygotsky's is that they both have Marxist origins. Bourdieu has been described as a cultural Marxist, interested in interpreting the relations of power between groups of people through the distribution of symbolic forms of human and social capital through social processes. While Bourdieu's ideas concern interpreting stasis, Vygotsky's ideas concern change, learning and intervention. Both sets of ideas draw on social, cultural and historical processes.

I illustrate these social processes with exclusionary practices around linguistic diversity, specifically demographics of language profiling, assimilation processes that work for monolingualism and against diversity in bilingual language development, and intervention. I start with a discussion of three key concepts of Bourdieu: field, social and linguistic capital and habitus, and how they relate to CLD and disability.

Field: Nested communities and practices

Society can be understood as nested communities that are related and juxtaposed to each other along axes of power. Some axes are gender, class, race, (dis)ability and, less frequently acknowledged, language. Communities may be any kind of system, such as institutions, or families that have shared social, cultural and language practices. Health and education services are two major provisions in most societies. They gather within them material resources, such as buildings, equipment, knowledge and expertise as well as social resources from people, such as knowing the neighbourhood, culture and language. Health and education are systems for providing services to clients, which are shaped by discourses and practices of enacting diversity and disability. Individuals also have resources, and they use these resources to access provision to meet their needs. In the UK, one aim of service providers is to allow everyone to have equal access to the resources. But not everyone comes with equal resources, or, rather, the resources that people bring are not valued equally.

Social and linguistic capital: Having resources

Bourdieu uses an economic metaphor to refer to these resources: 'capital', that is, social practice is a currency in the social market place. People can use the social, cultural and language capital that they possess to 'buy' or access resources from the systems and structures in society, so long as the systems recognise the value of the individual's capital. For example, knowing how to get a referral for your child to a service or a place for them in a school is a valuable resource and welcomed by service providers. Speaking English or the language of the provider, knowing how to ask questions about provision and respond to professional advice are individual resources that are also highly valued by service providers. Cultural knowledge, such as shared understanding of parenting skills and child–parent interaction between client and professional, punctuality and time keeping are valued by service providers. Individuals who do not bring this cultural and linguistic knowledge are seen as making additional demands on service providers, that is 'in addition' to the material resources already provided for their health and educational needs.

In the same way, language practices are also 'currency'. Linguistic capital refers to the capacity of the language as a carrier of knowledge. In monolingual communities, regional variations in spoken or written language that are associated with more education are attributed more value. Similarly, in multilingual societies, some languages are associated more with education and knowledge and, consequently, attributed more value than others. English as a global language carries high value, as do some European languages spoken by 'elitist bilinguals' (Skutnabb-Kangas, 1981). Linguistic capital also refers to the skills of language practices that are valued by service providers, such as communication and negotiation skills, literacy skills and knowledge of expert professional language practices. Against these criteria, speakers of minority languages are attributed low-value linguistic currency to the market place of health and education provisions, and construed as making demands on the linguistic resources of the provision. Transitory and refugee families, as in the case study, are also likely to be perceived in this way.

Service providers respond in different ways to providing 'additional resources'. They may resist on economic and assimilationist grounds, arguing that it is the individual's responsibility to develop relevant cultural and language knowledge. Modood's (2005) analysis is apposite: that society can tolerate CLD so long as it is managed privately. The contradiction of private diversity and public sameness is performed in contradictory practices. For example, it is not unusual in the UK to see health and educational establishments with public welcome signs in different languages and scripts, while hospital and school appointment cards advise patients/parents who do not speak English to bring someone who can interpret for them.

From the perspective of social capital, children entering school with languages and cultures other than the language of schooling may be seen as problems, demanding additional language and culture teaching resources. Schools draw unevenly on the cultural and language practices of pupils, which include language variations as well as other languages.

Particular practices towards authority, discipline, work and homework as well as language and literacy are more valued than others. For this reason, minority ethnic children from professional families often experience less difficulty settling into English schools than English children who are socially and culturally disadvantaged and poor. Nevertheless, the importance of the 'capital' metaphor is that it shows that the value of knowledge is *attributed* and it is not fixed. It can be changed by service providers and clients.

Habit(us): Knowing how to play the game of accessing provision

The recognition by service providers of individuals' and families' 'capital' is based on shared cultural assumptions and beliefs of knowing how to behave appropriately. To analyse this, Bourdieu uses another metaphor: playing the game, where the 'game' is social activity. An example would be an initial interview with parents who were concerned about their child's communication difficulties. From outside a culture, beliefs and assumptions appear arbitrary and 'given', rather than built up over time and experience by the group. Within the culture they are often unquestioned. Shared beliefs gives rise to dispositions about how to live together, which is shown in daily living habits (habitus), such as dress, food, tastes in music and fashion, attitudes to work, moral values, parenting practices, and also in shared social spaces, such as living together in neighbourhoods, language, literacy and communication practices. Within any cultural community, individuals play the game differently. The inner commitment to certain beliefs may be performed outwardly in different ways, such as wearing traditional dress, religious observance, bilingualism, or not. There are implications for service providers for understanding how individuals and families play the game.

Service providers must also place themselves in the game. They need to recognise their cultural assumptions and beliefs and who they share them with, which make them 'play the game' in a particular way. In addition, professionals are shaped by the *habitus* – cultural assumptions and beliefs – of their professional training and codes of behaviour. Cultural knowledge and beliefs differ within and across professional and practitioner groups. This is discussed later in the chapter on collaboration. Beliefs about one aspect of living can shape behaviour in another. For example, a teacher and a parent of a child with communication needs who both have strong religious beliefs, albeit from different traditions, may recognise they have shared values and beliefs around disability. The teacher may feel that she/he has more in common with the parent than with nonreligious colleagues, which may influence how she/he works with both.

This conceptual approach to the role of social representations in perpetuating unequal power hierarchies has been used to frame recent research in the UK context of policy, which emphasises partnerships between government and local communities in initiatives to reduce health inequalities. Campbell and McLean (2001) examined the impact of the social construction of ethnic identities on the likelihood of local community participation. They noted the way in which ethnic identities may be constructed in ways that undermine the likelihood of local community participation. Stereotypical representations of ethnically defined ingroups and outgroups (the ethnic 'other') constituted key symbolic resources used by informants in accounting for their low levels of engagement with local community networks. The construction of stereotypes is shaped by historical, economic and social forces, within the context of the 'institutional racism' that exist in England.

The lens of social theory affords a level of analysis and reflection not only on how clients are placed, but also how service providers, practitioners and researchers are placed. Bourdieu's metaphor of a market place where resources are exchanged explains the unequal value that some cultural and linguistic commodities are attributed. It also opens a way to consider how these commodities could be re-evaluated. The structures of service provision need to address this. Bourdieu's notion of 'playing the game' could be seen as diminishing important and central ideas in culture, such as religious and political beliefs. This is not its intention. Rather, it affords practitioners, researchers and parents a tool to understand positions that social groups take, and the movement of individuals within those groups around their belief systems as they negotiate to meet the needs and demands of life, in particular the needs of children who have language-related disabilities. Social analysis as a tool for reflexivity is essential for providers, practitioners and researchers working in the field of CLD and disability. Practitioners who show reflexivity and flexibility are more likely to be able to work successfully in these areas (see Chapter 10).

Tools for Social Practices of Exclusion and Inclusion

In this section, I make use of Bourdieu's ideas of social and linguistic capital to evaluate social practices of exclusion and inclusion in health and education provisions orientated by service needs rather than by culturally and linguistically diverse client needs. I take demographic profiling of ethnicity and language as a specific tool, which exemplifies processes for gauging linguistic capital, and examine two aspects that associate it with exclusionary and inclusive practices.

Language diversity as disabling

Disparities in the health care of racial and ethnic minorities mean that minorities do not always receive the same quality of health care or have the same access to health care, are less represented in the health professions, and have poorer overall health status than nonminorities. These disparities are recognised by many professions and governments and are the basis for policies and initiatives for eliminating racial and ethnic disparities in health care (e.g. American College of Physicians, 2004). A less recognised discourse of inequality of need and demand on health and educational provision is around linguistic diversity.

> Unmet language need is one of the key drivers of social exclusion, barriers to employment, education and training, and inequity in access to services. (Aspinall, 2005: 363)

Language is a key tool for access to and delivery of services in maintaining a healthy, educated and economically resourced population. Where service providers do not meet the communication needs of linguistically diverse clients, language practices are exclusionary.

Rationales for a national interest in language diversity are often based on legal and economic concerns. For example, there is a legal requirement in the UK to meet the needs of language diversity in health and education, set out in the Human Rights Act 1998 and the Race Relations (Amendment) Act 2000. Economically, ill health is a drain on a country's resources. Minority ethnic and migrant populations often have recognisable ill health characteristics that are linked to poverty, such as high infant mortality rates, high levels of childhood illness that require special education, high rates of mental ill health (as illustrated in the case study above) and, recently, high incidence and prevalence of HIV and AIDS (Nazroo, 1997, 2003). Language and communication disabilities are often associated with these aspects of ill health. Yet many aspects of ill health and disability are the *product* not the cause of exclusionary practices, such as poverty and discrimination.

Demographic profiling is an important tool used by majority groups in service provisions, often for excluding rather than including minority groups. Profiling largely seeks to inform provision from the perspective of the service providers' needs and to identify potential barriers for access to services. Monitoring usually surveys ethnicity, gender and socioeconomic status, but may not include language diversity. Profiling diversity is problematic at a variety of levels and can reveal social practices of exclusion.

Simplifying ethnic profiling

Conceptually, ethnic monitoring is in itself a deeply flawed structure and process for two main reasons. The tendency to use assumed categories of race-by-colour, monoethnicity and monolingualism avoids and prevents the complexities and dynamics of diversity being surfaced (Bonnett & Carrington, 2000; Hirschman *et al.*, 2000). Ethnic monitoring has been used for further exclusion of minority groups. Statistics suggesting supposedly large groups of ethnic minorities are traditionally used to raise fears of minorities 'swamping' the ethnic majority and making excessive demands on service provisions. Substantial increases in birth rates among minority ethnic populations may be used in a similar way. The association between ethnic monitoring and racist policies led the education department in the UK to stop collecting statistics between 1971 and 1979.

Monitoring linguistic diversity

Census data is a common way of obtaining information about national population' characteristics, including language, ethnicity and race, and many countries collect languages data. Of the countries in Europe, central Asia and North America, 76% asked one or more questions on first language, main language, most spoken language or knowledge of language(s) in the 2000–2001 round of censuses (Moss, 1999). Censuses in the USA (USCB 2000) and in Australia (ABS 2001) asked: 'Does the person speak a language other than English at home?' (and what language?) and 'How well does the person speak English?' with four categories of response. Canada asked five questions about language in its 2001 Census (2006), and New Zealand (2006) and South Africa (2003) also asked questions on language diversity.

The UK does *not* ask a census question about languages used by its citizens. Although strong cases have been made by business as well as for welfare reasons, the Office of National Statistics (ONS) did not include questions on language in the 2001 Census, and is reluctant to include such questions in the 2011 Census because proficiency in English language is among 'those topics where there is insufficient evidence of user demand to justify inclusion' (ONS, 2005, cited in Aspinall, 2005). The omission of language data has national and international implications. There is no recent national data in the UK for main languages spoken in the home, levels of proficiency in languages including English, and literacy skills in English and other languages. There is no comparative evidence nationally of changes over time or with other countries, which could inform responses to developing welfare provision in linguistically diverse contexts.

In the UK, health, education and social services use alternative sources of data on language diversity to inform planning, like national surveys such as the 1994 Fourth National Survey of Ethnic Minorities (Modood *et al.*, 1997), the 1999 national health survey and subsequent regular monitoring (Dolt, 2005). In education in the UK, national data in the 1990s show that 7–8% of the pupil population has minority ethnic heritage and a smaller proportion is from linguistic minority families. The proportions vary across urban/rural schools, with the more densely populated urban areas having the highest proportion (30%) of bilingual children in the country (DfEE, 1999). While at a local level, health and education services may collect data to inform local strategic planning. An important constraint on these alternative sources of data is that questions on language are not harmonised and there is no mechanism to compile them into a comprehensive source or to update information between censuses.

Monitoring linguistic resources

Surveying language proficiency monitors linguistic resources of clients. Depending on the orientation of questions, language profiling can be both an exclusionary and inclusive practice for linguistically diverse service users. Questions about service users' proficiency in the language of the provider, usually the majority language, primarily address service provider's needs. A focus on the percentage of users who have difficulty speaking the dominant language marginalises speakers of other languages from the service. On the other hand, language profiling questions inquiring about proficiency in all the languages and literacies of service users are inclusive and led by user needs. They provide information about how providers can develop optimum communicative access to users.

Without reliable language information, services in the UK use ethnicity, race and country of origin, as means for determining language diversity. According to the UK Census 2001, 51% of those described as

'Indian, Pakistani or Bangladeshi' were born overseas and might be considered to have English as their second language, but little more could be said of their language or literacy proficiency. Based on the 1994 Fourth National Survey of Ethnic Minorities, 400,000 (Carr-Hill *et al.*, 1996) and 1.7 million (Kirk, 2004) are estimated to have difficulties with English/limited English proficiency. Language skills in people aged 16–64 years were assessed and only 14% of Bengalis, 29% of Gujeratis, 26% of Punjabis, 41% of Chinese and 32% of refugees reached a 'survival level' of competence in English (Carr-Hill *et al.*, 1996). A study with 'African, Asian and Arabic' refugees in the UK found that a quarter understood spoken English and a fifth could speak English (Kirk, 2004).

Yet, information about ethnicity and nationality is insufficient to inform provision for interpreting and translation resources. The spoken varieties of the language in the home need to be identified. For example, Bengali, Punjabi and Chinese have different spoken varieties in the UK; Bengalis may speak standard Bangla, although most in England speak the Sylheti variety; Punjabi speakers may speak at least two varieties, Mirpuri from Pakistan and Indian Panjabi; Chinese people may speak Cantonese or Mandarin or regional varieties of each. Descriptors such as 'refugees', 'African' and 'Asian', offer little language information. Parents and families with limited basic skills in English need trained language support personnel to understand and participate in their child's time with professionals (see Chapter 10). In addition, cultural and religious information needs to be available to service providers to inform allocation of language support.

Identifying language diversity through race and nationality is not reliable. Language, culture and country of origin do not necessarily collocate. The professional association for applied linguists in the UK, the British Association for Applied Linguistics (BAAL), advises its members that:

> Language analysis cannot be used reliably to *determine* national origin, nationality or citizenship. This is because national origin, nationality and citizenship are all political or bureaucratic character-istics, which have no necessary connection to language. (BAAL 2004)

For example, in the case study at the beginning of the chapter, the family's language is Albanian, not 'Kosovan'. Furthermore, providers need to be mindful of the socialisation of language use, variations, dialects and cultural variations. Culturally and linguistically diverse service users and their families may not originate from another country, but may have links with a heritage country and belong to a cultural and linguistic diaspora.

There are three further social practices that affect collecting language diversity data and they are perceived as technical and administrative constraints. First, there is the technical complexity of collating the necessary range of metrics. For example, in the UK before 2003 it was not possible to know the distribution of students with characteristics of ethnicity, special educational need (SEN), gender and phase/type of schooling. A political decision by England's and Wales' Department of Education and Skills (DfES) meant that by 2003, the numerous local pupil datasets were brought together in the Pupil Level Annual School Census (PLASC). It offers comprehensive data on each pupil's phase and provision, achievement, gender and ethnicity, but not language diversity. The DfES uses PLASC data to analyse national trends, such as the relationship between ethnicity and SEN (Lindsay *et al.*, 2006).

Second, lack of knowledge by provision staff about ethnic and linguistic diversity can make demographic profiling sparse and inaccurate (Cline *et al.*, 2002). There is always potential for inaccuracy in language and literacy information at the point of inputting the information, such as knowledge of the accurate name of the language or variety spoken.

Third, service providers' questions about clients' language may be ambiguous to clients.

For culturally and linguistically diverse parents, there is a complex relationship between language and identity that may complicate service providers' questions related to allocation of language support for their child with language disabilities. One analysis suggests that multilingual speakers use their languages for perceived different sociopolitical purposes, such as languages for official purposes (vertical dimension) and languages for community, family and friendship purposes (horizontal dimension) (Nic Creith, 2000; Rassool, 2000; Martin, 2003). Enquiries about language use are likely to be understood along these dimensions, which may cause confusion for unwitting service providers. For example, parents may report to service providers (vertical dimension) that they speak Urdu, a language with high linguistic and cultural capital, signifying aspects of their identity – being Pakistani, Moslem and educated (LMP, 1985). The parent's response informs the service provider of the cultural and religious sensitivities required for working with the family, but not about allocating appropriate language support to providers concerned with a child's language development in the family (horizontal dimension). It would require more exploration by the service provider into spoken language at home, which in this example is more likely to be a variety of Mirpuri Panjabi, which does not have a written form and may, in addition, be perceived by parents as being less prestigious, with less linguistic capital.

How do we address these conceptual and politically driven social practices, which tend to exclude rather than include culturally and linguistically diverse services users from health and education through unmet language needs? Some social practices require political change and for others, professional development would address the risk.

Arguments for ethnic and language monitoring

While control and exclusion remain products of monitoring statistics, the argument to reinstate ethnic monitoring is based on human rights and equal opportunities for inclusion, which require information to enable provision and access for all. Demographic profiling can be developed from the clients' perspective to facilitate service provision to engage with CLD. In the UK and many countries, ethnic profiling increasingly seeks to avoid privileging 'default' categories of Whiteness and official nationality, preferring to offer hyphenated ethnic identities and open questions to identify languages and literacies use.

Sharing profiling resources at a local level, where schools collect information about language and ethnicity which health services and other services use, can inform the development and allocation of resources (Aspinall, 2005; Clark *et al.*, 1998). Several published sources describe the materials that health and education services can use to record local demography of ethnicity and language of service users (Baca & Cervantes, 1998, 2003; Hall *et al.*, 2001; Baker, 2001; Cline, 2000; Stow & Dodd, 2003). Information can be used to plan for the development and allocation of resources for interpreting and translation facilities, which underpin the provision of competent welfare systems to multilingual populations. Particular examples include identifying larger minority ethnic and language communities requiring substantial resources for language diversity and disability. Profiling can identify 'linguistically isolated' people and households whose needs can be easily overlooked, and educationally, schools may manage the needs of isolated bilingual learners comparatively well (Cline *et al.*, 2002). Survey data also identify itinerant people and families, such as Travellers, refugees and asylum seekers. The health, welfare and education needs of this group of people are usually substantial. Research shows that they find it particularly difficult to access services due to language differences (Harris, 2003).

Counting bilingual clients is an effective place for services to start in order to address these clients' needs. Steinstra (2002) noted that most research in the area of disability and ethnicity had this focus. As the majority of speech and language therapists in the UK have at least one or more bilingual children on their caseload (Winter, 1999), many speech and language therapy (SLT) services have recruited bilingual speakers as co-workers to support work with bilingual children and their families, to enhance access to the minority linguistic communities. One early indicator of the efficacy of offering community language support is in increased attendance and take-up figures (Winter, 1999).

Developing conceptual and material tools through professional development for practitioners who work with culturally and linguistically diverse service users could change some social practices, which construct language diversity and difference as a barrier to accessing health and education services. However, to change conceptually based practices about monitoring linguistic capital, such as census data collection and questionnaire orientation, for the purposes of developing language diversity in service provision will need more political responses.

In this section, I have made use of Bourdieu's ideas of social and linguistic capital to analyse social practices of exclusion and inclusion in health and education provisions orientated by service needs rather than by culturally and linguistically diverse client needs. I took demographic profiling of ethnicity and language as a specific tool that exemplifies processes for gauging linguistic capital, and examined two aspects that associate it with exclusionary and inclusive practices.

Social Processes Influencing Language Choice

In this section, I take Bourdieu's ideas of social and linguistic capital to interpret the social processes influencing service providers' choice of language for assessment intervention with language-related disability in contexts of linguistic diversity. The issue of choice of language for working with bilingual children with language disabilities mostly arises where service provision is monolingual. Thus, considerations about language choice in provision to culturally and linguistically diverse families are most often service needs-led, and bring about a form of coerced choice for families and clients. I discuss language choice as being shaped by processes interpreted by notions of *linguistic capital* and *habitus*:

(1) racism, racialisation of language and institutional racism/ linguicism;
(2) negotiating ethnic identity and language practices;

(3) language change and language choice;
(4) family's and child's bilingual dynamic: risks and resilience;
(5) language choices for present and future needs.

Racism, racialisation of language and institutional racism/linguicism

Monolingual service provision invokes the issue of language choice for culturally and linguistically diverse families involved in assessment and intervention for children with language delay or disability. Underpinning the absence of linguistic resources in monolingual provision is likely to be social processes, such as racialisation of language and institutionalised linguicism that marginalise minority languages. Racism can be understood as attributing inferior status to a race or racialised group (Blum, 2002). Racism is seen in the interaction between individuals where there is an uneven distribution of power and influence, discriminatory practices and the prejudiced belief and attitudes of individuals because of racial heritages. In the UK and many other countries, skin colour is taken as an indicator of race and a basis for racism. Racialisation is the imposition of racist attitudes on an issue. For example, (im)migration is racialised by linking movement of people to particular racial, inferiorised groups. The intrinsic dilemma and weakness in trying to define racism is that it is a term that is socially constructed differently by racial and racialised groups in society. Dictionary definitions try to define race as if it were a neutral issue. In defining race, we are both racially positioned as well as positioning ourselves racially in the debate. Definitions of race can only come from cross-race dialogue, where discussing the term 'race' is intrinsic to debating the issue, race, itself. Thus, in discussing race, we are always within the debate and cannot be outside it (Levinson, 2003).

Language can be racialised, that is, some languages are inferiorised by association with racial and ethnic groups. Where minority ethnic groups constitute linguistic minority communities, minority languages become a signifier of race and the minority language is racialised. For example, in the UK, Asian languages are racialised in comparison with European languages; in the USA, central and south American varieties of Spanish are racialised in a way that Iberian Spanish is not; in South Africa, indigenous African languages are racialised in comparison with English and Afrikaans; Romany in central Europe is racialised through its association with the stigmatised Romany people. Minority languages are not treated equally with each other or with English. Linguicism

(Skutnabb-Kangas *et al.*, 1995) is negative attitudes and stereotyping towards language diversity and to specific languages and language variations. I noted in the introductory chapter that monolinguals are the minority in a global context, nevertheless, monolingual speakers who are unfamiliar with bilingualism may express 'hostility' and 'sentiments more akin to class-related or racialist prejudices conveniently hidden behind a rationale of unilingual superiority' (Baetens-Beardsmore, 1986: 153). A Bourdieu reading on the social process of racialisation of language and linguicism concerns the power of linguistic capital.

Institutionalised racism/linguicism

In the UK, the Stephen Lawrence Enquiry (MacPherson, 1999) defined 'institutional racism'. It was the report of an inquiry into the death of Stephen Lawrence, a black youth who was murdered. The main finding was that the inadequate handling of the murder investigation by the police and the criminal justice system amounted to 'institutional racism'. Institutional racism was defined as:

> The collective failure of an organisation to provide an appropriate and professional service to people because of their colour, culture or ethnic origin. It can be seen or detected in processes, attitudes and behaviour which amount to discrimination through unwitting prejudice, ignorance, thoughtlessness and racist stereotyping which disadvantages minority ethnic people. (MacPherson of Cluny, 1999: 6.34)

Furthermore,

> There must be an unequivocal acceptance of the problem of institutional racism and its nature before it can be addressed, as it needs to be, in full partnership with members of minority ethnic communities. (MacPherson of Cluny, 1999: 6.84)

Drawing on Bourdieu's analysis, institutionalised racism is a practice within the nested service provision communities. This perspective moves the focus from individuals to a collective social process at an institutional level. The McPherson report recommended that every institution should examine both its policies and the outcomes of these policies, in order to ensure that any section of the community is not placed at a disadvantage. This should certainly apply to educational practices and to primary health care. Racial stereotyping and unconscious and unintentional racist attitudes among teachers have been exposed in research studies of pupils' views (reviewed in James & Woll, 2003).

Alongside institutional racism is institutional linguicism. Institutional linguicism may be one explanation for why well-intentioned practitioners advise culturally and linguistically diverse families to give up the minority language and to choose the service provider's language, often the country's majority language. Familiar arguments are that there is no professional support in the minority language for speech and language assessment. Second, the majority language is likely to offer the child access to education and employment. Both these arguments attribute low linguistic capital to developing culturally and linguistically diverse provision. While every child and family member has the right to access the language of power, this language right should not be at the expense of foregoing their heritage language. To paraphrase the MacPherson recommendation, in order to break the cycle of the reproduction of institutionalised linguicism, services and professional bodies need to recognise institutional linguicism in any of their practices by working with culturally and linguistically diverse communities.

Negotiating ethnic identity through language

An important approach to understanding identity is to explore the relationship between ethnicity and language practices. The relationship between identity, ethnicity and language has implications for service provision to culturally and linguistically diverse families. Language is a salient marker of ethnic identity and group membership, where ethnic identity is 'a subjective feeling of belonging' to a particular ethnic group (Noels & Clément, 1996: 214). Some research (e.g. Noels & Clément, 1996: 214) suggested a one-to-one correlation between ethnicity and language, but more recent research suggests that the identities of people from linguistic minorities are constantly constructed and reconstructed through their language practices. Their ethnic and linguistic identity is hyphenated, such as Italian-British, British-Panjabi, Hispanic-American, Australian-Greek (Pavlenko, 2004; LMP, 1985). The family's, parents' and child's construction of their identity and ethnicity are realised through their diverse language practices, which are negotiated differently by family members for different purposes. The relationship that each family builds between their ethnic identity and bilingual language practices informs their disposition for making a choice between their languages. Families who perceive that their ethnic identity may be diminished by adopting the majority language for their communicative practices at home, usually resist advice to use the L2 in the home.

Language change and language choice

The home language of many culturally and linguistically diverse families is unlikely to be a standard form of the language. Languages change in contact in linguistically diverse societies, particularly minority languages (see Romaine [1995] and Myers-Scotton [2006] for review). In multilingual societies, languages and language practices are hybrid, fractured and fluid, responding to the context and communicative demands. Minority languages are more likely to change as a result of influence from the majority language and maintaining 'pure' minority languages in a diverse society is unlikely. The dominant majority language, such as English in the UK, is less likely to change as a result of contact with minority languages (Martin *et al.*, 2003).

Bilingual speakers switch between languages (codeswitching). Codeswitching is a site for a great deal of research concerned with processes of language change and identity construction (e.g. Romaine, 1995; Myers-Scotton, 2006). Some key features are summarised here. Codeswitching is demonstrated when bilingual speakers borrow vocabulary across languages (lexical borrowing) and words and phrases are 'loaned' from one language and become established in another. Speakers may also change aspects of grammar structure in one language, with word order or word endings of the other. These changes may be used for situational purposes or they may become established and different language varieties emerge. Culturally and linguistically diverse young people use their languages, including the majority language, to create unique in-group language practices that rely on 'crossing' words, phrases, intonation patterns between languages (Rampton, 1995). 'Crossing' languages contributes to building identities. Codeswitching and language variation are not perceived as deficit forms of language nor do they indicate psycholinguistic disability, but are recognised as a pragmatic facility (Martin *et al.*, 2003, Myers-Scotton, 2006).

The implications of minority language change for language choice is that parents and families are unlikely to be able to use a 'pure' form of the language. They may never have had access to this form if they are first or later generations of the minority language community. Further, the language variation that the family speaks influences the recruitment of bilingual personnel and cultural and linguistic resources for working with the family. It is widely accepted that language variations can demonstrate all the characteristics of language in terms of structure, meaning and use, and should not be dismissed as inferior language forms, whether or not they have a written form.

Family's and child's bilingual dynamic: Risks and resilience

Resilience in maintaining CLD in bilingual families is largely due to varied and positive language practices. A Bourdieu reading is that where families attribute equal value to languages and develop collective communication practices, members can draw on individual resources to engage and maintain communication across languages. Bilingual and multilingual families use languages for different social purposes. For example, one language and literacy form may be used for religious practices, while another may be used for talking to particular members of the family, and a third language may be used with siblings and school friends. There is a body of research that documents the languages development of bilingual and trilingual children (e.g. Fantini, 1985; Cunningham-Andersson & Andersson, 1999; Zentella, 1997). These studies locate language development in a sociocultural context and offer an ecological approach to understanding the complexities and nuances of its development. Families may also have speakers who are monolingual either in the minority or majority language.

Becoming monolingual in the majority language is a risk for bilingual speakers. Language choice made intentionally or by default that results in loss of the home language is frequently driven by attributing low social capital to minority home languages. The social process of subtractive bilingualism is when the home language atrophies as the majority language develops, and is frequently a process of schooling (Cummins, 1984) and a choice in bilingual adolescents (Baker, 1992). One result of home language atrophy is that the younger generation cannot speak with their older relatives in the home, or to relatives and friends in the diaspora or on visits to the heritage country. Majority language choice can bring emotional sadness. Where children choose the majority language and not the minority language of parent(s), the choice is often a cause of concern and sadness to parents. Bilingual families report sadness and grief at their communicative loss with their deaf children who attend English-speaking school and learn English and English-based sign language. For some culturally and linguistically diverse Muslim parents, the loss of one of their minority languages, Urdu, is a concern because it means the loss of their child's religious development and identity (Ahmad *et al.*, 2002). The issue of language choice may not be discussed with parents and families, and reasons for not having sign language in the home are blamed on parents rather than exploring access/provider issues (Atkin *et al.*, 2002).

Genesee *et al.* (2004) present illustrative accounts of bilingual families in different sociolinguistic contexts making decisions about language choice. In Bourdieu's terms, the notion of *habitus* of the families being bilingual is central to this language decision. They identify three main areas of resilience/risks to a bilingual habitus for parents and professionals to consider:

- The requirement for two languages in the family's communicative repertoire.
- Stress to the child may be a risk in maintaining both languages.
- Language dominance of one language may deter intervention in the other language.

They argue that the sociolinguistic situation of families is a crucial determinant for language choice. For example, families who intend to stay only a short time in a country and intend to return to their homeland as soon as possible may not require the majority language of the country they are currently in. Genesee and his colleagues emphasise the importance that families maintain home languages and meaningful communication with their child who has communication difficulties. The more severe the children's communication needs and difficulties are, the higher the risk for choosing a monolingual option of the majority language. Two important aspects of the child's and family's communication habitus need to be considered for risks and resilience to bilingualism: communicative history and trajectory.

Communicative history and trajectory

Language choices for present communicative needs will impact on future needs. Current and future bilingual communication, *habitus*, is depicted in bilingual children's communicative history and trajectory. Bilingual communication history is the account of a child's development of receptive and expressive communication not only at the structural level of speech sounds, words and sentences, but also emotionally, socially and conceptually in different languages and cultures. Different language communities have different accounts of socialisation of language development (Schiefflin & Ochs, 1986). Children who are bilingual or/and with language disabilities can develop understanding of language even though they may not have demands made on them to talk or express themselves. Having receptive language only in the minority language is a recognised form of being bilingual (Romaine, 1995). Children with language disability, brought up in bilingual homes, can develop receptive and expressive language in both languages (Paradis *et al.*, 2003b).

Children with substantial communication needs are likely to have pervasive language difficulties into adulthood. The trajectory of communication needs and demands for the bilingual child with language disability needs to take account of the language practices of the community the child will be living in when she/he is a young person and an adult. Forms of communication and language considered for the future will inform decisions about language choice from early on in the child's communication development and intervention. Approaches that offer bilingual potential from the start need to be explored and implemented. Roberts and Gibbs (1989) gives an account of a child from a bilingual family with communication needs associated with cerebral palsy. She describes that the child used a symbols communication board in English at school and in Punjabi at home, with the necessary vocabulary changes for relevant communication in each context. This strategy maintained the child's communication in different language contexts. It met immediate communication needs for the child and others, as well having potential to develop into more sophisticated technological alternative and augmented communication systems as the child's needs determined.

Research into longer term management and communication trajectories involve collaborative work between professionals and parents. A three-year study, framed by capability theory, revealed how families drew on their resources to meet the needs and aspirations of the family and the young person with disability (Harry *et al.*, 1999, see Chapter 9). There is little research available into examining how communication trajectories are negotiated and performed for children with bilingual parents and with providers.

Conclusion

I set out to make the case that CLD contexts shape service provision for culturally and linguistically diverse people. Language diversity is recognised by providers as an important barrier for clients to access services. I have drawn on a theoretical frame of unequal valuing of languages to interpret aspects of inequalities in health and education service provision to culturally and linguistically diverse clients. I illustrated social processes of exclusion and inclusion through monolingual practices by service providers that are limited in their provision to culturally and linguistically diverse clients with language-related disabilities. I selected two practices: measuring the size of the language problem through language profiling and coercion of language choice.

Professional practice is not neutral or simply technical. Knowledge is not 'context free'. Technical knowledge, such as knowledge of stages of bilingual language development, assessment tools and intervention programmes for language-related disabilities, is mediated by social processes. Traditionally, provision and practice demonstrate an unequal valuing of the social, cultural and linguistic capital and resources that culturally and linguistically diverse clients bring, largely due to institutional racism and linguicism. This is demonstrated where client language profiling is largely orientated by the existing resources and needs of the providers, rather than by the language resources and needs of culturally and linguistically diverse clients. Where service provision does not have adequate language resources to meet client needs, there may be coercion practices on clients to choose the providers' language for management of impairment. Culturally and linguistically diverse clients with language-related disabilities and their families are at most risk in these contexts of having to curtail or abandon their diversity.

There are important tools to support change. The metaphor of social and linguistic 'capital' is based on the notion of attributing value to cultural and language knowledge. These values are not fixed and can be changed by service providers and clients. The metaphor of 'playing the game' is based on the notion that social groups can (re)position themselves and move on, informed by their beliefs, attitudes, habits and routines. The beliefs and routines of service providers as well as culturally and linguistically diverse clients can change. Acknowledging institutional racism and, by extension, institutional linguicism, can be acted upon by service providers by addressing their collective failure in partnership with culturally and linguistically diverse clients to provide appropriate professional provision for client diversity. Service providers, practitioners and researchers must take account of this challenge.

Chapter 3
Disability and Disabling Cultural and Linguistic Diversity

Introduction

The purpose of this chapter is to examine how disability, particularly language-related disability, is constructed in cultural and linguistic diversity (CLD) with reference to research literature and policies. Subsequent chapters sharpen the focus of the broad discussions introduced here. The line of argument is that difference is most often constructed as deficit. Differences of ableness are constructed as impairment and disability, and CLD is at risk of being perceived as disabling. The chapter explores drivers identified in the literature that 'disable diversity'. An important driver is determinist notions, which overarch understanding disability, race and ethnicity, and are also applied to language and cultural differences. This perspective also informs policies and services. A Vygotskian perspective of disability and diversity is one of development and potential capability, realised through personal and collective resources to meet needs.

This argument has four themes. The first theme evaluates from a Vygotskian perspective, four approaches that construct disability, impairment and special educational needs (SEN) through determinist and developmental discourses and draws implications for CLD. The second theme concerns 'diversity as disabling', that is, where practices construct CLD as impairing learning. There is a particular focus on language learning and communicative needs. I explore the confusion in conceptual and material tools that lead to practices of conflating racial, cultural and linguistic diversity with SEN, with examples of English as an additional language (EAL)/SEN confusion, underachievement and labelling practices. The third theme deals with 'racialising disability', where practices collocate disabilities with race/ethnic group, through disaggregation of social characteristics, such as disability, gender, race, ethnicity, culture and language. The fourth theme addresses implications of research that reconceptualises CLD and disability for provision led by service needs. Finally, I draw some conclusions.

Constructs of Disability

In this section, I evaluate from a Vygotskian perspective four current models of disability that are widely used in the literature, policies and practice. A determinist approach still permeates aspects of research and practice with assumptions that the nature and potential of our lives are determined by our genetic, biological and racial endowment, as well as our social and economic standing. Developmental approaches are presented in social models of disability and in relational approaches towards constructing SENs. An emerging model of disability derives from human and social capital theories. Understanding and managing disability grow from an individual's and family's capability in terms of social, human, material and linguistic capital and resources.

A central concern of Vygotsky's was the scope and speed of human development. How do humans advance so far beyond their initial biological endowment and in such diverse directions? (Wells, 2000: 53). His studies explored this concern in children with typical development and children with biological/cognitive impairments resulting in substantial difficulties in development and learning. This perspective on human development – both typical and atypical – enables a critical perspective on the determinist approaches to disability and impairment.

Biological model

The International Classification of Impairments, Disability and Handicaps (ICIDH) proposed by the World Health Organisation (WHO, 1980) defines disability, impairment and handicap from a medical/biological perspective. Impairment is an 'abnormality in the structure or the functioning of the body' due to disease or trauma; handicap is the 'restriction in the ability to perform tasks' due to impairment; disability is the 'social disadvantage' that could be associated with impairment, disability or both (Terzi, 2005: 199; Bury, 1996: 22). The concepts of impairment, disability and handicap are collapsed and become synonymous rather than being understood through different meanings. Difference from the mainstream is pathologised. The further dominant feature of the biological model is the individualisation of disability. From this perspective, disability is perceived as a personal tragedy for the child, parents and family. The main dimensions of this model concern identifying cause and causative factors and applying curative intervention that is centred in and on the individual, with an overemphasis at an individual level, in terms of person-fixing rather than context-changing. Research on disability within a biological model dominates many fields of impairment study, including specific language impairment (SLI) and, to a lesser extent, speech, language and communication needs (SLCN). The dominant research approach concerns phenotypes of SLI through experimental and positivist methodologies in psychological and linguistic fields (see Chapter 4).

The biological model of impairment is also recruited to pathologise race and ethnic difference. 'Deficit thinking' models, while held in disrepute by natural and social scientists, continue to be evidenced in educational thinking, policy and practice. They draw on three areas of study: genetics, poverty and culture. Current approaches to 'deficit thinking' draw on genetic bases as explanations of behaviour, particularly racial/ethnic differences in intelligence: 'inferior genes, inferior intelligence'. Genetic explanations are 'ultraconservative defeatist, determinist explanations of lower-class failure' (Pearl, 1997: 148). This 'nature deficit' model, which pathologises learning in race and ethnicities, gave way to the nurture argument, the 'cultural deficit thesis'. This thesis argues that linguistically and culturally diverse groups have deficit cultures and inadequate beliefs and value systems that lead to school failure. For example, deficit thinking was thought to be demonstrated in IQ testing. Valdes and Figueroa (1994) critically reviewed these studies and concluded that culturally and linguistically diverse children were effectively excluded from both linguistic and culture knowledge of IQ tests, and through the decontextualised testing environment in the dominant language (see Chapter 7).

Social model

Researchers with a social perspective argue that the WHO definitions are imprecise, contested and should be redefined. Disability refers to the stigma attached to individuals who have impairments, the pathologising of difference and the consequent marginalisation and discrimination experienced by people with impairments (Ahmad, 2000: 1). A social model of disability is concerned with how disability is constructed by others, in ways that can (dis)empower persons with the disability. It focuses on the social practices of 'making difficulties' at individual, institutional and national levels (Clough & Barton, 1995). This way of understanding disability and impairment moves the liability and burden of disability away from being the sole responsibility of the individual with the impairment, and their family, to society. Disablement is created by socially imposed barriers, so that 'disablement resides in ablest environments' and not within the disabled person alone. Research within a social model is not impairment focused, and is concerned with the social processes of constructing disability as the Other. Those who work within a social model of disability advocate that it is crucial to identify the fundamental argument that disability – the stigma of impairment – resides in the workings of an unjust society (Ahmad, 2000). They argue that the social construction of disability is a necessary aspect of an inclusive society and citizenship. The need to counter the marginalisation of people with impairment is as necessary as countering other forms of social exclusion, such as racism and sexism. There are implications for a social model of disability in contexts of CLD.

A relational approach: Special educational needs

A relational approach to disability is illustrated through the notion of SEN. It is an approach that constructs impairment as need, and need as negotiated by taking account of the interaction and potential for change between impairment and context. Evans (1995) examines a relational approach in the following way:

> Derived as it is from a medical approach emphasising "treatment", the category model implies that the learning problems lie within the individual child. On the other hand, the definition of SEN recognises that educational outcome is dependent on the interaction between the child, the education provided in the school, and the influences of the home and community. *Thus the teaching and education offered in any particular school may have a crucial impact on whether a child is identified as being in need of special provision.* The same child might be a candidate for special education in one school but not in another. In summary, it may be said that the first approach emphasises absolute characteristics while the second prioritises the relative aspects. (Evans, 1995: 203; my italics)

In the UK, SEN is currently defined in the way Evans describes, with the additional note that a child must not be regarded as having a learning difficulty solely because the language or form of language of the home is different from the language in which he or she will be taught. 'Lack of competence in English must not be equated with learning difficulties as understood in this Code' (DfE, 1994: 2.18, DfEE, 2001: 6.3).

In the UK, SEN is a legal and educational concept. Legal recognition of a child's SEN releases additional resources or changes in educational provision, such that the child's learning need is supported. Language-related disability, like many aspects of disability, is served by health and education services in most countries. The importance of a relational approach is that children's needs are relative to the context, the people around them, and the effectiveness of the interaction between them. For example, a deaf prelingual child in a family where no one uses sign language is communicatively disabled. The stigma of deafness isolates the child from the family. By contrast, where the child and family all use sign language, there is no communicative disability, although the child still has a hearing impairment.

Nevertheless, the concept of SEN is fraught with contradictions between biological, psychological and social models. Attempts to theorise the notion of SEN argue for a bio-psycho-social model (Norwich, 1990). Although SEN constructs children's needs in a more relational way, a medical approach continues to inform 'categories of impairment', resources and provision and specialist professionals. Furthermore, categories of educational difficulty are constructed and reconstructed in policy for resources. For example in the UK, over the last 20 years, the number of SEN categories have changed from 12 to 10 to 5, with some categories that required special provision disappearing, such as 'Delicate' and 'Epileptic', and others being recognised, such as 'Dyslexia'. Names of categories have also changed, such as from 'Speech defects' to 'Speech and Language Difficulties' to the most recent label 'Speech, Language and Communication Needs' (DfE, 1994; DfEE, 2001). Currently there are five categories of impairment recognised for resources: sensory (visual and/or hearing), physical, behavioural, cognitive, and communication difficulty along a continuum of severity and educational need.

The concept of SEN, despite the attempt to develop a social model of disability, continues to be informed by individualisation of need in terms of resources and pedagogy. Resources for educational needs follow and support individual difficulty rather than developing whole school approaches to disability and diversity. The notion of the continuum of SEN in severity within category types is not necessarily accompanied by a notion of a continuum of pedagogy, teaching and learning across all children's needs. Approaches, strategies, techniques and the practice of differentiation for individual children's SEN remain largely child-impairment focused (Lewis & Norwich, 2005) (see also Chapter 8). For EAL needs, the distinction made between educational needs that are additional language learning needs and special education needs (Tomlinson, 1982) is informed by the impairment category model. Recently, in Scotland, this distinction has been amended to a pedagogically informed and inclusive term: additional educational needs. Furthermore, in the UK and USA, recent policy agendas of 'personalisation' in learning may confound social models of disability and diversity.

A relational perspective could allow children's learning environments to be constructed across school and home, rather than dividing the child's learning environments along institutional lines. It accommodates multiple realities of bilingual learners with SEN, where children from minority culturally and linguistically diverse communities bring different cultures, religious beliefs and languages to school alongside the majority culture and language. A relational perspective is important for professionals who are not necessarily equipped to evaluate a bilingual child's learning difficulties because of a lack of conceptual tools and material tools, such as culturally and linguistically appropriate assessments and language development information.

A capability approach

A fourth approach draws on theories of human and social capital and economic capability (Sen, 1992, 1999). It emphasises the complexity of human capability and potential, rather than deficit in disability (Terzi, 2005). Some researchers interpret diversity, such as disability, cultural and linguistic differences, as *capability* for development (Harry *et al.*, 1999; Terzi, 2005). In the last chapter, human engagement and power in society was presented as resourced by different forms of capital: human, social, linguistic and material. Human capital is an individual's level of educational attainment embodied in their personal knowledge, skills and capabilities to act in certain social structures. Social capital is the social resources in the family and community that are accessible to the family, such as the social networks within families and between families. Material capital refers to the resources, such as income and wealth, which contribute to the family's socioeconomic standing. Linguistic capital refers to the communicative resources, spoken and written, of the family, both in the dominant and minority languages (Coleman, 1990; Li, 2007). A capability approach to disability argues that individuals' capability to manage their disabilities is interpreted not only through their own forms of capital and resources, but also through their family's and community's. Further, a capability approach explores ways of supporting the transformation of different forms of capital in the individual, family and community into resources to support the disability (Terzi, 2005).

While capability theory is drawn on to examine how different forms of social, human and material capital are used to develop linguistic capital (second language acquisition) in immigrant families (Li, 2007), it is less used to interpret transformation of capital into resources for disability in migrant families. Nevertheless, findings from other studies can be interpreted through this framework. Minority ethnic and linguistic families who care for members with disabilities are characterised by high levels of material deprivation and low levels of linguistic (second language) and social (family and community networks) capital (Hatton _et al._, 1997). Migrant families with low social, linguistic and material capital are also unlikely to produce the resources to access services that support disabilities (Harris, 2003). There are implications for service provision to orientate more to clients needs and seek ways to engage with the diverse social, linguistic and human capital of culturally and linguistically diverse families and individuals with disabilities.

Diversity as Disabling

In this section, I discuss with reference to research on practice, that conceptual confusions in practice construct diversity, particularly language diversity, as educationally disabling. I take three examples: conflating additional language learning needs with special learning needs, race and ethnicity associated with underachievement, and labelling as disabling. I draw on a Vygotskian perspective to interpret the examples as a lack of conceptual tools.

Children from culturally and linguistically diverse families may present educational and learning needs because they do not speak the language of instruction in school, or because they do not share cultural experiences with the majority of children, making it difficult for them to access and understand cultural-specific learning embedded in the curriculum. Culturally and linguistically diverse families may also respond differently to schooling, disability and language learning from majority language/culture families. In addition, some children from CLD backgrounds may have learning needs that are biologically based, social and emotional caused by trauma, and learning needs due to poverty. The importance of distinguishing between these two axes of educational need (diversity and disability) has been emphasised for over 20 years (Tomlinson, 1982; Frederickson & Cline, 2002). A small percentage of children have both kinds of needs, intrinsic sensory, physical, cognitive or language learning needs as well as having to learn through an additional language and/or culture. From a pedagogic perspective, the child is the most important person in a mediating process in teaching and learning (Moll, 2000: 262) and learners with additional educational needs demand specialised, personalised learning experiences.

Conflation of EAL/SEN

A serious conceptual confusion is evidenced when additional language learning needs and learning difficulties are conflated in educational practice with culturally, linguistically and racially diverse learners. Two explanations emerge from research: curriculum and economic. Troyna and Siraj-Blatchford's (1993) UK study showed that secondary school EAL students were assumed by their teachers to have language learning difficulties which predisposed them to learning difficulties across the curriculum and specifically for learning other languages. Evidence revealed that this assumption was unsubstantiated and most EAL students had primary school reports indicating satisfactory levels of English. An important outcome was that they were denied access to foreign language learning curriculum options, which their monolingual peers with SEN were allowed to study. Teachers' views indicated that their assumptions that shaped the educational management of these learners were based on 'common sense'.

A second study showed that schools working within economic constraints educationally manage learners with learning difficulties and learners with additional language needs in the same teaching groups. In an important study of two multiethnic secondary schools in the UK in the mid-1990s, Gillborn and Youdell (2000: 74–75) note that their findings of the practice of teaching pupils with EAL and SEN support earlier studies:

> Concentrating EAL pupils in certain of the "left-over" mixed ability classes immediately has the effect of barring them from any of the "fast groups". This is vitally important because it conflates EAL with lower "ability" in practice if not in principle. What we see here is a confirmation of the concerns raised in previous research that suggested that white teachers might sometimes misread Asian pupils' *language* problems as symptomatic of deeper-seated *learning* difficulties. (CRE, 1992; Gillborn & Gipps, 1996: 56–57; Troyna, 1991; Troyna & Siraj-Blatchford, 1993)

A further resource constraint may be a limited number of staff and/or limited staff expertise to manage the diverse educational needs of groups of EAL and SEN learners (Gillborn & Youdell, 2000). The implications for learners in undifferentiated groups are that their individual learning needs are glossed, and group needs are not individualised. Further evidence in a review of literature in the UK suggests that conceptual confusion and limited staff expertise underpin difficulties in identifying dyslexia (difficulties with literacy skills and print) in EAL learners (Cline & Shamsi, 2002). Staff may be unable to disentangle the language needs from learning needs.

Confusion and conflation of language disability (SLCN) and language learning (EAL) is also evident around specialist provisions, in referral practices and managing linguistic diversity. Referral practices by teachers and health workers, disadvantage the representation of minority clients in speech and language therapy provision in two ways. Minority linguistic preschool children in the UK are more likely to be referred later and more likely for language delay than intelligibility/speech difficulties, than their majority language peers (Stow & Dodd, 2005). Only a small percentage (although possibly in line with the national ratio) of school-age children attending specialist provisions for language and communication difficulties are from culturally and linguistically diverse backgrounds (Crutchley, 1999).

Specialist provision for children with substantial and severe SLCN is mainly at primary phase and there is little provision for children learning EAL with SLCN (Law *et al.*, 2000b). These provisions usually offer learning through English only and EAL learners leave the provision earlier than their monolingual peers, on the grounds that they can benefit from specialist EAL support in mainstream. Their diversity is managed better in provisions with head teachers and staff experienced with culturally and linguistically diverse pupils (Crutchley, 1999).

In the UK, for over 20 years (Swan Report, DES, 1985) learners with CLD and EAL needs have received language support in inclusive language provision from specialist professionals. The professional demarcation between language diversity and disability shows boundaried professional skills at risk of 'underlapping' services to meet culturally and linguistically diverse children's needs. Rather than argue for further segregated schooling for children with language disability from culturally and linguistically diverse families, there is a case for collaborative interprofessional working and learning together to improve knowledge, understanding and skills about the nature of language development and difficulties in bilingual children. (See Chapter 9 on collaborative work.)

There are other groups of culturally and linguistically diverse learners for whom professionals may not have the conceptual tools to meet their educational needs. New migrants, 'unaccompanied children', refugees and asylum seekers as new learners in schools present with complex social and emotional needs which profoundly affect learning (Rutter, 1994; Rutter & Jones, 1998). Studies of children traumatised by extreme social and emotional experiences, report that they are likely to demonstrate characteristics similar to language and learning difficulties for up to a year or more after arrival in school in the new country (Tolfree, 1996; Hamilton & Moore, 2004).

Race and ethnicity and underachievement

Diversity can be constructed as disabling through failure to achieve in school. Evidence in the literature on underachievement indicates low social expectations of educational attainment among many, but not all culturally and linguistically diverse groups.

Underachievement, or more accurately underattainment, is a focus of study in the 'effective school' and 'school improvement' literature rather than SEN or culturally and linguistically diverse studies. Pupils who underachieve or are low achievers, are thought to do so for reasons beyond the influence of schooling, such as poverty, date of birth, ethnicity and race, social class and gender. In recent studies in the UK, the role of the school system has become more central. The units of analysis of underachievement are usually based primarily on the Standard Assessment Tasks (SATs), which are public assessments at 6, 11, 14 and 16 years (Demie, 2001; Strand, 1999; Gillborn & Gipps, 1996; Gillborn & Youdell, 2000) and exclusions from school.

Recent studies in the UK indicate that there is a complex relationship between disaggregated factors of poverty, date of birth, ethnicity and race, social class and gender. There is no simple explanation for ethnic differences in educational achievement, and ethnicity does not presuppose educational underachievement (Demie, 2001). Many minority ethnolinguistic groups usually perform less well than their White English-speaking peers, e.g. Caribbean, Portuguese and African pupils, although some groups perform as well if not better, e.g. Indian and Chinese (Gillborn & Gipps, 1996; Strand, 1999; Demie, 2001). White working-class boys are the most likely to underachieve (Gillborn & Gipps, 1996). Gender differences are marked: girls outperform boys at all stages, except in maths (Strand, 1999; Demie, 2001). Poor children make comparatively less progress in all subjects (Strand, 1999). Early years EAL learners perform at very low levels, and reasonably proficient EAL pupils perform better than English-only speakers from 6 to 16 years (Demie, 2001). There was no school effectiveness difference noted.

The absence of a school effectiveness factor suggests that school failure is due to school practices, although the 'cultural deficit argument is mangled to deflect attention from school practices and lack of options to those locked in poverty' (Valencia, 1997). Socially determinist explanations, such as poor parenting, trauma, abuse in early years, assert that school cannot impact on the internal individual development with its pessimistic trajectory into an adulthood of failure. Schools are relinquished of the responsibility to examine other obstacles to success that may have been 'put in the path of students'.

> When school failure persistently correlates with class, race and ethnicity, an exhaustive examination of the school practices is vitally needed before conclusions about student deficiencies can be advanced. Belief in deficit theories inhibit and deter this examination of inequitable school practices. (Pearl, 1997: 148)

School practices with minority ethnic and linguistic pupils have become more central to studies of underachievement in the UK (Blair & Bourne, 1998; Gillborn & Mirza, 2000). They identify concerns among parents about teachers' discriminatory practices and racism towards them and pupils, and concerns about ineffective communication between home and school. These studies along with school inspection reports (OFSTED, 2002) identified school improvement strategies, the most successful being strong leadership on equal opportunities and social justice from the head teacher and education authority.

The most negative evidence of attainment is school exclusion figures. They show that predictors for exclusion are ethnicity and race, gender and disability. In the UK, the highest number of excluded youngsters have Caribbean heritage (Osler, 1997; Osler & Hill, 1999; DfES, 2001b). Pupils of White and Black Caribbean descent are at risk of underachieving and are proportionally over-represented in school exclusions, yet little is known to date about the barriers to their achievement (Parsons *et al.*, 2004). A high proportion of students with identified social, emotional and behaviour difficulties (SEBD) are Caribbean heritage boys (Cooper, 2006). When these finding are read together, it suggests that in UK schooling this group of learners continues to be problematic due to a complex interaction of socioeconomic disadvantage, low teacher expectation linked to misunderstandings of mixed heritage identities and backgrounds, and behavioural issues and attitudes towards achievement.

In the USA, Hispanic and African American youngsters are the highest ethnic groups for exclusions and drop out from school (e.g. Krezmien *et al.*, 2006). In the UK, there is long-standing evidence that more boys are excluded than girls (York *et al.*, 1972), and more recently that over four times as many boys are excluded than girls (84.5:14.5%; Gallagher, 1997). Although the number of disabled children who are excluded is low, there are seven times as many children with statements of SEN excluded as children without statements (0.61% compared with 0.09%; DfES, 2001b).

In the USA, explanations for underachievement and school failure of minority ethnic and linguistic students also look to school effectiveness, socioeconomic and sociocultural studies. Many studies acknowledge the limitations of evidence of educational achievement obtained only from SATs and other tests, as the UK studies tend to do. Measures such as exclusion and drop-outs are also crude negative indicators of low achievement. Some studies examine social behaviour with more sensitive indicators of compliance to schooling, such as punctuality, work habits, school meals. They are concerned to fracture homogeneous notions of culturally and linguistically diverse students, in particular Hispanic students, and to identify why some culturally and linguistically diverse pupils are more successful in school than others. While over-riding concern and explanation are found in language differences, other avenues for exploration are cultural concerns. Strategies that develop culturally and linguistically diverse students' biculturalism and identity are also likely to enhance their attitude towards school and academic work (Rumberger & Larson, 1998; Cummins, 1994, 2000).

Yet, the several domains of knowledge and skills implicated in teaching and supporting minority culturally and linguistically diverse students with SEN are separated by professional and research specialisms with implications for fractured educational management of culturally and linguistically diverse learners who are not succeeding with traditional classroom instruction (Gersten & Woodward, 1994). The notion of distributed cognitions (discussed in Chapter 1) is helpful here: 'knowledge is... a collective resource... in the routines we build and use together' (Mercer, 2000: 190). Developing highly specialist knowledge is a recommended whole school strategy (Blair & Bourne, 1998; OFSTED, 2002) that necessarily involves specialist knowledges distributed across several professions. Such a strategy needs a shared focus, not only to prevent children with multiple learning needs slipping between service provisions, but also to develop new and more effective practice. The implications for collaborative work practices, assessment and teaching and learning approaches for practitioners who work in schools with culturally and linguistically diverse learners with SEN are examined in later chapters.

Diversity as disabling through labelling

The third example in the literature where diversity is perceived and performed as disabling, is labelling impairment, migrants and culturally and linguistically diverse communities. Specifically, diagnosis is a cultural practice, labels impact on identity, and metaphors of disease are used to describe diversity. A further example is the silence of disabled and culturally and linguistically diverse people in naming their own needs.

Labelling and diagnosis are cultural practices (Duchan & Kovarsky, 2005) that operate at a macrolevel of policy, professional and ethnic social groups as well as at a microlevel of families and communities. Labelling and diagnostic practices are informed by beliefs and values about what counts as salient behaviour belonging to a particular category of impairment. For example, *speech* impairment rather than hearing impairment is what historically has been counted as evidence of deafness in Nicaragua (Polich, 2005).

Traditionally 'labelling theory' in disability studies is concerned with two main issues, accuracy and entitlement. In language-related disability, labels seek to be medically, linguistically and/or psychologically accurate. Given that language disabilities are dynamic and change with development, accuracy of language impairment category labels may be contested where they suggest a static problem rather than indicate the changing nature of children's needs. For example, a speech difficulty may resolve while the underlying difficulty with processing phonological knowledge may emerge later as a dyslexia-type difficulty; a label of 'autism' in early childhood may need to change to a label of Asperger's syndrome in adolescence in line with the development of the young person's strengths, difficulties and needs. This approach is from the perspective of the cultural practice of professionals rather than clients. From a client perspective, parents may choose to use a more popularly known label, such as 'autism', rather than a less familiar but more technically accurate label, such as 'pervasive developmental disorder not otherwise specified' (PDDnos) (Foster-Galasso, 2005: 19).

For clients, labelling disability is both a stigma and a portal to entitlement and resources. Educational segregation follows when labels become a tool in the practice of segregating children through special schooling and nurturing the stigma of impairment. In the UK, the use of specific labels, such as dyslexia, dyspraxia, autistic spectrum disorders (ASD), are necessary to access specific funding. In the USA, labelling of educational needs for CLD may also bring educational segregation.

Bilingual special education provision may carry negative perceptions and present some linguistic minority parents with a quandary for their children (Baca & Cervantes, 1998, 2003).

Diagnosing and labelling inform the construction of identity. Labels invoke cultural premises about who we are and our potential relationships with others (Duchan & Kovarsky, 2005: 5). One negative effect is social exclusion. More positively, individuals and families report being able to identify and feel more included with others in that impairment category (Foster-Galasso, 2005). They are able to use impairment labels as tools for inclusion that enable them to engage with research evidence and to access resources, as well as engaging with others in the disability community, which facilitates developing identity.

Two important discourses that construct perceptions and practice in the field of disability and diversity are 'bad mouthing' of race and disability, and the disease metaphor for bilingualism. Cummins (1984) opens his discussion of bilingualism and SEN on the close relationship of race, ethnicity and language diversity with intellectual ability in the practice of 'labelling' migrants. He discusses the discourse of documents in the late 19th and early 20th century that describe new immigrants to the USA and Canada in terms of intellectual impairment, such as 'feeble minded'. In this way racial, cultural and linguistic diversity were constructed as disabling.

Historically, children and adults with disability have been called variously: *retarded, spastic, subnormal, disordered, deviant, delayed, handicapped, impaired,* and more recently they are referred to as having *special educational needs* and *difficulties in learning and language.* Many of these terms continue in use, although there are some differences across countries. For example, in the USA the term *mental retardation* is used to distinguish between 'moderate learning difficulties' and 'specific learning difficulties', while in the UK, the term 'mental retardation' has been replaced by 'severe/profound and multiple learning difficulties' in academic, policy and professional discourses (Daniels, 2000: 50).

In the UK, many impairment labels are in colloquial usage as offensive forms of insult and abuse. They perform the role of stigmatising disability. Corbett (1996) describes these discourses of disability as 'bad mouthing'. In the same way, terms for ethnic and CLD groups are used colloquially for abuse to stigmatise minority ethnic and linguistic groups. There have been two main responses to 'bad mouthing' in the UK. Racist verbal abuse is constrained in the UK by racial discrimination legislation. The response to 'bad mouthing' disability has been a form of verbal hygiene, driven by the social model of disability to erase the stigma of disability. This is enacted in various ways, such as traditional and colloquial labels are replaced by impairment descriptors: deaf/hearing impaired, mute and dumb/speech and language difficulties, and positive descriptors are employed, such as wheel chair users. There are implications for verbal hygiene in labelling practices across cultures and languages, particularly for translation/interpretation in work practice. Conceptualising social models of disability is also evidenced through changes in labels.

A 'disease' metaphor (Nelson, 2005: 277) is commonly used to depict CLD. The metaphor constructs bilingualism as schizophrenia, and 'being bilingual' or developing additional languages and cultures, as schizophrenic. The strength of metaphor over simile is discussed in the first chapter; metaphors re-present and re-form real objects and lived experiences. Disease metaphors that link bilingualism with severe and pervasive mental illness have considerable potential negative impact. Such that advice, guidance and education constructed within this metaphor and orientated towards monolingualism are perceived as curative, healing and disease prevention.

Labelling is also a practice of subordination. In some accounts of constructing SEN, the ability continuum is privileged as being the main axis of difference

> with other systemic axes of difference being race, ethnicity, religion, nationality, social class, gender, sexuality, physical appearance and command of the English language. (Benjamin, 2002: 9).

Benjamin (2002: 4) discusses the complexity of labelling 'students who have been formally identified as having SEN', yet who are not identified as 'intellectually impaired' nor do they describe themselves as having SEN. With reservations, she chooses the label 'intellectual subordination' for the youngsters in her study (Benjamin, 2002: 140). Benjamin has two concerns. The precarious position she is in of being a 'labeller' of a group of people of which she is not a member. Furthermore, this label suggests homogeneity of the group and does not allow for the range of 'differential learning ability' based on the learning differences within the group. She argues that while much of the intellectual subordination is socially and politically produced through inappropriate and inadequate assessment procedures, they are a group of learners 'who are potentially made vulnerable because of their intrinsic intellectual limitation' (Benjamin, 2002: 140).

Culturally and linguistically diverse learners are often 'linguistically subordinated' in monolingual, e.g. English-only, educational environments.

They are potentially vulnerable socially and academically because of their developmental linguistic limitations in English. Bilingual learners of EAL with alleged speech and language difficulties are doubly subordinated. They are potentially vulnerable to 'double discrimination' (Baxter *et al.*, 1990). In terms of educational needs, some bilingual learners may have learning needs due to 'intrinsic intellectual limitation', while others may have needs based on 'intrinsic and specific language learning limitations', learners who would be described as having SLI in both/all their languages.

Labelling is also to do with the silence of the individuals themselves in offering descriptions and labels of their own disabilities. An impetus to change talk and thought about disability is driven by the fact that labelling discourses are not generated by disabled people themselves.

> These definitions have always been conceived of by others, never are they the expression of a group of people finding their own identity, their own history. The assertion of difference between people is seldom neutral, it almost always implies some kind of social distance or distinction. (Ryan & Thomas, 1980: 13, cited in Armstrong *et al.*, 2000)

According to Ryan and Thomas (1980) and Armstrong *et al.* (2000), discourses about disability that are not multivoiced – are not authentic voices from a range of perspectives – raise issues of power asymmetry between disabled and 'abled' people. They are discourses of 'oppression and exclusion', which primarily exclude people who are disabled as well as those who try to change the discourse towards diversity and inclusion.

In the field of disability, there is an increasing body of research by disabled scholars who place the perspectives of being disabled at the centre of researching disability (Barnes & Mercer, 1996; Oliver, 1990, 1992). They draw from sister discourses in feminism and race in taking a critical line of enquiry based on egalitarian and democratic approaches, which challenge dominant ideas and offer new directions for understanding disability. There are only a few studies in the field of disability and bilingualism/race conducted by disabled scholars from diverse ethnic and language backgrounds, and they admit that their race identity is marginalised by the need to 'negate the issues of their race in order to "fit in with" the rest of the Disability Movement' (Hill, 1994, in Ahmad, 2000: 3). There are also studies conducted by able-bodied ethnic and bilingual scholars, which offer fundamentally important insights and perspectives on understanding and developing a discourse about diversity in ethnicity and language (e.g. Mirza, 1998; Diniz & Usmani, 2001). These voices contribute to redressing the power asymmetries in constituting new discourses about disability in CLD.

Racialising Disability

This section examines the evidence from the literature concerning 'racialising disability', through the notion of over- and under-representation of Black and minority students with SEN in education. Monitoring practices collocate categories of impairment with race/ethnic group to reveal practices that racialise disability.

Coard (1971, 2005) was among the first to write about the phenomenon of over-representation of Black pupils in schools of 'educationally subnormal' children in the UK, a practice which racialised disability. Over- or under-representation of racial or CLD groups in educational disability racialises disability. Coard identifies three social processes that shaped the educational management and placement in special education of Black children:

- Low teacher expectation for Black students.
- Low motivation to succeed academically by Black students.
- Low expectations about Black students' performance.

Low expectation to achieve is evidenced when practices of 'streaming' and 'setting' place Black and culturally and linguistically diverse pupils in classes where curriculum learning is limited in comparison with their White peers (Gillborn & Youdell, 2000; Gillborn & Mirza, 2000). There is evidence of practices that racialise learning and disability by individual teachers as well as at the institutional level of the whole school (Daniels *et al.*, 2000b). Daniels *et al.*'s study (2000b) indicated that SEN category was a function of colour, ethnicity and gender as well as school resources. Thus, Black African Caribbean boys were more likely to be identified as having behavioural difficulties and less likely to be identified as having dyslexia than Asian or White boys, and boys more than girls.

Until the mid-2000s in the UK, it was not possible to know the comparative representation of minority ethnic pupils with SEN. The Department for Education and Skills (DfES) has begun to collate these data, partly in response to concerns about over- and under-representation of ethnic minority pupils with SEN. An early analysis of the first year's data indicates key findings resonate with existing findings (Lindsay *et al.*, 2006).

(1) Poverty and social disadvantage is the most important influence on the incidence of SEN for all minority ethnic groups.

(2) The majority of pupils with SEN are from the dominant White British ethnic group, about four in five SEN pupils.

(3) 'Black Caribbean' and 'Mixed White and Black Caribbean' pupils are about 1.5 times more likely to be identified a having SEBD than White British pupils.

(4) Travellers of Irish heritage and Gypsy/Roma pupils are 2.7 and 2.6 times more likely to have SEN in comparison with White British pupils.

(5) Bangladeshi pupils are nearly twice as likely to be identified as having a hearing impairment than White British pupils, and Pakistani pupils are between 2 and 2.5 times more likely to have profound and multiple learning difficulties, visual impairment, hearing impairment or multisensory impairment than White British pupils. The authors in the report attribute this 'to a greater incidence of genetic factors related to consanguinity (parents are blood relations)'. A recent review of literature (Mir *et al.*, 2001: 7) adopts a different starting point:

> in the case of learning difficulties consanguinity [first-cousin marriages] has effectively been ruled out as a single explanation.

Mir *et al.* (2001: 10) emphasise the established link between certain impairments, such as hearing loss and learning difficulties, and socio-economic deprivation that is widespread among the Pakistani population in the UK.

(6) Asian and Chinese pupils are less likely than White British pupils to be identified with moderate learning difficulties, specific learning difficulties (dyslexia) and ASD. Chinese children are the only minority ethnic group over-represented in SLCN. Categories of under-representation are explained in the report by possible professional difficulties in disentangling learning difficulties from EAL.

> The over-representation of Chinese pupils with SLCN requires attention... The suitability and accuracy of assessments and intervention by speech and language therapists and education-ists requires further research to ensure that different needs arising from children having EAL compared with or in addition to developmental language difficulties are recognised and addressed appropriately. (Lindsay *et al.*, 2006: 120)

This analysis also echoes the earlier discussion that language diversity can be constructed as disabling learning opportunities.

These findings suggest evidence of practices that 'racialise disability', in that they link racial/ethnic groups with SEN categories in very familiar ways: African Caribbean with exclusion and behaviour difficulties, EAL with language disability, Roma and Travellers with very low attainment and much higher SEN identification. The links between Pakistani and Bangladeshi pupils and the higher incidence of profound complex needs and deafness is also familiar through existing consanguinity studies. The findings raise questions again about professional knowledge and expertise around identifying SEN, as well as the influence of the distribution of additional resources.

Two main implications emerge from these findings. The majority of resource allocation continues to go to the White majority ethnic group. Yet, there are strong arguments and evidence that culturally and linguistically diverse pupils with additional educational needs for sociocultural reasons require additional resources in mainstream education. Not least of these resources is developing professional knowledge and expertise in working with these learners, and their families and communities.

Under-representation could also indicate a resistance to linking developing EAL knowledge and skills with language difficulties, and to racialising language disability. Nevertheless, similar discriminatory social practices and structures may underpin under- and over-representation practices. For example, Coard (1971) in his study shows that high levels of over-representation of Black children in schools for pupils with learning difficulties were the result of discriminatory social and professional practices. Also, Diniz (1999) in a brief review of the literature on SEN and race in the UK, argues that institutional racism, particularly among the research community, is an explanation for the dearth of evidence, analysis and argumentation in the field.

Reconceptualising Disability and Diversity

This section draws on reconceptualisations of disability and diversity in the literature. Steinstra's point in the introductory chapter is revisited to move from a notion of disaggregated categories of race, ethnicity, gender and impairment, to a more unitary phenomenon of disabled, racial, cultural and linguistic diversity. The section also explores implications for provision.

Steinstra (2002) opens a review of literature on disability, race, ethnicity, language and religion by noting that

> The lives of people with disabilities are shaped by their racial and ethnic status, their religion and their first language. Yet little research has been done on these intersections. (Steinstra, 2002: 1)

Her review of literature demonstrates important features that have implications for provision. First, she notes that the majority of studies reviewed are from North America, which may not only demonstrate the small body of evidence available, but may also reflect a bias in her search. Nevertheless, the findings of the review are similar to a much smaller review based on UK research literature (Diniz, 1999). Diniz found less than 20 studies (although it was not an exhaustive search) reported in the literature over the 1990s. He noted that several categories of impairment had no research evidence around race and CLD. The two reviews of the literature take slightly different perspectives. Steinstra focuses on the interstices of disability and cultural and ethnic diversity, while Diniz takes a more categorical approach to disability and diversity. Nevertheless, the two reviews find similar processes operating in research on different sides of the Atlantic. In their conclusions, Diniz finds that the lack of research in the field supports a claim for institutional racism among the dominantly White/monolingual English research community. Steinstra advocates a more self-conscious research community and one that works more with communities who experience life at the intersections of race/ethnicity/heritage languages/religion and disability. They both assert the need for much more research in the field. A cause of concern is that Steinstra's and Diniz's reviews show that there is almost no research at all on the interstices between disability and heritage language/bilingualism.

Service needs-led provision

Most research in the field is policy and provision driven (Steinstra, 2002). Most studies take the dominant agent's perspective, that of the service provider, which constructs the purpose of the research to inform about providing better 'culturally competent' services. Research in the UK shows that when community language support is available, for example through trained interpreters, there is more take-up of speech and language therapy services (Winter, 1999) and parent involvement in school activities, such as parents' evenings (Blackledge, 2000). Service providers understand that meeting the needs of minority ethnic and linguistic children with disabilities and their families requires setting up community outreach work, interpreter and translation services, culturally sensitive educational and therapeutic work, as well as giving voice to subordinated narratives (Dwivedi, 2002). In addition, professional development needs to incorporate perspectives of difference and diversity, aiming to raise not only cultural awareness by gaining knowledge, but also cultural sensitivity through experiences that challenge one's respective cultural identities and their understanding and acceptance of others (Dwivedi, 2002: 30).

Client needs-led provision

Yet, research that focuses on improving 'culturally competent' services assumes that the service being offered is universally required and is unable to examine the sources of cultural difference and inequalities in provision. Steinstra (2002) advocates that more research is needed from a participatory perspective, involving minority ethnic and linguistic people, in order to explore the processes of their participation. Research from this perspective produces knowledge about how impairment and disability are lived realities, situated in local talk and beliefs of the individuals, families and their communities, and their approaches to service provision. Some research in this vein is at the intersection of disability, minority cultures and languages and poverty (e.g. Ahmad *et al.*, 2000; Atkin *et al.*, 2002; Hatton *et al.*, 2002).

An alternative to provision determined by service needs, is provision informed by social justice, agency of the providers and the needs of clients. A theory of social justice must be based on a shared cultural understanding of fairness. Rawls (1999) argues that an unequal distribution of wealth is only good in a society if the least advantaged benefit. Wealth can be understood not only as material goods, but also cultural and linguistic capital that underpins human capital. We know that unequal distribution of material goods and social and linguistic capital are not advantageous to all. Poverty, ill health and disability are highly correlated and probably mutually causative. They are also highly correlated with minority ethnic and linguistic communities (Hatton *et al.*, 1997; Fujiura & Yamaki, 2000). Structures of service provision can change through the action and agency of people. Two factors need to be in play: an awareness of social justice by the service providers and sufficient demand from clients. Developing sufficient demand, that is agency, is often difficult to achieve among culturally and linguistically diverse client groups, who are underserved by the dominant social, cultural and linguistic providers. It can be achieved through sheer size of client numbers. It can also be achieved by a desire (agency) among service providers to meet this need and to change service provision structures to meet the needs of clients. Strong drivers to develop customised service provision include national initiatives, such as race relations legislation, service policy initiatives and professional guidelines (e.g. the McPherson Report, 1999; Every Child Matters, 2003; No Child Left Behind Act of 2001 (Public Law 107–110), USA; RCSLT, 2006; ASHA, 2008) (see Chapter 9).

There are calls for research to reconceptualise the relationship between disability and diversity other than through causative mechanisms, to inform client needs-led provision:

> ethnic inequalities in health are important because they might point to a wider understanding of mechanisms producing inequalities in health. However, a concern with mechanisms in health inequalities research can lead to a focus on technical interventions along causal pathways, with the roots of health inequalities, wider social inequalities, being ignored. (Nazroo, 1998: 1)

Nazroo's point can be applied to education inequalities as to health inequalities. Research findings point to practices which continue to link racial groups with impairment, and to draw on determinist causative models to interpret impairment, such as biological causes such as race, biosocial causes such as consanguinity, and social causes such as poverty, culture and language. To what extent could these findings be read through a social model or capability model to understand disability in relation to other social inequalities and in the interaction between individuals and diversity, context and sociocultural influences? If, from these findings, we interpret that additional educational need is (re)constructed through social behaviours that marginalise diversity, race, culture and language, we would need to address wider sociocultural relationships of clients and service providers, such as poverty and institutional racism, rather than only target particular minority groups and impairment categories.

Conclusion

This chapter has demonstrated, with reference to research studies, that fundamental questions are raised by the literature about the complex relationship between disability and diversity in ethnicity, race, culture and language. The main argument from a Vygotskian perspective is that while determinist models of interpreting disability and diversity are widely used, they are misleading. They not only support highly individualised approaches to impairment and intervention, they can also construct diversity as deficit and disabling. Examples are found in social and educational practices that confuse and conflate language development with learning difficulties (EAL with SEN) and in the consistent patterns of educational underachievement linked with particular, but not all, ethnically and linguistically diverse groups of pupils. In a wider sense, labelling discourses construct linguistic diversity as disease and linguistic subordination.

Determinist models do not link to development, transformation and learning. Developmental models are better equipped to address the development of conceptual tools to understand the phenomenon of CLD and disability. Recent reviews of literature presented in the chapter indicate that research approaches that disaggregate individual traits of gender, race, ethnicity and impairment categories, to reveal practices of disabling diversity and racialising disability, are driven by service needs. Providers respond to findings by seeking out causal pathways and developing technical expertise, rather than engaging in the more intransigent underlying processes that generate social inequalities in health and education (Nazroo, 1998).

Alternative research approaches focus on exploring clients' perspectives that can inform client needs-led provision. One such approach is through 'identity studies' although it has yet to achieve its promise in changing provision and practice. There is research, using a capability model of disability and diversity, which interrogates the assumption by the providers that provision, as it is currently constructed, meets the needs universally of clients. Further studies orientated by perspectives of social justice need to explore how providers and culturally and linguistically diverse clients reinterpret, renegotiate and customise provision much more to the needs of culturally and linguistically diverse clients.

The approaches in research and provision to conceptualising impairment and disability in contexts of diversity introduced here are the basis of the following chapters. Several issues are revisited in the next three chapters on categorical needs: speech and language difficulties, dyslexia and deafness.

Chapter 4

Bilingual Speech and Language Development and Difficulties

A Case Study

A 5 year old boy is referred to a speech and language therapy service and the speech and language therapist meets the parents for an initial interview. They are concerned because he is showing behaviour problems and becomes frustrated when he is not understood at home. The parents speak Tiv, a Nigerian language, at home. His father or mother frequently returns to Nigeria for two or three months at a time. They came to Britain when the child was aged three and half years. They say that the child speaks a mixture of English and Tiv with his younger brother. His parents report that the boy is not using Tiv appropriate for his age and that his speech is not clear. (Duncan, 1989: 119)

Introduction

The purpose of this chapter is to examine the phenomenon of speech and language difficulties, also known as disorders, in bilingual children with reference to research literature. My specific aim is to clarify the issues considered as central to speech and language difficulties in dual language development and to discuss the implications. There are three caveats. As there is a small body of research on these difficulties in bilingualism, we usually have to extrapolate from theories and studies of monolingual children about what may be pertinent for bilingual children. Speech and language difficulties are understood mainly from perspectives that construct the problems as within the child, rather than as co-constructed phenomena between speaker and listener. Studies concerned with distinguishing substantial language learning difficulties from features of bilingual/second language development through assessment are explored in Chapter 7, and studies of intervention and support are explored in Chapter 8.

In this chapter, I explore four themes. I begin by looking at terms of description and causes of difficulties. I use the second section to examine approaches that represent knowledge of language and knowledge of processing language as indices of bilingual language development, delay and difficulties. In section three, I examine three categories of language difficulties that have been researched cross-linguistically and in bilingual children: language delay, grammar difficulties and speech difficulties. The fourth section deals with bilingual and second language development, and I draw some conclusions with reference to the case study.

Terminologies and Causes

Some bilingual learners, like monolingual learners, have difficulties learning language, speech and communication, and demonstrate delays and difficulties in comparison with peers that go beyond what is typically encountered in learning a second or additional language and get in the way of effective communication. The case study at the start of the chapter captures a fraction of the concerns of bilingual children with speech and language difficulties and their families. Typically, features of difficulties are presented as: speech is difficult to understand or unintelligible, delayed language development in comparison with siblings and in this case a younger sibling, language 'mixing', and all within a bilingual environment. Furthermore, the scenario showed that communication difficulties might be related to other concerns, such as social and emotional behaviour.

There is a categorical typology of speech, language and communication difficulties (e.g. Adams *et al.*, 1997). Most terms describing speech and language difficulties are deficit-focused and specific to one language level. An important focus of research is on specific difficulty with grammar: specific language impairment (SLI). Other aspects of language difficulty researched in the literature include specific speech impairment (e.g. Grunwell, 1987; Dodd, 1995; Stackhouse & Wells, 1997); language impairment (LI); specific speech and language difficulties (phonological-syntactic impairment) (e.g. Fletcher & Hall, 1992); lexical and relational semantics (e.g. Ellis Weismar & Hesketh, 1996); semantic and pragmatic impairment (SPI); pragmatic (language) impairment (PLI/PI) (e.g. Rinaldi 1992a, 1992b, 2000; Norbury & Bishop, 2002; Adams *et al.*, 2005). Terms indicating more global language difficulty include developmental language disorder and developmental language delay. A newer term, derived from an educational perspective, is more inclusive and focused more on learning needs: speech, language and communication needs

(SLCN; Dockrell & Lindsay, 1998). Children's communication difficulties also include stammering and voicing problems, which are not dealt with here.

Description

Learners with a specific difficulty in developing language as their primary educational need are often defined normatively, that is in comparison with normally developing peers. Bishop (1992) defines specific language difficulty across four broad criteria. Language development is 'abnormal or delayed' despite sufficient exposure to the ambient language, a normal capacity to perceive language, a brain which is adequate for learning in the nonverbal domain and intact articulatory structures. These criteria have become more exclusive for research and provision purposes, so that measured language ability is below 1 standard deviation, nonverbal IQ is above 85, hearing is not problematic, there is no neurological dysfunction, oral structures and motor function are not problematic and social and physical interactions are not restricted (Leonard, 1998: 10).

Compared to their age-level peers, children with SLI have difficulties mainly developing grammar/syntax of language (Bishop, 1992; Leonard, 1998). Cross-linguistic studies show that some children demonstrate these difficulties in other first languages, such as Italian, Hebrew, Greek, Panjabi[1] (Leonard & Bortolini, 1998; Duncan & Gibbs, 1987; Pert & Letts, 2003; Rice, 1994).

These problems exist in the absence of global learning difficulties or neurological, sensory or psychosocial and environmental factors, which might adequately explain the extreme difficulties these children show in developing language (Fey et al., 2003: 3; Adams et al., 1997). The specific difficulty is not due to hearing difficulties/loss, general learning difficulties, emotional problems, although they may be associated (Bishop, 2006).

Applying Bishop's (1992) and Fey and colleagues' (2003) definition of SLI is problematic for culturally and linguistically diverse children, for at least two reasons. We do not know enough about the development of other languages, particularly developing bilingually, to be able to claim that 'language acquisition was abnormal'. An IQ of 85 can be a criterion for identifying SLI, which is intended to exclude children with speech and language difficulties associated with global learning difficulties. However, it also excludes bilingual children, as IQ tests, verbal and nonverbal, usually have cultural and linguistic biases. For this reason, Swedish researchers of bilingual speech and language difficulties argue that they cannot use the term 'SLI' and opt for the term 'LI' (Salameh, 2003).

A main focus of research attempts to identify a universal phenotype, set of characteristics, for language deficit, so-called SLI (Tager-Flusberg & Cooper, 1999). Despite the focus of research, there is little uniformity in definitions and measures used to identify preschool children with SLI and no consensus about identifying it in older children, adolescents and adults (Conti-Ramsden & Botting, 1999). Comparison of case history questionnaire data versus individual testing can show a high proportion of disagreement in the classification of SLI (Tallal *et al.*, 2001). Observable behaviours and test scores may appear similar, but underlying processing difficulties and compensatory behaviours can be different (Constable, 1993, 2001).

Having typical overall development except in learning language identifies children with SLI. Nevertheless, they constitute a heterogeneous grouping, which makes it more difficult to identify SLI in practice (Leonard, 1998). Monolingual and bilingual children with these difficulties have problems, varying in severity, with speech and/or grammar, both understanding and producing language. They have smaller vocabularies and often atypical ('deviant') patterns in understanding and expressing speech and grammar in comparison with their typically developing peers. These patterns may appear similar to patterns of second language development, with implications for assessment and intervention (Håkansson & Nettelbladt, 1996; Håkansson *et al.*, 2003).

Monolingual studies show that language difficulties usually develop in early childhood when language fails to develop at the expected rate. Most children outgrow this, although a substantial proportion continue to show difficulties in oral language, reading and literacy skills (dyslexia), numeracy and maths throughout their life, especially if not identified and supported (Snowling & Stackhouse, 2006; Clegg *et al.*, 2005). More boys are identified than girls, in line with gender distribution over special educational need (SEN) (see Chapter 3, discussion), although in the nonidentified population, the gender distribution is nearly equal (Tomblin *et al.*, 1997).

Causes

Speech and language difficulties are usually thought to have a cause, although bilingualism does not cause speech and language difficulties. Although there are early publications that link multilingualism with speech pathology, more recent research shows that bilingualism/dual language development is a positive experience for bilingual children with language learning difficulties (e.g. Paradis *et al.*, 2003b).

Causes of speech and language difficulties are constructed in a biomedical model of knowledge. Language-based difficulties are usually explained by the relationship between genetic and social predispositions. While there is not a single 'grammar gene', SLI is thought to be genetically complex (SLI Consortium, 2002, 2004). Family studies show a hereditary link with these difficulties (Pembrey [1992], Gopnik & Crago [1991], and see Stromswold [1998, 2000] for a comprehensive review of family studies). Studies of twins support work that suggests most clinically significant language difficulties in children do not result from acquired brain lesions or adverse environmental experiences, but from genetic factors that presumably influence early brain development. They argue that this work indicates that early language delay is a distinct disorder and that shared environment is significantly less important (e.g. Dale *et al.*, 1998). This research approach is based mainly on testing aspects of language development. Some aspects of language processing, such as nonword repetition skills, are claimed to be highly heritable and provide a phenotypic marker for SLI (Bishop *et al.*, 1996; SLI Consortium, 2002, 2004).

The relationship between heritable and social influences is often more obscure. A frequently cited cause of speech and language difficulties is mild or fluctuating hearing loss (Bishop, 1986), which may be hereditary or from the social environment, such as poor housing or nutrition, and often associated with linguistic minority communities (Ahmad *et al.*, 2000a; Mir *et al.*, 2001). Some monolingual and bilingual children may present with communication difficulties, which on further investigation are due to substantial social trauma and deprivation. These experiences can inhibit the development of cognitive functions in children and disrupt language learning (Bishop & Mogford, 1993). For many monolingual and bilingual children with speech and language difficulties, no known cause is identified. Nevertheless, whatever the cause of speech and language disabilities, the associated difficulties for communicating have far-reaching effects on social and academic learning.

I use the next section to discuss, with reference to the literature, the dominant ways of representing bilingual first language and understanding speech and language difficulties, which focus on internal cognitive activity and may not account enough (or at all) for external practices.

Ways of Knowing About Language Learning and Difficulties

Models are useful conceptual tools for managing knowledge about language learning, difficulties and breakdown for research and practice in therapy and education. It is generally accepted that we have a biological and cultural predisposition to learn language. Our brains are predisposed to learn knowledge about language and to learn knowledge about processing linguistic information, for one or several languages. Language develops through engagement with the social world, so that children build communication practices that relate socially constructed meanings to the content and form of language knowledge. As yet, there is no generally agreed model of knowledge for bilingual language development and difficulties.

Research of language development is usually represented through linguistic, psycholinguistic and sociocultural frameworks, while research of language disability is also represented though linguistic and psycholinguistic frames, but to a much lesser extent through sociocultural approaches – which is the purpose of this book. Currently, psycholinguistic approaches are the dominant discourse for language development and difficulties. Advocates propose that children apply powerful cognitive strategies to make sense of their complex language environments (Bates & McWhinney, 1987; Tomasello & Brookes, 1999). The relationship between two types of knowledge – knowledge of language and knowledge of cognitions/processing language information – is regarded as central to understanding children's developing language, as a first or additional language, and children's language difficulties. Cognitive knowledge, such as children's implicit and explicit knowledge of organising and managing language information (e.g. phonological awareness), is understood to be important in formal language teaching, literacy teaching and intervention in speech and language difficulties.

I look at two important theories in bilingual development, Dual Language System hypothesis and Processability theory. They posit that the structural aspects of each language in a bilingual child develop relatively independently of each other and in similar forms as for a monolingual learner. Meaning, though, is likely to develop differently.

Dual language system hypothesis

It is generally acknowledged that languages in bilingual development grow separately. However, there was some controversy about how to explain language mixing in the early years of bilingual first language development before 'talk' became differentiated into two separate language codes. One approach argued that early knowledge about organising language was undifferentiated and accounted for by a unitary language system that later bifurcated into two separate language codes (Volterra & Taeschner, 1978). More widely accepted now is the Dual Language System hypothesis (Genesee, 1989), which posits that children develop knowledge about two separate language codes from the start of bilingual development, informed by a predisposition about how to organise language. Evidence to support this hypothesis comes from numerous studies, for example: reanalysis of the data for the unitary language system hypothesis (Genesee, 1989); longitudinal bilingual child studies show separate grammar and morphology development (e.g. Meisel, 1989; De Houwer, 1990) and discrete phonology development (e.g. Zhu & Dodd, 2006a); and studies of infant auditory discrimination show differentiated responses to stimuli from two different languages from as early as 4 months of age (Bosch & Sebastián-Gallés, 1997).

An important feature of bilingual development is 'language mixing', particularly vocabulary mixing as codeswitching. Codeswitching is usually understood as communicative skills demonstrating pragmatic proficiency (Myers-Scotton, 2006). It is not usually interpreted as an indicator of difficulties or disorder in bilingual children (Martin *et al.*, 2003). Codeswitching and lexical borrowing and mixing as a form of codeswitching are discussed further in Chapter 2 as aspects of pragmatic proficiency.

There is a growing body of research on first language early development of grammar and morphology across a range of languages that indicate that structural forms of language are unique and specific to each language (see Pienemann [2005] and colleagues for German, English, Swedish, Japanese, Arabic, Chinese, and Thoradottir [2005] for French and English). Analysing the language of bilingual children shows that, regardless of the child's other language, structural aspects of each of the two languages emerge very much like those in monolingual children (Meisel [1989] for French and German, e.g. for L1 English, Dulay & Burt [1974], Fathman [1975], Krashen *et al.* [1979] and Paradis *et al.* [2003b]). Comparisons of development across languages show that profiles of morphology and other structural development are different. The increase in information about first language development has implications for informing assessment and intervention practices.

Processability theory

Another way of understanding monolingual and bilingual language development uses Processability theory. Processability theory (Pienemann, 1998) is a theory of language development that has been used in cross-linguistic studies to explain bilingual language development. It views language development in a similar way to models of first and second language learning that build on the computer metaphor, a model of language processing (Levelt, 1989). In this approach, language development for the child is driven by a maturational linear dynamic. Even though it is not the same line of development in each language, variation in development is predictable across children and contexts (Pienemann, 2005). According to Processability theory, languages in bilingualism (multilingualism) develop relatively independently of each other.

> The target language is developed according to certain principles, where progress builds on previous steps. The model is not language-specific which makes uniform descriptions of increasing complexity possible even in typologically different languages. Processability theory indicates the degree of grammatical processability and consequently also the order of acquisition between different grammatical structures, such as tense marking, plural agreement and word order. This theory also spells out the processing prerequisites needed for the developmental levels. (Salameh, 2003: 15)

Processability theory also claims to explain interference and interlanguage. While little cross-linguistic transfer of grammar and morphology has been noted in children's bilingual first language development, there is some transfer, or interference, which is sensitive to the developmental state of the learner's language (Pienemann *et al.*, 2005). That is, structures that are earlier emerging in one language may be used in the other language. Pienemann and colleagues have looked in a similar way at the influence of languages developing together in interlanguage. Interlanguage is a term usually used to describe the emerging language of an adult/adolescent as she/he progresses in developing a target language (Selinker, 1972). Three drivers usually orientate interlanguage: the gradual predictable development of language-specific knowledge of the new language, as well as knowledge of the learner's first language, and idiosyncratic language learning.

Within Pienemann's framework, difficulties in speech and language development are explained as forms of variation due to lack of, or problematic, knowledge of language-specific information and processing knowledge. A group of researchers in Sweden have used Processability theory to describe and explain typical and atypical bilingual language development in Arabic–Swedish children (Håkansson, 2005; Håkansson *et al.*, 2003; Salameh *et al.*, 2004). Based on developmental data from over 1000 adults and children with Swedish as a second language, a stage model with milestones has been suggested for Swedish as a second language (Pienemann & Håkansson, 1999), which has been applied to Swedish children with and without speech and language difficulties (Håkansson, 1997, 2001).

I introduce some key concepts about the psycholinguistic approach, which is the dominant paradigm in research and practice in speech and language difficulties. The concepts inform the discussions that follow on speech and language difficulties in bilingual learners.

Psycholinguistic approach: Key concepts

Psycholinguistic approaches, as exemplified by Processability theory, posit that there are two types of knowledge about language: knowledge about language and knowledge about organising and processing language. Language knowledge is language-specific and is constructed in a hierarchy of increasingly complex phrase and sentence forms. Language development is hypothesised as the child's gradual acquisition of *lemmas* and grammatical knowledge from simple to more complex forms, through a hierarchical trajectory towards the adult form of target language performance. In psycholinguistic approaches, grammars are thought to be lexically driven. That is, words have phonological and semantic/conceptual information as well as grammatical category information attachments, such as noun, verb, and are referred to as lemmas. For example, lemmas with noun category information are processed to build noun phrases with appropriate word-level grammar (morphology), to link with verb phrases to form sentences that are shaped by information for clause formation and word order.

Psycholinguistic approaches also posit knowledge about organising grammar information. One idea of how children learn to use the three kinds of linguistic information in words is through *bootstrapping*. Bootstrapping is a hypothesis about how children, in particular, might use linguistic knowledge to interpret the information afforded by one kind of linguistic information to help access another kind. There are three forms of hypothesised bootstrapping. For example, take the utterance *Sarah is feeding the rabbit*: a child may draw from the physical scene the meaning of the utterance and work out the relationship of the participants to the utterance (semantic bootstrapping; Pinker, 1989), notice from the rhythm and stress in the utterance the important words that go together (phonological bootstrapping; Clark, 1993; Chiat, 2000), and perceive the grammatical connection, particularly the verb, with the related words to establish the verb argument and understand the meaning of the proposition (grammatical bootstrapping; Fisher *et al.*, 1994). Children in CLD contexts, learn different language knowledges, simultaneously or one later than another depending on the context, through 'bootstrapping' different language knowledge into different patterns.

A problem with a bootstrapping hypothesis is that agency of language learning is obscure. The perspective is of language development from within the child with a focus on a genetic predisposition to learn language that drives a maturational development. The critique is that in the absence of specific agency, agency and intentions are ascribed to devices and mechanisms of cognitive language learning (Pavlenko & Lantolf, 2000: 175). Shifting the ground to a sociocultural (Vygotskian) interpretation of bootstrapping, children learn language primarily through social engagement, others scaffold for the child the salience of cultural relationships and scaffold how they are represented in linguistic relations, and the different aspects of linguistic information are scaffolded through repetition, modelling and recasting. Clearly, both perspectives are needed, particularly considering bilingual language development.

Researchers who use a computational metaphor posit a knowledge of processing language information as highly specialised, task-specific, autonomous and automatic (Pienemann, 1998). Chunks of language are processed immediately and incrementally build on each other. Knowledge of processing output is linear, although it may be mapped onto meaning differently. An important aspect of organising knowledge is memory, both for content information and for grammatical information. Knowledge about grammatical memory is highly specialised and task-specific to automatically process information about grammar. There seem to be similar memory knowledges for phonological and semantic information. Knowledge about working memory, on the other hand, is the resource for very short-term attentive processes, which include conceptualising and monitoring (Baddeley, 1990). These two memories are also known as 'procedural memory' and are thought to process other motor and cognitive skills. Everything that can be represented at conscious level, such as awareness of language learning and conceptual learning, is thought to be processed by 'declarative knowledge/memory'.

Procedural and declarative knowledges are familiar constructs in second language research (Towell & Hawkins, 1994).

A psycholinguistic approach, particularly Processability theory, is a 'learnability' theory rather than a 'learning' theory. The child is constructed as an active problem-solver of the language puzzle, where predetermined maturation engages with the linguistic environment, in what Pienemann (2005: 2) describes as a personal 'logico-mathematical space'. There are echoes of a Piagetian account of cognitive development, where adults are facilitators of maturational development rather than involved in transforming children's development. In some accounts, the psycholinguistic processing system is anthropomorphised, that is, the system itself is imbued with abilities to select, reject and decide on aspects of language to process (Pavlenko & Lantolf, 2000: 176; Potter, 1996). Learnability theories (Pinker, 1994) take little account of learning language with others in a co-construction of language knowledge. How are young bilingual learners to be engaged to change and transform their slower or unusual language development, which marginalises them from communication and academic learning? This is the question that Vygotsky asked about children with severe learning difficulties and one that is addressed for bilingual children with speech and language difficulties in the chapter on intervention.

In the third section of the chapter, I look particularly at aspects of language form that present challenges for monolingual and bilingual children vulnerable to language difficulties.

Core Difficulties

Difficulties in morphology and grammar are both a core feature of speech and language difficulties and a research focus. In this section, I examine morphology and verb grammar, bilingual speech difficulties, and core difficulties at a phonological level, in particular nonword repetition skills.

Morphology and verb grammar

Language-specific morpheme development

Language-specific developmental information about morphology in bilingual children is important for identifying language difficulties. There seems to be a developmental sequence of morphology and early grammar that is language-specific, which most learners follow on their way towards a target language, whether they develop the language as a first or additional language (for review, see Bialystok, 2001). In English, for example, it is generally accepted that the function morphemes of word grammar (morphology), identified as early emerging in first language English by Brown (1973), also emerge early in L2 English regardless of learners' first language (Dulay & Burt, 1974; Fathman, 1975). It seems there is a language-specific constraint on this aspect of language development. What would such a constraint look like?

Function morphemes (determiners) and bound morphemes (prefixes, suffixes, concord) contrast with content/lexical morphemes (nouns, verbs), and are more difficult to detect in speech. Phonologically they are unstressed and often omitted in child language and contracted in adult speech; semantically they have abstract, or almost no, meaning, yet grammatically they are obligatory. Emergence does not depend on conceptual knowledge. Cross-linguistically, similar function morphemes emerge in children's talk at different stages across languages, depending on the position they have in grammatical sequences. The example often cited is the emergence of spatial relations morphemes 'in/on' in the speech of children simultaneously bilingual in Hungarian and Serbo–Croatian. In Hungarian, the morphemes are suffixed and in Serbo–Croatian they are prepositioned before the noun. Children developed the suffix morpheme in Hungarian before Serbo–Croatian (Slobin, 1973, cited in Chiat, 2000: 199–200). Morphemes in more highly inflected languages may develop earlier (Duncan & Gibbs, 1987). Morphosyntactic errors have not been found to be as prominent in children with SLI in highly inflected languages (Leonard, 1998). Explanations include that forms following nouns are easier to perceive/learn than structures before the noun. Post-positioning offers a more salient connection between the morpheme and the noun it is semantically associated with. Alternatively, functional morphemes in highly inflected languages may carry a higher semantic load. Other salience markers are phonological, such as rhythm stress in word order, although they have no semantic salience.

Language-specific grammatical complexity

Surface patterns of language development and difficulties are language-specific, thus bilingual children have different emerging profiles in each language. Two examples come from morphology and grammar development. A distinguishing characteristic of language difficulties for English-speaking children (e.g. 5+ years) is persistent difficulty with verb vocabulary and verb morphology (see for review, Eadie, 2004b). However, children with SLI have less difficulty in other languages that have different verb structures (Hebrew: Dromi *et al.*, 1999; Spanish: Bedore & Leonard, 2002; Italian: Bortolini *et al.*, 1998).

Grammatical complexity is sensitive to language-specific variation. Monolingual English-speaking children with language difficulties have more difficulty than same-age peers, understanding increasing grammatical complexity than sentence length (Ellis Weismar *et al.*, 1999; Montgomery, 2000). In a cross-linguistic study, English and Hungarian children with SLI show that they have less difficulties understanding longer simple sentences and more difficulties understanding short (or long) complex sentences (Marton *et al.*, 2006). However, it was for different reasons in each language. In English, lower accuracy was associated with grammatical (syntactic) complexity and in Hungarian it was associated with morphological complexity. The implications for assessment are that children's language difficulties need to be assessed in each of their languages. There are implications for teaching/learning, particularly practitioner talk, with children with these kinds of difficulties, where even short sentences can make high demands on children's understanding if their structure is not simple.

Language-sensitive phonological and morphological links

Children with language difficulties seem to have less difficulty with functional morphemes that have robust (stressed) phonological information. That is, the more auditory saliency the morphemes have, the more likely they will be learnt correctly. In Italian, bound function morphemes that are usually unstressed, such as the direct object pronoun and third person singular 's', are highly likely to be omitted by preschool children with SLI (Bortolini *et al.*, 2002). In these circumstances, it would seem that there is too little phonological information for children with SLI to learn the morphemes (phonological bootstrapping). Bortoloni and colleagues (2006) claim that these features are 'strong clinical markers' to identify SLI, although the third person singular 's' was a slightly less reliable marker because the children sometimes used it correctly. These studies with children with SLI in Italian show the connection between language-sensitive phonological information, grammatical knowledge and performance. These studies may also indicate that language-sensitive phonological (syllabic and prosodic) information plays a role in determining the suitability of nonword repetition as a clinical marker of SLI. Nonword repetition is discussed later.

I now turn to speech, and introduce a typology of speech difficulties, which I discuss with reference to bilingual and cross-linguistic studies of the organisation of phonological knowledge in other languages and children's phonological difficulties.

Bilingual speech difficulties

Speech difficulties affecting intelligibility are categorised by four subgroups: motor articulation difficulties, delayed phonological development, consistent and inconsistent patterns of phonological difficulty, including childhood apraxia of speech (CAS) (dyspraxia) (Dodd, 1995). Bilingual studies indicate separate development of phonology information across languages (e.g. Pienemann, 1998; Zhu Hua & Dodd, 2006a). Speech difficulties arise from difficulties organising phonological information. Cross-linguistic and bilingual studies support a similar typology of speech difficulties, suggesting that they arise from difficulties in cognitive knowledge of organising and processing language-specific information (e.g. Italian: Bortolini & Leonard, 1991; Cantonese: So & Dodd, 1994, 1995; Turkish: Topbas & Konrot, 1996; Spanish: Goldstein, 2005; German: Fox & Dodd, 2001; Swedish: Pienneman & Håkansson, 1999; Punjabi: Stow & Pert, 2006).

Speech difficulties are currently understood through a psycholinguistic framework, and particularly through the notion of a 'speech information processing chain' (e.g. Dodd, 1995; Stackhouse & Wells, 1997). Our understanding of knowledge of phonological information focuses mainly on organisation within single words. The sequence of processing speech knowledge is auditory perception and discrimination, meaning and grammar, motor programming and planning, and articulating speech is the final executive stage. Cross-linguistic studies with bilingual children show that surface speech errors reflect similar difficulties organising phonological knowledge regardless of the language-specific phonological system. For example, deleting unstressed syllables affects both phonologies. Zhu Hua and Dodd, (2006b) summarise, from a collection of studies on bilingual speech difficulties, shared characteristics and noticeable differences of speech difficulties in bilingual children.

Speech difficulties in bilingual children

Children tend to demonstrate similar types of surface difficulties in both languages, although not identical, which suggests that there is a single underlying difficulty in processing knowledge affecting both phonological knowledges. For example, difficulty in phonological memory affects development in both surface phonologies of Welsh/English bilingual children (Ball *et al.*, 2006), with implications for assessment and intervention.

Articulation difficulties

Articulation is a motor function, and difficulties in articulation of speech sounds and sequences are not at a level of linguistic meaning. It is the final aspect of the speech chain. Thorough motor assessment of movements for speech reveals organic/maturational speech motor difficulties, which affect articulation of speech sounds in both languages. Intervention in one language for speech articulation difficulties transfers to the other language (Holm *et al.*, 1997). Learning new motor speech patterns of a second language is still developing between 4 and 9 years (de Bot, 1992).

Bilingual phonological development

The developmental sequence of speech sounds is shaped by maturation, such as speech motor development, auditory acuity and mental capacities, across languages. In bilingual first language, syllabic and segmental (consonants and vowels; CV) phonological information develops simultaneously and language specifically across both languages. Bilingual phonological development is different compared with monolingual phonological development (Holm & Dodd, 1997). Transfer of phonological knowledge across languages is unlikely (Holm & Dodd, 1999), although it has been noted across Arabic/Swedish sequential bilinguals (Salameh, 2003). Holm and Dodd (1999) suggest that bilingual children may show 'normal interference between [their] languages' where the confusions in speech sounds are typical of bilingual children speaking those two languages and resolve themselves relatively quickly as children develop the two speech sound codes. Confusion of aspects of phonological systems and speech sounds is a developmental characteristic of bilingual learners. In older learners and adults, these confusions may remain and become recognisable as features of a foreign/second language accent. Salameh (2003) notes the importance of recognising developmental aspects of second language phonology that improve with engagement with the language, over at least one and half to two years. This finding has assessment implications. They need not be considered as speech difficulties unless they persist and prevent intelligibility. Persistent severe speech difficulties have other explanations.

Delayed phonological development

When phonological development is not age appropriate and shows consistent patterns of 'errors' similar to that of younger children, it is said to be delayed. Typically, the delay resolves when speech becomes age appropriate, but sometimes it can continue (Dodd *et al.*, 2000). The development of surface speech patterns can be analysed by 'natural processes' (Stampe, 1979; Ingram, 1989). These processes affect syllabic and segmental information by reducing the meaningful contrast between words. Syllabic processes simplify the shape and prosody of the syllable (e.g. cluster reduction, final consonant deletion, weak syllable deletion). Segmental (speech sounds) information is simplified when speech sounds are articulated near the same place of articulation as the target sound and/or in a similar manner, such as 'fronting' process (velar/alveolar) and 'stopping' process (fricative/plosive). Homonyms are a feature of developing and delayed speech: e.g. 'tofy' is said for both toffee and coffee, 'tik' for stick and tick; 'tar' for guitar, tar and car. As children become aware and are made aware of the potential communicative confusion, 'errors' can resolve. These processes are evident in monolingual and bilingual phonological development.

How do we know when a bilingual child's speech and language delay/difficulties have resolved? Evidence for 'growing out of it', that is the *normalisation of speech variations*, indicates that speech difficulties in monolingual English children typically resolve at about 7 years of age and difficulties after that, particularly after 9 years, will persist (Shriberg *et al.*, 1999). However, researchers of languages other than English are hesitant to identify 'normalisation' of speech development because of dialect variations and other sociolinguistic factors (Goldstein, 2005). There is no research evidence about typical 'normalisation' of speech development in learners of English as an additional language (EAL) or other languages to inform referring policy and practice and assessment practice. Such research would need to consider the phonological developmental trajectories of both languages, as well as the regional variations of local speakers. Perhaps it would be more feasible to involve sociocultural implicit knowledges about typical acceptable speech practices.

Consistent 'deviant' speech difficulties

Children whose speech is characterised by systematic use of atypical (nondevelopmental) phonological patterns are described as having consistent deviant phonology, e.g. deleting all syllable initial consonants (Leonard, 1985; Ingram, 1989). It is thought to be due to difficulties organising and abstracting relevant phonological information from the speech of others. Consequently, children with these types of speech patterns have difficulties with phonological awareness tasks, such as segmental, syllabic-based tasks of alliteration and rhyme, and tasks on judging legitimate sound sequences (legality awareness) across languages. These difficulties are evident in both/all languages because of difficulties organising internal phonological information in the speech information processing chain. Assessment and intervention would need to address the phonologies of both languages.

Inconsistent 'deviant' speech difficulties

Children with 'inconsistent speech disorder' produce variable pronunciations of the same words or phonological features not only from context to context, but also within the same context. Their speech has unpredictable variation between a relatively large number of speech sounds. They have an unstable *phonological* system because of difficulties in planning and organising the selection, and sequencing, of phonological information for speech sounds, syllables and word sequences. This difficulty may be explained by the child's phonological knowledge being 'underspecified or degraded' for word production. It is further explained by the child having *phonetic* programmes with articulatory parameters that are too broad, leading to additional articulatory (phonetic) variability even when the correct speech sound (phoneme) is selected (Dodd & McCormack, 1995; Crosbie *et al.*, 2005). In these psycholinguistic accounts of speech difficulties, the 'agent' of these difficulties is not always identified, although it may be implied it is the anthropomorphised processing system. It is, in fact, the child, and their biopsychological maturational predisposition (see Chapter 8). As both phonemic and phonetic organisation is confused, assessment and intervention would need to be language-specific. There is little research evidence of bilingual children with these difficulties.

Childhood apraxia of speech

Children with CAS are different from children with inconsistent speech disorder. Although all have speech marked by inconsistency, children with CAS

- are worse in imitation than in spontaneous production (in contrast with children with inconsistent speech disorder who are better at imitation than spontaneous speech);
- have different cues to elicit production of words;
- have oro-motor difficulties.

CAS (also referred to as dyspraxia) is controversial because of the conflicting ways it has been discussed in studies. Nevertheless, there is agreement that it is a severe speech difficulty with a neurological basis, which is generally described in speech information processing terms. CAS is described as 'a multilevel speech disorder characterised by disturbed programming and planning of speech movements that cannot be attributed to neuromuscular weakness' (Ozanne, 1995; Moriarty & Gillon, 2006). Children's speech is characterised by a limited number of speech sounds, inconsistent speech patterns in CV, difficulty sequencing articulatory movements, prosodic inconsistencies, difficulties with other aspects of expressive language, phonological processing difficulties and reading and writing difficulties (Stackhouse & Snowling, 1992a, 1992b; Ozanne, 1995). As with inconsistent speech disorder, it is thought that CAS results from difficulties organising phonological information, particularly in storing, selecting and retrieving information to inform articulation. A distinguishing feature of CAS is that articulation is also affected, in that the intimate and symbiotic relationship between articulation and phonology of speech is disturbed due to the inconsistent feedback from motor patterns in the realisation of speech (Dodd, 1995). Related aspects of language, such as vocabulary learning, reading, writing and spelling are likely to be affected, with implications for educational success (Stackhouse & Snowling, 1992a, 1992b; Lewis *et al.*, 2004; Marquardt *et al.*, 2002). There are likely to be several professionals involved with the educational management of learners who are identified with dyspraxia, with implications for collaborative work (see Chapter 9). There is little published evidence about bilingual children with CAS. Both (all) languages will be affected in complex and multilevel ways.

There is research evidence about delayed phonology and consistent phonological difficulties from a Swedish study of bilingual children with a cohort of children with speech and language difficulties. A study (Salameh, 2003) of Arabic–Swedish sequential bilingual children aged between 3 and 6 years with less than 3 years engagement with L2 Swedish, compared the phonological development of a group of typically developing children with children who had identified language difficulties. The important findings were that profiles of the surface patterns of the two groups were qualitatively similar, but quantitatively different. The typically developing group showed an expected asymmetry in development between the two languages, with more syllabic and segmental processes of simplification in L2 words than L1. Children with language difficulties showed significantly higher incidence of syllabic simplification across both languages than the comparison group, with similar processes operating across both languages.

The profiles of phonological information (syllabic and segmental) across L1 and L2 were relatively symmetrical for the group with language difficulties. The profile for the typically developing sequential bilingual children suggests that organisational knowledge of phonological information was more developed in L1 language, and less in L2 language. The profile for the sequential bilingual children with language difficulties suggests that the children's surface speech pattern difficulties arose from applying similar, inadequate organisation knowledge to the phonological information of both languages. Salameh (2003) also reports that the lexical development of the bilingual children was slower in comparison with their monolingual Swedish peers. In addition, vocabulary development in the bilingual children with speech and language difficulties was even slower. There are implications for literacy skills and educational success.

Analysis of surface patterns presented by phonological processes need to be supplemented by information about consistency in and across contexts. Information from assessment of tasks that reflect the organisation, processing and management of the two phonologies is also necessary, to inform therapy intervention as well as educational support.

Core difficulties at phonological level: Nonword repetition

Research studies are interested in looking at phonological information in nonword repetition as a core characteristic of speech and language difficulties. Nonword repetition reflects abilities to learn new phonological sequences for new words. This task appraises knowledge about organising phonological information without support from semantic information or prior rote learning of the word (Kamhi, 1998; Gathercole & Baddeley, 1996). Difficulties impact on vocabulary learning, comprehension and production of language. Nonword repetition seems to be a strong distinguishing feature between bilingual language difficulties and slower SLA, which needs to be further researched.

Nonword repetition abilities are independent of language-specific information, but need to take account of surface features and permissible phonological (phonotactic) patterns of the language. For example, the base unit for phonological form is syllabic, with segmental and prosodic knowledge. English is a language with numerous syllabic possibilities (e.g. CV, VC, CVC, CCVCC), while other languages, such as Cantonese, are syllabic with a smaller number of syllable possibilities, possibly because form is also constituted through tone. Cantonese-speaking children with SLI performed as well as their peers with typical language development on a nonword repetition task (organising phonological knowledge) because the Cantonese syllabic form is easier to organise with a more limited inventory of CV (Stokes *et al.*, 2006). There are implications for designing assessment tasks. When prosodic information (weakly stressed syllables) was included in testing Italian monolingual children with SLI, they showed that they were highly likely to omit unstressed syllables in nonword repetition tasks of polysyllabic non-words with Italian phonology (Bortolini *et al.*, 2006). These findings have implications for assessment and learning new words in educational contexts.

A critical reflection on understanding speech difficulties and nonword repetition shows that research evidence has been generated within a cognitive paradigm with little or no account taken of context. Bilingu-alism is depicted as a cognitive construct. Implications for assessment and intervention are indicated, but clearly require further theoretical work to interpret how they would be enacted. Studies in second language learning draw on Vygotskian approaches to teaching/learning in group and classroom contexts to examine and understand intervention processes, and are discussed further in Chapters 7 and 8. In the next section, I deal with second/additional language development in school-aged children with language difficulties.

Second Language Development (L2, SLA): Interference, Transfer, Interlanguage

There is a large amount of literature on second language development. I narrow my focus here to an aspect of L2 development that is a site of potential confusion with speech and language difficulties. There are four stages of typical L2 development (Tabors, 1997).

(1) Home language use.
(2) Nonverbal period in L2 contexts, which can be confused with difficulties in understanding and pragmatics in L2.
(3) Telegraphic and formulaic use, which may be confused with delayed and 'disordered' L2 language development.
(4) Productive language use.

When linguistic minority children enter school, generally they rapidly develop the surface patterns of the additional language for social communication, usually within 1–2 years. Yet, they have considerable difficulties managing the language demands for academic learning. It may take a further 5–7 years for them to develop the complex grammar and vocabulary associated with curriculum learning (Cummins, 2000; Thomas & Collier, 1997). Second or additional language development shows more variation than bilingual first language, but development appears still to follow the Dual Language System hypothesis. L2 development depends on the quality and amount of exposure as well as engagement with the language. L2 learners demonstrate 'interlanguage' – a unique language system produced by the learner evolving over time towards the second language (Selinker, 1972).

A second language learner may be mistakenly identified as having speech and language difficulties, or 'impaired language learning'. Patterns in developing grammar and morphology in a language can be similar for children with speech and language difficulties, language spoken by younger children or even for children in the early stage of learning a second language (interlanguage). However, there are aspects of language development that are different from that of younger learners and second language learners, specifically verb grammar and morphology development (Genesee *et al.*, 2004: 19). Researchers and practitioners working with this group of learners need to be familiar with descriptions of sequences of second/additional language development.

Another type of language mixing is shown by 'nontarget grammar forms' in the developing languages, that is, when grammatical and morphological features of the first language are transferred unintentionally to the other language. This phenomenon may be called transfer and is a typical feature of development of bilingual and second language learners. It may be a strong feature of second language development as children develop an emerging evolving form of the language, an interlanguage (Selinker, 1972). It indexes a complex relationship between languages. Interlanguage, while appearing full of 'errors', is a demonstration of systematic development and learning towards the target additional language, through language-specific information being organised by processing knowledge. The second language learner usually has difficulties learning L2 morphology, particularly verb grammar, and phonology. Hence, the surface language patterns of talk by children developing second/additional language can appear similar to those of children with speech and language difficulties.

Pienneman's Processability theory contributes to conceptualising the interference or transfer phenomena across languages. Transfer is only likely to occur when two similar forms in the hierarchies of language structures in each language emerge at the same time. The L2 structure appears influenced by the L1 form and like an L2 'error'. In this interpretation, language learning is more determinist and the role of the learner seems passive.

Another interpretation of the pace and errors of second language learning, particularly in the early period, is that children use their knowledge of their first language to scaffold learning of the second language (Genesee *et al.*, 2004). When structures between the L1 and L2 differ, the learner relies on L1 language-specific information to inform learning L2 structures in grammar or phonology, which usually results in L2 'errors'. Second language learners aged 4–5 years, who have already developed a phonological system, have internal phonological knowledge that they are likely to draw on to 'scaffold' learning the phonology of the second language. For example, they may categorise the phonological knowledge of the second language like their established first language, or they may use metacognitive knowledge and phonological awareness to develop phonological learning strategies. Here, the learner, whether L2 or with speech and language difficulties, is constructed as agentive.

Conclusions

In this chapter, I have examined aspects of speech and language development and difficulties in bilingual children. Bilingual first language development shows a similar sequence of speech and language development in each language as language-specific monolingual development. Development of sequential bilingualism shows similarities in the monolingual developmental sequence and, depending on the age of the learner, may show transfer of language information from the first language to the second/additional language in the process of development. Bilingual speech and language difficulties are generally constructed in research and practice through the speech-processing chain. They are understood to arise from difficulties with knowledge for organising phonological information. Bilingual children are likely to show slightly different surface level difficulties in their languages, with implications for assessment and intervention in both languages. This chapter speaks to Steinstra's notion of how we construct bilingual disability: either/or, or and/and. Bilingual children with and without speech and language difficulties develop structural aspects of language as independent systems: and/and: Arabic and Swedish, German and French. This is further evidence that either/or choices are constructed socially rather than by the child's speech and language difficulties.

How would the information in this chapter help us to understand the difficulties with language development for the sequential bilingual Tiv/English child whose case was presented at the beginning of the chapter? First, the child is developing bilingually and shows pragmatic proficiency in codeswitching across his languages even though he has language difficulties. This is in line with evidence discussed in the chapter, that children with language difficulties become bilingual when they have to engage with contexts of CLD. Further, we see that his difficulties in one area of language development do not prevent him from developing social language proficiency using both his languages. His speech may be an important indicator of where his language difficulties lie. Evidence indicates that surface speech difficulties are usually linked with difficulties organising phonological information, which can have a widespread effect, delaying language development. Speech difficulties are also associated with difficulties developing literacy skills in school. It would be important to examine more closely these difficulties in language performance across both languages. The child's move to England and the alternate absence of one or other of his parents may have a social and emotional impact on his bilingual language development. This aspect may also need to be explored. Chapter 7 looks at issues concerning assessment of speech and language difficulties.

Note

1. There are two spellings of Punjabi/Panjabi. They are often interchangeable. Here, the spelling is the same as in the article's title.

Chapter 5

Literacy, Biliteracies and Difficulties with Printed Language

Case Study

Three English–Panjabi children aged 7 years of age have speech difficulties in both languages and are receiving therapy bilingually. They are learning literacy skills in school in English only. P had severely delayed phonological development but now has only a specific confusion with one pair of speech sounds; his literacy skills and practices in creative writing and documentation are developing well; he is progressing slightly ahead of his class peers and is self-confident. T had delayed speech and receptive and expressive language development and he still has one atypical speech articulation; some of his literacy skills are delayed; he spells phonetically and relies on copying new words; he is good at creative writing although slow at documentation and is self-confident. K's speech was unintelligible and she had difficulties with other language levels; she has improved and can make herself understood; she has limited sight vocabulary; she prints and copies all words; her progress is slower than her peers and her self-confidence is low. (Martin *et al.*, 1997)

Introduction

This chapter is about literacy, literacy practices and difficulties with printed language in contexts of cultural and linguistic diversity (CLD). Some children and adults, both monolingual and bilingual, have more difficulty than their peers in learning to handle print – to read, spell and write, despite having similar nonverbal intelligence measures, life experiences and teaching and learning opportunities and experiences. Difficulties with printed language are often called dyslexia or specific learning difficulties (LD). The purpose of the chapter is to examine inter-relationships across psychological and critical sociocultural approaches to literacy for educational practices with bilingual children with literacy disabilities.

Dyslexia is also associated with speech and language difficulties. The case study at the beginning of the chapter shows profiles of three bilingual children who have speech, language and literacy difficulties. Although two of them seem to be overcoming difficulties with literacy skills, the third child continues to have substantial difficulties. The relationship between speech, language and communication difficulties and dyslexia is not straightforward. Evidence from monolingual children supports the view that specific language impairment (SLI) and dyslexia are distinct but potentially co-occurring developmental language-related difficulties. Difficulties in phonological processing are closely associated with dyslexia, but not with SLI when it occurs in the absence of dyslexia (Catts *et al.*, 2005).

The chapter explores four perspectives. I use the first section to contextualise studies of literacy, literacies and difficulties in literacy development concerning dyslexia and multilingualism. The second section evaluates the insights and constraints afforded by psychological and linguistic approaches to dyslexia and CLD. The third section examines sociocultural and critical anthropological perspectives on literacy and biliteracies, and highlights the significance of a critical perspective for bilingual learners. The fourth section examines the implications of research findings for educational practices for culturally and linguistically diverse learners with dyslexia. Finally, I draw some conclusions.

Approaches to Researching Literacy, Literacies and Dyslexia

In the introductory chapter, I introduced the idea that researching bilingualism and disability is a boundaried zone of study, with different disciplines 'underlapping' in research, and cited Cline and Reason (1993: 30–34):

> it seems strange that the research traditions on specific learning difficulties (dyslexia) and social and cultural differences have remained in different compartments.

Literacy skills and dyslexia are mainly researched through cognitive psychological and psycholinguistic approaches, while bilingualism and biliteracy are researched through sociocultural and critical anthropological perspectives. Cummins describes researching biliteracy and difficulties developing literacy skills as 'parallel discourses' that mirror a similar dualism in wider debates about effective education for culturally and linguistically diverse learners (Cummins, 2000: 247). Rassool conceptualises literacy research as a *regionalised field of enquiry* of four overlapping areas of study that represent the dialogic relationship between literacy knowledges and subject disciplines: linguistics, sociological and cultural theory, social anthropology and social history, and psychology (Rassool, 2002: 34–35). Hornberger constructs the relationship across research disciplines for biliteracy as an inter-relationship of nested continua (Hornberger, 1989), which reflects ideologies of literacy (Hornberger & Skilton-Sylvester, 2000). An important site in this chapter is the inter-relatedness of research for educational practice for bilingual learners with literacy disability.

Different levels of analysis of literacy across the disciplines of study add to the multidimensional aspect of the field. Psychological approaches focus on technical knowledge skills, e.g. phonemic awareness, single words and sentential meaning, assessment and 'diagnosis' of difficulties. Linguistic and psycholinguistic studies explore sense and meaning making in literacy texts and reading comprehension for learning. Sociocultural approaches focus on social routines involving literacy, such as religious practices, which contribute to developing shared cultural cognitions. Anthropological approaches examine literacy as a site of social organisation, distribution of power and privilege, and a site of ideological agency and struggle, and negotiation of individual and collective identities.

Research from these disciplines informs practice: social practice, ideological practice, cultural practice and educational practice. 'Crossing boundaries' between research disciplines creates overlapping knowledges that inform practice about literacy (Rassool, 2002). For example, educational practice for literacy is informed by psychological knowledge of processing language and orthography, linguistic knowledge of forms and structures of text; sociocultural knowledge of situated meaning making, (in)equities in distribution of literacy knowledges; and critical anthropological knowledge of empowerment and subordination of vernaculars, languages, literacies and literacy practices, and the impact on learners' agency and identity. The chapter examines the emerging evidence base from inter-related research that informs educational practice for literacy with bilingual learners. It also reveals the little inter-related research evidence that informs educational practice for bilingual learners with dyslexia, and highlights it as a specific site for further study.

Where do the difficulties lie?

Literacy is often used as a barometer for schooling and educational success at national and individual levels. Low achievement with reading among additional language learners is a concern in the UK. The international study, Programme for International Student Assessment (PISA;[1] OECD, 2001) investigated language spoken at home and achievement levels on reading literacy, mathematical literacy and scientific literacy. In the UK, students who did not speak the language of assessment or other national language were nearly twice as likely to be among the lowest 25% of performers in reading skills compared to those who spoke the language of the assessment most of the time (OECD, 2001; West & Pennel, 2003). Similar findings have been identified in two major studies that examined reading in schools in the USA (Snow *et al.*, 1998; Snow, 2002). In the UK, literacy and attainment in bilingual learners is an area of increasing interest in policy and practice, yet it remains largely under-researched (Soler *et al.*, 2002).

With reference to the research paradigms, at least three possible interpretations emerge. A psychological interpretation would be that the problem lies in individual learners' difficulties in learning literacy, including dyslexia. Alternatively, from a sociocultural perspective, the problem lies in the teaching/learning approaches to literacy for culturally and linguistically diverse students, where bilingual learners in particular are at risk of being 'pedagogically disabled'. From an anthropological perspective, the problem lies in the coercive and discriminatory educational structures that privilege the dominant language and literacy and subordinate and marginalise others. The inter-relatedness of literacy perspectives offers a powerful lens to study educational practice that addresses difficulties developing literacy in multi/bilingual learners.

While bilingual and English as an additional language (EAL) learners are mainly referenced in this chapter, an important constituency is foreign language (FL) learners. Children's dyslexia may often only become obvious when they engage with print in other languages, for example, FL learning in school. This issue is becoming increasingly important as English as a foreign language (EFL) becomes more widespread as the medium of curriculum instruction for primary school aged children in many countries.

Psycholinguistic Approaches to Dyslexia and Literacy in Bilingual Learners

I use this section to present a psychological perspective of dyslexia. Developments in research and provision indicate moves away from exclusive decontextualised understandings of dyslexia to more inclusive contextualised approaches that seek to accommodate CLD. I discuss three substantive aspects of psychological and linguistic dyslexia research: dyslexia as a flaky concept, core difficulties associated with dyslexia, and reading comprehension difficulties, and offer a critical perspective for bilingual learners with dyslexia. I begin with a review of studies that indicate that bilingualism has a positive effect on learning cognitive tools for literacy skills.

A traditional psychological approach constructs literacy as a cognitive tool that can be applied to any text in any situation. From this perspective, literacy is a homogeneous entity, a learnt set of 'autonomous' cognitive skills, not dependent on social, cultural or language context. This is the dominant approach to research on development and difficulties in reading, spelling and writing. Research done in the 1980s showed that preliterate children who had phonological awareness, that is, showed metalinguistic awareness of speech sounds and syllable formation in words, went on to be more successful readers than their peers who did not have phonological awareness (Bradley & Bryant, 1983). Thus approach has become the basis for policy and practice of literacy teaching in the UK and USA, illustrated by literacy curricula that emphasise the development of phonological awareness to facilitate phoneme-grapheme correspondence skills and orthography skills and knowledge.

Research on EAL and literacy development also has a psychological orientation. Preschool and primary school bilingual children perform similar to, and often better than, their monolingual peers on preliteracy and literacy tasks (Bruck & Genesee, 1995; Campbell & Sais, 1995; Frederickson & Frith, 1998). Psychological research indicates that bilingual languages and literacies are cognitively *inter*dependent (Bialystok, 2001; Cummins, 1984, 2000). Learning and cognitive skills are transferable across languages and literacies, for example, words and letters with the same orthographic representation across languages are read in either language by young bilingual learners (Durgunoglu *et al.*, 1993). Interdependence across languages and literacies is a positively enhancing and essential aspect of learning in bilingual contexts, and links with findings of cognitive flexibility associated with bilingualism (Cummins, 1984; Bialystok, 2001). Psychological research explores the cognitive tools that learners need to develop for literacy skills and practices. From a Vygotskian perspective, the important criticism is that studies are not contextualised sufficiently in the sociocultural meaningfulness of literacy and its practices. There are implications for educational practice.

Dyslexia: A flaky concept

Increasingly, researchers recognise the 'flakiness' of the boundaries between dyslexia, dyslexia-type difficulties and 'common or garden variety' reading difficulties. There is a move away from exclusive definitions that depend on a discrepancy between children's reading level and their general cognitive and academic functioning (Stanovich, 1998; Stanovich & Siegel, 1994). There are other poor readers with inadequate phonological processing skills as well as poor oral language or low general cognitive abilities, who are often referred to as 'common or garden variety' poor readers (Castles & Coltheart, 1993; Stanovich, 1994). Slow progress developing literacy skills despite the usual experiences of teaching and engagement with literacy is also taken as a marker for dyslexia.

Individual dyslexics show noticeably varied patterns of visual and phonological difficulties in their reading (Seymour, 1986). Variations in literacy difficulties (mild, moderate, severe) are more likely due to quantitative differences in risk factors rather than qualitative differences in subtypes of difficulty. That is, dyslexia difficulties are on a spectrum of severity modified by risk and protective factors (Bradley & Bryant, 1985; Snowling, 2001). Risk factors lie in the balance of strengths and weaknesses in compensatory factors, such as visual memory, perceptual speed and exposure to print. Protective factors are better oral language skills (Snowling, 2001) as well as early identification and appropriate intervention (Pumphrey, 1991; Snow et al., 1998).

Identifying causes of dyslexia has been an important strand of research in the medical/psychological discourse. Dyslexia has been attributed to neurological differences, phonological processing difficulties and poor teaching (Stanovich, 1994). The extent to which neurological differences are a correlation or a cause of dyslexia is not clear. People with dyslexia may have cerebellum and medulla differences in brain development (Perani et al. [1996] in Schneider & Crombie [2003]) as well as neuronal asymmetries in the visual cortex in comparison with people who do not have dyslexia (Jenner et al., 1999). Some children with persistent reading difficulties may have spatial cognition problems (Del Giudice et al., 2000). There is no evidence that dyslexia is due to difficulties with vision and eye problems; children may have difficulties in reading due to visual acuity problems, but these reading difficulties would not be classified as 'dyslexia'. Studies may also include adults with acquired neurological problems involving print difficulties. Neurological studies with bilingual people with dyslexia are rare.

Different terms are used to describe dyslexia, which contributes to the permeable boundaries ('flakiness') of the concept of dyslexia:

- *Dyslexia* usually refers to difficulties with print and literacy skills – usually reading and spelling, and writing difficulties may also be involved or identified separately as *dysgraphia*.
- Dyslexia may include numeracy difficulties or they may be referred to separately as *dyscalculia*.
- The majority of education psychologists in the UK prefer the term *specific learning difficulties* (SpLD).
- In the USA, SpLD in literacy are called *learning difficulties* (LD) and contrast with global LD, which are called mental retardation (MR).

Often children with dyslexia may also show associated difficulties:

- hyperactivity and low levels of attention for learning (attention deficit and hyperactivity disorder, ADHD);
- higher level difficulties in social language use (Asperger's syndrome);
- motor coordination difficulties (dyspraxia) often shown in fine motor coordination difficulties or major handwriting difficulties;
- difficulties with numeracy may be due to not understanding how the number system or place values work (Simmons & Singleton, 2007);
- low self-esteem and social, emotional and behaviour difficulties (Riddick *et al.*, 1999; Alexander-Passe, 2006).

Furthermore, despite evidence to the contrary, assumptions can be made that learning literacy skills for additional languages is a cause of dyslexia. The coincident emergence of dyslexia-type difficulties with late second language learning can lead to *blaming bilingualism* for the difficulties. Since the early 1990s, Ganschow and Sparks have been researching students in higher education who are learning a second language for their college degree. Students who demonstrated no difficulties in their first language, English, could show dyslexia-type difficulties in literacy tasks in the second language. They identified three major findings. Linguistic interdependency between languages for both understanding and expression means that weaknesses in processing L1 also transfer to L2/curriculum modern foreign language learning (MFL or FL) at all language levels (phonology/orthography, grammar, vocabulary) (Ganschow & Sparks, 1993). A hierarchy of vulnerability of processing skills in the additional language suggests that phonology/orthography processing skills are the most likely to be affected, followed by grammar and syntactic processing skills. Semantic processing skills are least likely to be affected. Students with these difficulties may have a strong emotional response through loss of confidence, leading to a negative attitude to L2/EAL/MFL learning. This, in turn, is likely to be a consequence of identified linguistic processing weakness rather than the initial cause of poor L2/EAL/MFL performance, and they need personal and pedagogic support.

These findings support what Ganschow and Sparks (1993) call the Linguistic Coding Differences hypothesis (LCDH). Their findings go beyond phonological processing explanations for dyslexia. They identify the probability that other language levels are implicated and need to be included in assessment, intervention and teaching. They identify semantics and meaning making as the least affected resource, and a protective factor to be built on in intervention. They construct the social-emotional dimension as a casualty rather than a cause of difficulties in additional language learning.

In a study of higher education students in the USA, Schwartz (2000) showed that up to 10% of an annual cohort of university/college students had dyslexia difficulties in EFL learning. Both avenues of research offer interpretations of findings that are pedagogically orientated. L1 may appear unproblematic due to years of teaching and over-learning so that automaticity has been achieved. Schwartz argues that students need direct explicit teaching of encoding and decoding second language/EAL and FL skills along a continuum of language processing. Since dyslexia-type difficulties seem only to show for these students in contexts of learning L2/EAL/FL, it is possible to see how assumptions that the additional language causes dyslexia may be mistakenly constructed (Cline *et al.*, 2001).

Core difficulties

From a psychological perspective, dyslexia and difficulties managing print for monolingual and bilingual children are due to two core difficulties: auditory phonological processing difficulties and visual orthographic difficulties. As a consequence, there are difficulties with rapid processing of print information and in reading comprehension.

Dyslexia is linked to speech and language difficulties through a shared theoretical and research interface, speech processing set out in the previous chapter, and both are based on models of single-word processing.

A core difficulty of dyslexia is the Phonological Deficit hypothesis, which concerns phonological processing and speed of processing language (Stanovich & Seigel, 1994; Yopp, 1992; Snowling, 2001). Children, who also have literacy difficulties, usually show difficulties with phonological awareness knowledge in processing phonological information and segmenting phonological representations of words at the level of syllables and speech sound sequences. Segmentation skills are described as nonlinguistic cognitive skills for manipulating word level phonemic information. Thus, phonological processing difficulties, including segmentation, are thought not to be language-specific and are likely to affect the child's skills across her/his languages. Difficulties at this level also affect the speed of processing auditory language as well as language in print. Assessment in educational practice explores this aspect, since slower work has implications for understanding instructions, joining in discussion, individual progress, keeping up with class work, and fatigue.

Meanings of words play no part in typical phonological processing tasks. When children do invoke meanings, it is explained through the model as a compensatory semantic route for children with difficulties in processing phonological information. For example, when asked in a rhyming task which is the odd one out: 'egg, leg, chicken', instead of responding 'chicken', a child with difficulties processing phonological knowledge may respond 'leg', reasoning that egg/chicken are semantically linked (Stackhouse & Wells, 1997).

Orthography-phonology correspondence presents the second area of core difficulty, demonstrated in research in alphabetic and logographic scripts. Children show problems with the alphabet principle, that is matching speech sound to letter: phoneme-grapheme correspondence. It seems that children need a level of phonological processing skills to 'crack the alphabet code' to learn phoneme-grapheme correspondence. Alphabetic writing systems with more transparent (shallower) phoneme-grapheme correspondence, such as Italian, Spanish, Greek, Hindi, seem easier for children to crack the alphabet code, suggesting that orthographic difficulties are language-specific (e.g. Castle & Coltheart, 1993). In the psychological literature, it may be referred to as the 'hypothesis of granularity and transparency'. Languages where orthography-to-phonology mapping is transparent, not granular and languages whose orthographic unit representing sound at a whole character or word level (logographic) are unlikely to produce a high incidence of developmental phonological dyslexia (Wydell & Butterworth, 1999).

Two features of 'deep' orthographies have been identified as making additional visual learning demands: (in)consistency of phoneme-grapheme correspondence (e.g. in English /f/ is spelt f, ph, gh) and redundant letters (e.g. in English 'k' and 'e' in knife). English orthography has a strong showing of both these factors (Goswami, 1992). Studies of children learning English orthography show there are children with satisfactory phonological processing skills who, nevertheless, have substantial and persistent difficulties handling print, particularly spelling. This suggests that visual learning demands over and above transparent phoneme-grapheme correspondence make some orthographies more difficult to learn and particularly challenging for some children. This finding is also evident in other language orthographies.

Most research in the psycholinguistic paradigm on dyslexia is conducted in and on English, and some other alphabetic languages. There is a small but growing body of studies looking at the implications for different logographic literacies, e.g. Chinese, Japanese languages/scripts (Durgunoglu & Verhoeven, 1998). One monolingual study on naming responses with nearly 2000 Japanese middle and high school learners claimed that Japanese Kanji orthography induces dyslexic-type errors, including semantic errors and visual errors, due to a very weak and unstable association between Kanji and phonology (Jun Yamada, 1998).

It would be possible for bilingual children to show difficulties with print in one language but not in another, where one language has a 'deep' orthography and the other a 'shallow', transparent orthography. Case studies illustrate this dissociation phenomenon, for example two cases of developmental dyslexia learning to read English as compared to Kannada and Hindi (two Indian scripts) were differentially affected (Karanth, 1992). Like most of the other Indian writing systems, Hindi (Devanagiri) is phonologically transparent, nearly always regular, while English is considerably irregular. A study of a 16-year-old English/ Japanese bilingual boy, showed reading/writing difficulties in English only. He was born and went to school in Japan and his spoken language at home is English with highly literate L1 English parents. Unlike the learners in Jun Yamada's study (1998), he performed at a superior level in reading in logographic Japanese Kanji and syllabic Kana. In contrast, his performance in various reading and writing tests in English as well as tasks involving phonological processing was very poor, even when compared to his Japanese contemporaries. Yet, he had no problem with letter names or letter sounds, and his phoneme categorisation was well within the normal range of English native speakers. The 'shallow/deep' relationship between phonology and orthographies could account for the bilingual learner's dissociation between his ability to read English and Japanese (Wydell & Butterworth, 1999).

Within the psychological perspective, studies attribute learning phoneme-grapheme literacy skills to learners' intrinsic difficulties matching across phonologies and orthographies. Yet, literacy skills are taught and success or difficulty in developing literacy skills, particularly shown in the two studies in Kanji, could be attributed to effective teaching and learning practices at school. These findings have implications for educational practice.

A study that looked at penmanship skills in older and younger groups of Chinese literate children found differential effects of spatial movement, visuospatial and stroke sequence information on finger-tracing tasks of Chinese characters. The authors note that

> Studies with Chinese children with dyslexia (Woo & Hoosain, 1984) showed that readers of logographic languages greatly relied on visual information processing for word recognition. Therefore these readers are likely to constitute a significant subgroup of dyslexia of visual deficit origin (Slaghuis *et al.*, 1993). For them, using the proprioceptive channel may be an augmentation to their deficient visual processing route and finger tracing may be a useful intervention method to alleviate reading [and writing] difficulties. (Yuet-Yee Yim-Ng *et al.*, 2000: 569)

The findings of this study together with the two studies cited in the quotation, suggest a higher reliance on visual information processing for word recognition than is the case for alphabetic orthographies. Further, the authors suggest that a multisensory approach would be useful for Chinese children with logographic literacy difficulties. However, in the absence of a comparison of performance between Chinese and another logographic or nonlogographic language, we cannot draw firm conclusions. The authors posit that the findings suggest different subtypes of dyslexia across language and orthographies. However, Snowling (2001) challenges the notion of subtypes, arguing for a spectrum of dyslexia difficulty moderated by risks and supportive influences, albeit from an evidence base of English and alphabetic orthographies.

There are implications for educational practice with learners developing orthographic knowledge of an additional language for schooling, such as English. Assessing the components of reading and orthographic skills in bilingual learners' first language literacy needs to be informed by knowledge of the 'transparency' and visual demands of the language/ orthography, before making comparisons and anticipating transfer to English orthography. Learning to read and spell in English is likely to be demanding for all learners, with implications for educational practice (Cline & Frederickson, 1999).

Reading comprehension

Reading comprehension is a further site of difficulty in developing literacy skills, and warranted a major review of research and educational practice in the USA (Snow, 2002). Understanding reading has implications for primary and secondary school attainment. Three levels of analysis of reading for meaning are analysed here: word level meaning, meaning of language form, and meaning of genre.

Understanding word level reading can be problematic in several ways. 'Reading' words accurately but without understanding, so-called 'barking at print' (hyperlexia), occurs when structural 'decoding' reading skills develop in advance of sense and meaning making. This may be problematic in some contexts, although it is a literacy practice in other contexts and communities, such as rote-learning Koranic scripture (Rassool, 2002). Learners with limited language, particularly with language-related difficulties, and also learners of an additional language, may read nonwords, new or unfamiliar words as a familiar word (Stackhouse & Wells, 1997), which interrupts sense-making of new words in print. A study of 8-year-old bilingual EAL learners in the UK explored their understanding of short texts that had been read to them (Nelson, 2006). Children misunderstood the texts because of misunderstanding vocabulary. For example, 'matchstick men' was understood as 'firemen', and a protective 'film' covering a wound was associated with television. Further interviews showed that they had difficulty with polysemy in EAL, suggesting that language and literacy are still limited tools for learning/thinking for them, after 3–4 years of English schooling (Cummins, 1984; Thomas & Collier, 1997).

Speed of processing print is recognised as an issue affecting word level reading comprehension (Stringer & Stanovich, 2000). Older learners with dyslexia may have developed a substantial sight vocabulary, but find reading new texts, particularly for curriculum learning, a slow, demanding and tiring procedure. They decode unfamiliar specialist words at the expense of making sense and meaning of the wider text, such as the main idea in a paragraph, making predictions, identifying implications or understanding inferences (Goldfus, 2001).

Making sense of academic texts is jeopardised by difficulties developing knowledge of language form and meaning. Smith (1971) referred to making meaning in reading as a psycholinguistic guessing game to learn new vocabulary and develop concepts and higher thinking skills. Texts for curriculum subject learning have specialist vocabulary and grammatical constructions (Perera, 1986), which present additional challenges for learners with literacy difficulties. Monolingual and bilingual learners with difficulties developing literacy often read less than their peers and not for enjoyment, with consequences for vocabulary and grammar development (Goldfus, 2001). Furthermore, cultural embeddedness of reading comprehension may disadvantage bilingual and EAL learners (Cline & Frederickson, 1999).

Reading comprehension is enhanced when readers recognise the features and style of the language of the text that serve the communicative function, so-called genre (Halliday, 1989). Identifying the genre and context of use of the text helps readers to scaffold their understanding and learning from texts (de la Mata & Santamaria, 2001). Genre concerns communicative function and is culturally sensitive, and consequently is likely to be a source of difficulty for some culturally and linguistically diverse students. The genre of textbooks is usually expository, in contrast to the narrative genre of stories and novels (Goldfus, 2001). Possibly as a function of these many aspects, the role of genre in reading comprehension for monolingual, bilingual and EAL learners with language difficulties is under-researched.

A critical perspective

Research in the neurological, psychological and psycholinguist paradigms is the main evidence base of research for dyslexia and substantial literacy difficulties; sociological paradigms tend not to identify dyslexia as a site for study. While the vast majority of this research is with monolinguals, mostly English, there is an emerging body of research on dyslexia across other languages and orthographies. Furthermore, there is a small body of research that attempts to examine the inter-relatedness of research in bilingualism and dyslexia (Frederickson & Cline, 1990, 2002; Cline & Frederickson, 1999; Martin, 1999; Martin *et al.*, 1997; Ganschow & Sparks, 1993), with implications for educational practice and professional development.

Nevertheless, a psychological account of dyslexia in CLD contexts is constrained by a lack of critical self-awareness, both conceptually and for its application to educational practice. It offers knowledge about difficulties developing literacy components and skills, orientated towards diagnosis through testing, and implications and applications for intervention/pedagogy tend to be instrumental. The paradigm has a determinist orientation, constructing dyslexia as a pervasive developmental difficulty in particular language contexts. Research offers a highly individualised account of literacy LD, which decontextualises learners and their learning from wider contexts as well as families, peers and teachers. There are critiques of research within the paradigm, but the paradigm offers no critical perspective of itself, its positioning as one discourse among several on difficulties developing literacy in culturally and linguistically diverse contexts. Studies tends to be reductive in that they seek to identify core difficulties and do not usually draw on the resources of the bilingual learners' other languages/orthographies for learning support. I turn now to more sociolinguistic approaches.

Sociocultural and Anthropological Approaches

In this section, I discuss sociocultural and anthropological approaches to dyslexia and substantial literacy difficulties in contexts of bilingualism and biliteracy. These approaches shift the focus from a psychological paradigm, to give a critical social account of literacy disability in context. The section first considers research on literacy from a Vygotskian, sociocultural perspective, to examine notions of situated meaning and learning, with particular reference to the literature of home and school biliteracy practices for linguistic minority children. There are few studies though in this paradigm on dyslexia-type needs. Recent research in an anthropological paradigm critically frames the different perspectives through the lens of power, privilege, agency and identity. I draw on the continua of biliteracy (Hornberger, 1989) to discuss studies. The implications for educational practice for literacy are discussed in the next section.

Researchers in this paradigm critically engage with traditional perspectives of psychological and anthropological approaches to learning literacy. They critique the psychological position on individual learning, arguing against human thinking being reducible to individual properties or traits, and for social learning as a notion of *distributed cognition*. An important exponent is Moll (1992, 2000; Moll & Gonzalez, 2005).

Thinking is usually considered as taking place solely within the mind of the individual, what some psychologists refer to as *solo* or *in-the-head cognition*. Schools accept this notion, testing students to determine their presumed individual ability or intelligence, which is considered an immutable, fixed attribute or trait of the individual... [but] human thinking is not reducible to individual properties or traits. Instead, it is always mediated, distributed among persons, artefacts, activities and settings. (Moll, 2000: 265)

A sociocultural approach places learning within cultural worlds. The information-processing activity that children do within their heads to make sense of the structural aspects of print and other forms of literacy is embedded in meaning making through cultural artefacts and practices for literacy. The implication for teaching and learning is that sense making is inseparable from meaning making. Children with difficulties developing literacy skills (dyslexia) are at various times unable to engage with meaning-making aspects of print because of difficulties making sense of the printed word.

A sociocultural approach also critically evaluates traditional normative anthropological perspectives of literacy. Normative concepts of culture are often used in education and psychology, but are of little use in teaching and of little relevance to everyday lives of children or their families. Moll (2000) argues that for educational purposes, a more refined notion of culture is needed if it is to be useful for mediated learning.

The purpose is for teachers to develop both theory and methods to identify and document cultural resources found in the immediate school community, as represented by the children's households that could be used for teaching [...]. This applied project, then, contains two elements that are essential within a Vygotskian theoretical formulation: It seeks to understand culture as practice and to harness its resources to transform social (educational) reality. (Moll, 2000: 258)

Moll and colleagues conducted an important ethnographic analysis of culturally and linguistically diverse households by classroom teachers (Moll, 1992). He argues teachers need to find out about the literacy practices and 'funds of literacy knowledge' in culturally and linguistically diverse families. However, parents' and families' literacy practices may only partially include the child, and he advocates the importance of exploring the bilingual child's own literacy practices and the development of the child's identity through those practices, and to include them in schooling.

Developing biliteracies

The relationship between home literacy practice and development of literacy skills in school is well established (Tizard & Hughes, 1984; Wells, 1986; Hannon, 1995). The advantages for bilingual children are that, before coming to school, they may well have experienced a diversity of literacy practices and been introduced to different literacies and orthographies; for example, letter writing to family members in the diaspora, newspapers, religious and cultural stories, songs and poems (Bhatt, 1994; Saxena, 1994). Bilingual learners bring many literacy knowledges to learning and becoming literate (e.g. Gregory, 1997; Kenner, 1997; Datta, 2007).

Educators and other professionals may be unaware of literacy practices in the homes of bilingual children. They assume that minority linguistic parents are not bilingual/biliterate in the language of schooling and that bilingual children come from literacy deprived environments (Gregory & Biarnes, 1994; Blackledge, 2000). Teachers may act on these assumptions and not encourage home literacy practices in English; for example, they may not send reading books home with bilingual children, or send reading books home that are not at the child's reading age (Blackledge, 2000). Other studies report encouragement between teachers and parents in literacy endeavours (Sneddon, 2000). Parents with limited spoken English and English literacy skills can and do successfully support their children's English literacy development (Tizard *et al.*, 1982; Blackledge, 2000) and may also involve older siblings to support the literacy development of younger ones (Gregory, 1996, 1998). In the USA, work done by Moll (1992) and Delgado-Gaitan (1991) with teachers and Hispanic families shows similar findings.

Studies on biliteracy skills and practices indicate the role of scaffolding across languages and literacies, building on prior knowledge in the home language and literacy practices, to develop language and literacy in the additional language of schooling and enhance academic achievement (Sneddon, 1993, 2000). Sneddon and others draw theoretically on the idea of common underlying proficiency (Cummins, 1984) to explain two-way transfer of cognitive and linguistic skills between languages (see also Verhoeven, 1994). Even though bilingual children's languages and literacies are supported by parents, family and community, over time and by the beginning of secondary school, home literacy practices can decrease or even disappear (Sneddon, 2000).

Literacy knowledge and practices that bilingual children bring to school either from their homes or from attending complementary language schools, can be used productively by teachers to develop literacy skills and practices in English (Moll, 1992; Kenner, 2000). Kenner's study shows how teachers can facilitate bilingual learners by working through both languages to encourage scaffolding of cognitive and linguistic knowledge across their languages. She demonstrated that literacy practices afford important opportunities for young children and older learners to construct their identity as bilinguals and biliterates.

Sociocultural research draws on the Vygotskian ideas of distributed social cognitions, and cognitive tools of building on prior learning to develop both languages and literacy skills. There are implications for differentiated use across age with home language and literacies as tools for learning for bilingual children. This research further underscores the need for educationists to be familiar with home language and literacy practices to inform classroom pedagogies. While dyslexia is not addressed, failure to develop literacies for school purposes is analysed through social processes and the contextualised nature of language and literacy practices, and studies identify the need for a critical frame to analyse privileging language and literacy practices.

A critical anthropological paradigm

The critical anthropological paradigm in literacy research is developed by New Literacy Studies (NLS) (Street, 1984, 1993; New London Group, 1996; Barton & Hamilton, 1998). In a schematic representation of approaches to literacy study, NLS is oppositional to the traditional psychological perspective of literacy skills and dyslexia. NLS tries 'to shift the ground on which we consider issues of language and literacy' (Street, 2003: 79) from literacy as a learnt set of cognitive, psycholinguistic and motor skills, and literacy development as stages and phases of incremental knowledge and ability of skills, individually centred. Sociocultural perspectives, including NLS, conceptualise literacy in expanded and expansive terms, as heterogeneous, situated, social and cultural practices. They also introduce a level of analysis that examines the role of power and privilege in language and literacy practices.

Researchers in NLS often use the term 'literacies' partly to distinguish the concept from the traditional homogenous 'autonomous' notion of literacy. Multiliteracies, as defined by the New London Group (1996: 63), refer to the multiplicity of communication channels and media in our changing world, as well as to the increasing saliency of CLD. The concept extends literacy beyond reading and writing to other domains, such as the visual, audio, spatial and behavioural (Kress & van Leeuwen, 1996;

Hornberger & Skilton-Sylvester, 2000: 107). People engage in literacy practices in ways that are not necessarily dependent on their literacy skills. For example, the fall in numbers of people purchasing daily newspapers is not related to a decrease in literacy skills, but to the rise of other sources of news and comment, such as 24-hour news on radio, television and the internet. Multiliteracies are a means to transform social and educational exclusion for people with difficulties with print. There seems to be a gradual thawing of attitudes and practices towards multiliteracies for students (with dyslexia-type needs) in assessed work in higher education.

A sociocultural and critical approach to biliteracy is developed in the continua model of biliteracy (Hornberger, 1989). This framework can be used to situate research, teaching and language planning in linguistically diverse settings. Hornberger argues that the more their learning contexts allow learners to draw on all points of the continua, the greater are the chances for their full biliterate development. She describes the model thus:

> The model uses the notion of intersecting and nested continua to demonstrate the multiple and complex interrelationships between bilingualism and literacy and the importance of contexts, media and content through which biliteracy develops. Specifically, it depicts the **development** of biliteracy along intersecting first language-second language, receptive-productive, and oral-written language skills continua, through the **medium** of two (or more) languages and literacies whose linguistic structures vary from similar to dissimilar, whose scripts vary from convergent to divergent, and to which the developing biliterate individual's exposure varies from simultaneous to successive; in **contexts** that encompass micro- to macro-levels and are characterised by varying mixes along the monolingual-bilingual and oral-literate continua; and with **content** that ranges from majority to minority perspectives and experiences, literary to vernacular styles and genres, and decontextualised to contextualised language texts. (Hornberger, 1989; Hornberger & Skilton-Sylvester, 2000: 96)

This model offers several levels of analysis for biliteracy development, across aspects of context, media and content, and within each aspect there is a continuum mediated by power and privilege. From a critical anthropological perspective, literacy is an axis for distribution of power (Hornberger & Skilton-Sylvester, 2000). Attention is not usually given to all points on the continua, and movement along the power continua may well be contested with an implicit privileging of one end of the continua over the other. For example, literacy is privileged over oral language, majority language over minority language, L2 (school) over L1 (home), decontextualised media (academic texts) over contextualised (magazines), and orthographic scripts that are similar to the orthography of the dominant language, over dissimilar (Hornberger & Skilton-Sylvester, 2000). In the same manner, 'readers' are privileged over 'nonreaders' which in this model usually refers to those who are excluded from access to literacies due to gender, race and poverty. However, although not necessarily intended, it could also refer to those bilingual and monolingual readers marginalised with dyslexia-type difficulties and language learning disabilities.

Individuals with dyslexia may be excluded from important social knowledge and practices, such as health education, that depend on literacy skills. Women's magazines are regarded as a primary source of information and education on health and relationship matters and serve a didactic need, for example concerning breast and ovarian cancers, mental health and child-rearing practices (Giddens, 1992). There are implications in accessing this information for women with limited language/print skills and dyslexia. Yet, there are increasingly available alternatives to print for accessing information, such as audiotapes and cassettes, CDs and videos. Through multiliteracy practices, lack of literacy skills may be become less exclusionary.

Hornberger and Skilton-Sylvester (2000) analyse the tensions and dilemmas enacted as social marginalisation and exclusion surrounding literacy/biliteracy within a model of biliteracy. They use the framework to make visible the ways in which policy discourses, mainstream school practices and assumptions surrounding literacy and bilingualism have acted to disempower students from marginalised communities (Cummins, 2000: 272). Power relations can be changed and the challenge for educationists is how to transform them (Street, 1994), particularly in the field of bilingualism, biliteracy and language and literacy disabilities. Critical reflection on daily lived experiences to examine the sources and patterns of implicit privileging can be a route to transforming power relations (Street, 1996). Next, the implications for educational practice are discussed.

Educational Practice

This section concerns educational practice for dyslexia and literacy disability in contexts of biliteracy and bilingualism through the lens of

Vygotskian ideas and critical pedagogy. I discuss, with reference to the literature from the psychological and sociocultural perspectives of multiliteracies and dyslexia, two areas of inter-relatedness that inform educational practice, namely assessment and pedagogy. The argument that I make is similar to that of Snow and colleagues:

> There is little evidence that children experiencing difficulties learning to read, even those with identifiable learning disabilities, need radically different sorts of supports than children at low risk, although they may need much more intensive support. Childhood environments that support early literacy development and excellent instruction are important for all children. Excellent instruction is the best intervention for children who demonstrate problems learning to read. (Snow *et al.*, 1998: 3)

Key concepts

Key ideas in a Vygotskian framework draw on cognitive psychological and sociocultural tools to inform educational practice with learners with dyslexia in contexts of multiliteracies. Research from the psychological and sociocultural perspectives of biliteracies indicate that individual cognitions and socially distributed cognitions derive from and are embedded in meaningful social, cultural and historical literacy practices. Effective assessment practices and teaching/learning explore and build on prior knowledge and learning in order to scaffold new learning.

Contact with the social and physical world through direct experience affords learning through experience in daily life. More abstract higher cognitive learning is indirect and 'mediated' through tools that may be signs, including language and literacy, as well as conceptual/psychological and material tools, artefacts and activities. Bilingualism and biliteracies offer potentially more tools and avenues for mediation with culturally and linguistically diverse learners with dyslexia. Everyday experiences/concepts are transformed into 'scientific'/curriculum concepts through informed teaching and learning methodology. 'The process of appropriation of psychological tools is determined by the nature of the disability and correlated modifications [differentiation] of teaching methods' (Gindis, 2003: 209).

Mediation through tools affords two routes to learning about literacy skills, 'knowing how' and 'knowing what'. 'Knowing how' to learn literacy skills involves teaching/learning cognitive and metalinguistic strategies, and 'knowing what' of literacy involves teaching/learning the substantive content, e.g. phonological–orthographic correspondence, texts of curriculum subjects. We develop appropriate tools to solve problems and the neatness-of-fit of the tools (concepts, materials, activities) and the interaction between the tool and the task enhances learning:

> Through the use of tools we become aware of the very activity we are engaged in. So we become an agent of change through changing ourselves. It is a personal revolution – a cognitive one – with a social origin. (Negueruela, 2008: 223)

Pedagogies based in psychological perspectives are instrumental in their approach, focusing on 'remediating' aspects of the diagnosis, and helping learners to catch up with their peers. Critical literacies are concerned with raising learners' awareness of their own process of learning which enables them to transform themselves and their environments and realities.

Critical pedagogy for multiliteracies

The New London Group (1996) set out a critical pedagogy of multiliteracies, building on the knowledge and experience of extended multiliteracies of bilingual learners. There are four components for the 'how' of and 'what' of pedagogy, which are presented with application to bilingual learners with literacy difficulties: *situated practice*, *overt instruction*, *critical framing* and *transformed practice*. Critical pedagogy is potentially relevant and inclusive for bilingual learners with difficulties with print. In the following discussion, I inter-relate sociocultural/anthropological perspectives of critical pedagogy with evidence from psychological perspectives in order to make them relevant pedagogically to the needs of bilingual dyslexia learners.

Situated practice

Situated practice entails immersing classroom teaching and learning of literacy in the experiences of literacies and literacy practices of the learners and builds on the notion of prior knowledge and learning. The 'what' of pedagogy is oriented by the central notion of design, that is, the making and remaking of meaning from literacy resources. Resources include forms of media, such as vernaculars, grammars, genres, visual representations of multiliteracies (Hornberger & Skilton-Sylvester, 2000). Pedagogy encourages making and taking meaning from knowledge resources ('designs') available to the learners, so that individuals/groups create their own literacies and re-present personal meaning making from designs available to them in languages and literacies they engage with.

Evidence from the psychological paradigm indicates that good oral language skills are a supportive factor for learners with specific difficulties learning 'basic skills' for literacy (Snowling, 2001). Developing and enhancing first/home language proficiency as preparation for, and throughout, teaching literacy with bilingual, EAL and FL learners supports scaffolding and transfer between language and literacy knowledges (e.g. Snow *et al.*, 1998). Literacy practices of minority linguistic children benefit from home language practices (Moll *et al.*, 1992).

A continuum of privilege is reflected in local and national policy contexts that prescribe, to different degrees, 'standard' literacy designs for monolingualism and monoliteracy (Hornberger & Skilton-Sylvester, 2000). Prescribed standard designs place major constraints on teachers who may wish to work with all students along a continuum of awareness, knowledge and facility, including those with dyslexia-type difficulties and with multiliteracies. Nevertheless, educators can respond to policy contexts through critical pedagogy. Hornberger and Skilton-Sylvester (2000) submit that teachers' own learning through preparation of materials in the process of engaging with critical pedagogies becomes a teaching resource in their classrooms for bilingual learners. Multilingual literacy practices and 'funds of knowledge' offer teachers and other professionals a resource to mediate teaching and learning literacy skills for schooling for all children (Moll, 1992).

Situated practice for identification and teaching practices.   From a psychological perspective, a major concern for educational practice with additional language learners is 'disentangling' specific literacy difficulties from slower learning of literacy skills and additional language skills (Cline & Frederickson, 1999; Lindsay *et al.*, 2006). This concern reflects the basic Vygotskian tension between within-child cognitive difficulties and sociocultural differences that cause difficulties in schooling. From a psychological perspective, problems lie with individual bilingual learners, and the case study at the beginning of the chapter is typically framed in a psychological paradigm. Individual profiles are presented of three bilingual children who have speech, language and literacy difficulties, with information only about the dominant language, English, text-based school practices. From a sociocultural perspective, dyslexia assessment practices need to be embedded and situated in learners' multiliteracy practices. From a critical perspective, assessment practices are often situated along the more privileged end of the continuum, usually within professionals' monolingual, monoliterate practices.

Research instruments used to identify the within-child nature of preliteracy and dyslexia-type difficulties have been adapted for educational assessment, and for bilingual learners, e.g. Phonological Assessment Battery (PhAB; Frederickson et al., 1997). They focus on phonological awareness and processing, carried out across specific phonological segmentation tasks. Most tasks are conducted on single words and single syllable words that require children to show awareness and processing skills through tasks of recognition as well as generating new forms. There is a substantial body of research on these skills in English, and a growing body of studies in other languages (e.g. Verhoeven, 1994; Gupta, 2004), but limited transfer into assessment tools.

There is further evidence to suggest that identification and assessment practices for bilingual learners in the UK may be unsatisfactory in terms of instrumentation and professional practice. Testing culturally and linguistically diverse children on monolingual standardised tests is unfair and inadequate. Reading tests are often standardised on populations that have excluded statistical representation of bilingual groups. Restricted access to contextual and cultural knowledge that is embedded in the additional language and informs reading comprehension, disadvantages and makes vulnerable to exclusion bilingual children/ additional language learners (Cline & Frederickson, 1999) (see also Chapter 7). Assessment of processing phonological knowledge is seen as fundamental in the identification of dyslexia-type difficulties. There is critical awareness within the psychological approach that this avenue of exploration alone is problematic because it leaves unexplored learners' knowledge of other levels of language, meaning making, and other languages and orthographies which are particularly important for the older learner (Schneider & Ganschow, 2000). Furthermore, it focuses on learners' difficulties rather than on their strengths.

A Scottish study (Deponio *et al.*, 2000), building on previous research carried out for the Commission for Racial Equality (CRE, 1996, Special Educational Needs Assessment in Strathclyde), showed that professionals did not always know how to assess and identify dyslexia in bilingual children. The evidence presented significant under-representation of bilingual children among pupils assessed as having specific LD/ dyslexia. Children were not always assessed in their first language and the process of assessment tended to be lengthy and inconclusive. The report's conclusions recommended caution when considering dyslexia in the early stages of second language development. These practices go some way to explaining the low numbers of bilingual learners who are officially recognised as having dyslexia in English special educational needs (SEN) statistics (Lindsay *et al.*, 2006). The study illustrates that in the absence of appropriate conceptual tools, there is disempowerment both for professionals and bilingual learners with alleged literacy difficulties in their care.

The critical evaluation offered here highlights the constraints of operating only within a psychological paradigm for educational practice with bilingual learners with dyslexia-type difficulties. A focus on decontextualisation, segmentation and literacy skills inhibits situating teaching, learning and identification practices of dyslexia difficulties within the prior knowledge and experience of bilingual learners. There is potential for building on sociocultural conceptual tools afforded by both languages and literacies.

Overt instruction

A pertinent criticism of critical pedagogy is that it is strong on developing knowledge of the relationship between power and literacy practices, but less strong on integrating pedagogies for formal features of the language and literacy skills of schooling.

Overt instruction of the 'what' of language and literacy skills pedagogy involves scaffolding learners' progress through explicit teaching not only of content of standard literacy designs, e.g. the alphabetic principle, spelling rules, punctuation, genres for academic writing, but also teaching a conscious understanding of the systems and organisation of language and literacy. This approach is distinct from traditional explicit teaching of grammar, through drills and repetitious practice, which is not meaningful, although may be recommended by evidence from the psychological paradigm for learners with dyslexia. There are publications documenting intervention programmes and advice for supporting children with dyslexia (e.g. Peer & Reid, 2000; Reid & Peer, 2000). Few programmes are explicitly orientated to meet bilingual learners with (bi)literacy needs. Evaluation of these programmes is under-researched, with little critical interrogation of the psychological or traditional approach they adopt.

Overt instruction also includes the 'how' of pedagogy, teaching cognitive strategies and metalinguistic knowledge. Bilingual, EAL and EFL learners, including those with dyslexia-type difficulties, benefit from this approach (McWilliam, 1998; Goldfus, 2001; Nelson, 2006). A critical dimension can be built into overt instruction programmes. Discussion of patterns of meaning that work in different social and cultural contexts encourages a contrastive linguistic perspective that replaces teaching grammar and standard forms (Kalantzis & Cope, 1999: 272). Teaching understanding and meaning in print through experience-text-relationship have been developed for minority groups (Au, 1979; Al Sheik Abdullah, Sarimah, 2005).

Multisensory methods, as part of overt instruction for learners with dyslexia, can be formulated theoretically as tools in Vygotskian ideas concerning the neatness-of-fit between tools and specific conceptual learning, that is, tool-and-result. One programme developed for learners with dyslexia has also been used with L2 learners (Serrano-Lopez & Poehner, 2008). It uses learning activities mediated through the creation of 3-D clay models to represent difficult concepts, which include spelling and grammatical forms (Davis, 1997). Davis' method does not explicitly refer to Vygotskian theory, but it does focus on developing conceptual knowledge underpinning language knowledge through a series of stages, using materials that present abstract language knowledge to learners in a physical form; for example, learners model in clay the relational concept of a preposition, or an event, and key words may be spelt out in clay 'worms'. Discussions between teacher and learners make explicit the zone of proximal development that learners and teacher are working within.

Motor skills for penmanship in writing are not language-specific and can be transferred across similar orthographies. For different orthographies, such as English/Arabic and Chinese as discussed earlier, different motor skills would need to be learnt. Intervention programmes for penmanship skills include multisensory strategies:

- finger tracing with the index finger of the preferred hand, of the alphabet characters in textured substances, such as sand or salt, promotes proprioception, visuospatial and stroke sequence information about the characters;
- verbalising the movements in the stroke patterns;
- supportive artefacts, such as thicker finger grips on pencils, lined paper, textured alphabet forms.

However, these strategies are rarely theorised in published programmes, even in Vygotskian terms, as tools for conceptual learning of orthographic skills.

Situated practices and overt instruction are familiar in teaching and learning practices that are socioculturally and critically aware of learners' needs beyond instrumental literacy skills. In Vygotskian terms, these practices both surface and value prior learning as a basis for future learning of languages and literacies. They develop learners' awareness of the psychological, social and material tools that they are implicated in learning conceptual knowledge. The next two components of a critical pedagogy for literacies address relationships of power and identity in contexts of multiliteracies and dyslexia.

Critical framing

Critical framing is pedagogy that develops learners' critical awareness of the roots and values of the literacies that they engage with. Learners appreciate not only the immediate meaning of their literacies, but also contextualise the cultural histories in terms of social and political value and privilege that are attributed to their languages and literacies by their communities, school, wider society and themselves. They become aware of whose interests are served by particular literacy practices, for example, by exploring comparative family literacy practices, e.g. religious literacies, within their class, school and across groups in wider society. They can investigate the prominence and influence that their languages, literacies and orthographies have locally and in wider society – through literature, novels, magazines, theatre, plays, films, radio and TV – and produced by/for whose interests. Critically framing the social management of literacies engages various literacy knowledges: experiential, literal, personal meaning as well as a critical understanding of different literacies and orthographies in their own community and in wider society (Cummins, 2000).

Critical framing practices include bilingual learners with dyslexia. Students can be encouraged to explore the exclusionary practices surrounding 'nonreaders' whether for dyslexia or 'illiteracy'. In many societies, processes of exclusion across gender and disability exclude girls as well as those with dyslexia and other LDs, from important social knowledge and practices, such as health education, accessible through literacy skills. When literacies, their practices and processes of exclusion are rooted and framed by critical understanding of social and cultural values and privilege, learners are more likely to be prepared to use literacy as a tool for change.

Transformational pedagogy

Transformational pedagogy aims to put transformed meaning to work in other contexts and cultural sites, by empowering learners to make changes in their world by transforming traditional and familiar ways of understanding and meaning. Learners develop voice and identity through agency, and agency enhances second language development in demonstrable and durable ways (van Lier, 2008: 178). New identities are shaped by ongoing struggles and reconciliations and these can reflect resistance as well as conformity (van Lier, 2008: 177). Resistance, as an expression of agency, can be conducive or disruptive to learning, for example, Canagarajah's (1999) work on using home languages in the EFL classroom. Also Baugh (1999, cited in Cummins, 2000: 277) notes that African American students resist any behaviour that could be considered as 'acting white', including in language and literacy practices. Bilingual adolescent learners with literacy difficulties, who have experienced years of ineffective educational practice for meeting their needs, may adopt non-cooperative, disruptive or 'clowning' behaviours to avoid failure by resisting engagement with literacy skills that are based on instrumental learning (Goldfus, 2001).

Transformational pedagogy is an under-researched area for bilingual learners with language and literacy needs. An important site that is emerging in disability studies is research in pedagogies of self-advocacy for learners with difficulties, which would be a rich site for transformational pedagogies for bilingual learners with literacy and language-related needs.

Critical motivation

Learners' personal motivation is an issue that is brought to the fore in programmes for bilingual learners with learning needs. One approach is a 'simplistic focus on self esteem' based on a notion of 'a unitary concept of a psychological construct' of motivation (Nieto, 1999: 208). Motivation, or lack of it, is often cited as a cause for literacy difficulties. However, as Ganschow and Sparks (1993) note, becoming demotivated to read is a casualty of reading failure rather than a cause. Students' persistent failure with print is demotivating. Kozulin (1999) explains higher achievement between groups on cognitive learning programmes by stronger motivation in one group.

From a more critical perspective, self-esteem is relational and situated, depending on the positioning of the individual and context on a continuum (Nieto, 1999). Contexts where students are discriminated, undervalued and marginalised create learners with low self-esteem. Minority ethnic and linguistic students are more likely to experience learning in these contexts and they learn (internalise) the negative messages taught in these contexts. Pedagogic approaches that actively include learners' participation and build on and integrate learners' knowledge into curriculum reading and learning motivate learners and learning. Cummins (2000: 278) notes that 'we see the positive effects of integrating students' sense of self with active language use and engagement with literacy ... than one who is confined to a passive role within the classroom'. A study of a metacognitive approach to reading comprehension with adolescent learners described as having persistent reading difficulties showed that improvement in reading comprehension and attainment had a positive social and emotional effect on learners' approach to literacy and learning (Goldfus, 2001). Personal and collective agency in engaging with language and literacy learning is central to critical pedagogies. Beyond school, families and communities play key roles in mediating more positive and self-affirming self-perceptions for culturally and linguistically diverse learners with literacy difficulties.

Critical focus on language and literacy

Cummins' (2000) framework lends itself more readily to integrating evidence from the psychological paradigm with critical pedagogies to support learners with substantial difficulties with print. Cummins (2000) sees critical pedagogy as representing a significant advance on literacy research in the psychological paradigm for school effectiveness/improvement. He develops a framework for pedagogy that promotes second language learners' linguistic and cognitive development, and encourages growth of critical literacy skills to infuse cognitive challenge and intrinsic motivation in the interactions between teachers and students. His framework for academic language learning has three components. Focus on Meaning focuses first on a *literal phase* of reading comprehension, and embeds critical aspects of literacy pedagogy in *experiential, personal, critical* and *creative phases*. Focus on Language develops knowledge of linguistic forms and uses and critical analysis of them. Focus on Use is where language is used to generate new knowledge, create literature and art and act on social realities (Cummins, 2000: 273–280). Critical pedagogy that aims to increase critical awareness of language and literacies on the continuum of privilege orientates teaching and learning for literacies in multilingualism across all of these components of instruction.

Conclusion

This chapter, with reference to the literature, explores the inter-relatedness of psychological and sociocultural understandings for educational practices with learners with dyslexia in CLD contexts. Psychological approaches offer insights into dyslexia, assessment and intervention support, and increasingly across languages, but do not contextualise learning about literacy, literacy skills and the uses and purposes of multiliteracies that bilingual learners engage with. Sociocultural and critical perspectives take account of multiliteracies and the diversity of language and literacy practices that help shape learners' identity and agency, but this research does not attend to the specific educational needs experienced by monolingual and bilingual learners who have substantial and persistent difficulties with print.

Discussions about bringing together research from two different paradigms raise concerns about legitimacy of knowledge. We need to be cautious about linking two parallel paradigms that generate very different kinds of discourses and findings, particularly when there is little research on their inter-relatedness or conceptual overlap. Yet, educational practice for bilingual learners with difficulties with print, needs to be informed by both paradigms. Drawing on a Vygotskian framework for teaching and learning, the chapter has sought to identify the inter-relationships across findings from psychological and critical sociocultural approaches for educational practices with bilingual children with literacy disabilities. Development of new educational practices for this group of bilingual learners becomes itself a conceptual and material tool for teachers' learning, so that teachers themselves are changed. At a material level, Vygotskian theoretical formulations for existing multisensory teaching approaches to literacy skills for bilingual learners afford new understandings about cognitive strategies used by bilingual learners developing biliteracies.

From a sociocultural perspective of educational practice, a main criticism of psychological approaches to teaching and learning is that they are instrumental rather than critical. Critical pedagogy concerns practices of teaching and learning that intend to interrupt particular historical, situated systems of educational coercion in order to bring about consciousness of learning. Exponents of critical and Vygotskian pedagogy submit that transformation of consciousness in teaching and learning takes place at the intersection of three agencies involved: the teacher, the learner and the knowledge they aim to produce together. From this perspective, teachers, learners and programmes for bilingual learners with dyslexia in contexts of subordinated languages and literacies would be expected to change to accomplish successful multiliteracy learning.

The case study at the beginning of the chapter presents three bilingual children's literacy skills from a psycholinguistic perspective. Our focus is drawn to the relationship between the children's spoken language skills, particularly the development of phonological knowledge and phonological processing knowledge, and their literacy skills in the language of schooling. The development of the children's skills with orthography in their additional language, which is the language of schooling, is emphasised with no attention to their knowledge and practices in other aspects of literacy practices in their home and school languages. This approach is familiar in school reports. It is worth considering how the case study might be re-presented to give a more inclusive account of the bilingual children's developing literacies, and their additional needs.

Note

1. Programme for International Student Assessment (PISA) is a triennial world-wide test of 15-year-old school children's scholastic performance, the implementation of which is coordinated by the Organisation for Economic Cooperation and Development (OECD).

Chapter 6

Deafness in Culturally and Linguistically Diverse Communities

Case Study

D is a 45-year-old man. He was born in England and as a neonate acquired profound hearing difficulties, severe visual difficulties, learning difficulties and motor and co-ordination difficulties due to muscular spasticity associated with cerebral palsy. He moved with his family to Dublin, in the Republic of Ireland when he was aged 1 year. It was difficult to find educational provision to meet his multisensory needs and he went to a school for the deaf when he was 5 until he was 10, where communication focused on oral/aural methods rather than sign. He then moved to a school for children with profound and multiple needs in Belfast, Northern Ireland, a province in the UK, until he was 17 years old. Oral communication was used for four years and then Makaton (Walker, 1973; Walker & Armfield, 1981; Walker, 1996) was introduced, which is a modified form of British Sign Language (BSL) for people with hearing and learning difficulties. His family also learnt Makaton. At 17, he returned to live at home in the Republic and attended a Training Centre daily, where Lamb (pronounced Lawve) is used, a modified version of Irish Sign Language (ISL). For the past three years, he has been learning ISL, as have his family. Learning to communicate has been a life-enhancing experience for him and his family. (My extended family)

Introduction

This chapter concerns children and young people with hearing loss and impairment, from culturally and linguistically diverse families and contexts. It explores research and practice issues, with reference to the literature, from a sociocultural and historical perspective. The main issues concern causes of hearing loss, the bilingualism of oralism and sign for communication, identity and belonging to community, all of which are made more complex in culturally and linguistically diverse societies. Distinct research methodologies are evident across aspects of the field, yet Deafness and hearing loss at the interface with cultural and linguistic diversity (CLD) is under-researched. Like dyslexia, d/Deafness may be contested as a disability (Lane, 2002, 2005) and it is considered an important area to be included here.

Mahon (2007) describes how deaf children from a CLD background are likely to have had a complex exposure to languages before starting school. They are exposed to their family's first spoken language(s) and to the majority language of the region, country or education from siblings. For second and third generation migrant families, the majority language may be spoken most alongside other languages used by older family members or for religious or cultural purposes. In addition, some parents of deaf children, as the case study illustrates, begin to learn a sign language, such as BSL, ISL or American Sign Language (ASL), or learn some signs, while many families develop their own system of home signing, and all will use a great deal of nonverbal communication. Early intervention from specialist professionals influences the child's engagement with language, and their advice to culturally and linguistically diverse families varies. Supporting home language development encourages patterns of socialisation and development similar to typical development. Yet, families may be advised to speak only the dominant language of professionals, such as English, which they may speak with different levels of proficiency. Developing the language of schooling, particularly for deaf children from culturally and linguistically diverse families, may present more challenges for parents and children and their teachers than for other children for whom the language of home and schooling are the same (Mahon, 2007: 9).

The case study illustrates aspects of communicative experience that are typical of many deaf individuals and their families who move between countries and educational provisions. Sign languages are a unique linguistic and communicative response to the impact of deafness by the Deaf community. The case illustrates that sign languages are generated within social, historical and national contexts, signified by two or more sign languages functioning across borders, within one small island nation. The extent to which different sign languages contribute to producing and reproducing distinct ethnicities and cultures in Deaf communities is an area for research. From an individual perspective, the young man's cognitive and motor difficulties did not seem to have a determinist effect on his communication. The communities he became part of, engaged him in learning and communicating through their sign languages. Relationships between service providers and client families, particularly through the issue of agency in families around using sign language for culturally and linguistically diverse families, is under-researched and is discussed later in the chapter.

I argue that, increasingly, approaches to research and practice in the field of hearing loss are reorientating to include a sociocultural dimension of ethnic, cultural and linguistic diversity. From a Vygotskian perspective, this analysis is framed as a move from determinist constructs of hearing loss to identifying avenues for developmental intervention through sociocultural change. The chapter comprises four sections. In the first section, two distinct lines of enquiry into deafness and bilingualism are examined. I use the second section to review studies on causes of hearing impairment and associated difficulties, particularly behaviour, to surface the importance of taking account of race/ethnicity, and cultural and language diversity. In the third section, I look at new understandings offered by studies, which examine the construction of identities in Deaf people from diverse backgrounds. The fourth section focuses on studies from 'hearing' and 'deaf' perspectives among bilingual communities and the educational and environmental implications for inclusion of hearing disability. The chapter is guided by questions such as: to what extent does research and practice in the field of deafness explore the intersection of CLD? How is the research used and how is it discussed and reported? What are the implications for education and for equity and access to health and education? Finally, I draw some conclusions.

Researching deafness and Deafness

In this section, concepts and frameworks that orientate research in hearing loss are discussed. Usually the term *Deaf* with a capital 'D' is used to refer to people who are born deaf or become deaf (or 'deafened') in early childhood. They are more likely to communicate through sign language and see themselves as part of the Deaf Community and Deaf Culture, which is a relatively close community – for example, Deaf people often marry other Deaf people or have Deaf partners. They do not usually see themselves as having a disability, but a difference. Where *deafness* is used with a small 'd', the term refers to the wider, all-inclusive deaf population, where the majority uses spoken language and a written form. This includes hard of hearing people and people who have become deaf in adulthood or in later life, many of whom also have considerable difficulties in communicating with hearing professionals. In addition, people with multisensory disabilities (deafblind) who are born deaf or are deafened in early childhood tend to identify with the Deaf Community, whereas the majority of people who are deafblind, and who are deafened later in life, identify with the blind hearing community (Sign and Mental Health Foundation, 2006: 1).

This convention of using lowercase and uppercase letters is used in other areas of language study to distinguish between technical and critical approaches. Notably, Gee (2005) distinguishes '*discourse* studies' which is research focusing on technical, empirical analyses of language in use, from '*Discourse* studies' that stress the connections between language, identities and ideologies (Gee, 2005: 7). Could this distinction between technical-empirical and critical-interpretative approaches be applied to approaches to researching hearing loss? There is a degree of self-awareness in research on Deafness that is not so visible in research in other impairments. Studies of *deafness* could be said to refer to the historically dominant research strand of the technical study of the bio/medico/psychological approach to hearing impairment. Using upper-case 'D' in the term *Deafness* could be used to indicate a more critical, sociopolitical methodology, examining critically the connections between hearing loss, ideologies and identities.

The strand of research in deafness-as-impairment is orientated by the bio/medical model. Studies typically look at occurrence (incidence) and frequency (prevalence) of type, causes of, and interventions for, deafness across race/ethnicity and bilingual populations. These studies tend to take a determinist view of deafness, by linking ethnicity (pre)dispositions to predisposing environmental factors, such as cultural practices and poverty. This view has implications for future research, policy and practice at the intersection of deafness, race, ethnicity and bilingualism. Prominence to genetic predispositions or life practices positions minority groups as vulnerable to, and marginalised by, deafness. Caution is needed using findings to explain or to *justify* that deaf CLD groups are marginalised.

Research in Deafness-as-disability is orientated by a social model of disability and is less interested in finding cause–effect relationships for different aspects of impairment. Studies explore identity, education, employment and social and communicative practices among Deaf people and their families, including those who live in minority ethnic and multilingual contexts. This strand of research also examines social and linguistic practices that marginalise Deaf people in minority ethnic and CLD groups and how they and their families manage marginalisation. There are many moving accounts by deaf people about how their interaction with hearing others is severely limited by hearing people's monolingualism in speech, and inability to communicate through sign. They argue persuasively that it is as much the responsibility of the hearing person as it is the deaf person to become bilingual in sign and speech. Similarly, culturally and linguistically diverse parents and families narrate stories of loss about their children growing up without the language, culture and religion of their home and community (Ahmad *et al.*, 2000b).

As the Deaf community establishes its cultural distinctiveness, it identifies itself, and increasingly becomes recognised, as a linguistic minority using sign language. In several countries, the national sign language is one of the official/national languages (e.g. South Africa, Sweden, Thailand). In the USA, ASL is recognised as a legitimate, distinct language. In some states, such as Ohio and Texas, hearing high school pupils may study ASL for their foreign language requirement (Burch, 2000). However, in the European Union (EU), half a million people use a sign language, yet sign languages are excluded from EU minority language statistics, laws and reports, indicating that sign language has no/low official status (Krausneker, 2003)

In the UK, sign language is the first or preferred language of around 70,000 people, although exact figures for minority ethnic deaf people are not available. Among individuals of Hispanic descent living in the USA in 1990–1991, 4.2%, or over 900,000 individuals, had hearing impairments (Ries, 1994, cited in Steinberg *et al.*, 2003). As the case study at the beginning of the chapter indicates, even countries that are geographically, politically, culturally and linguistically very close, may develop distinct sign languages. As the case showed, while deaf learners can become bilingual in sign languages, there are implications for their families and education.

Bilingualism is a term shared by linguistically diverse communities and the Deaf community. There are shared issues, similarities and differences in research on bilingualism across signing/oralism and diverse cultural and linguistic communities (Cline, 1997). For example, there are arguments put by both sign language and English as an additional language (EAL) movements that advocate one language in the classroom to learn concepts and higher thinking skills. Issues of assimilation and normalisation of minority linguistic groups into mainstream majority language society are of concern to both oralists/signers in deaf education and bilingualism researchers. Bilingual deaf educationists and EAL/bilingual educationists are concerned about the role of two languages in the child's development of learning and socialisation practices. Yet, there is a lack of research evidence on the merits of working with children in lipreading, auditory training and signing in contexts where there are at least two spoken languages, such as for Hispanic and Asian children (Steinberg *et al.*, 2003).

Impairment Studies of Deafness in Linguistically Diverse Communities

Researchers of hearing impairment distinguish between the types of deafness they investigate, across cause, type and severity of deafness. In the intersection of race/ethnicity and culture/language, studies focus on the occurrence (incidence), frequency (prevalence) and type of hearing impairment that occurs in different communities in different countries, and in minority groups in one country, e.g. the UK or USA. These studies, underpinned by determinist notions, look for genetic predisposition in minority groups as well as cultural practices. More critical approaches link the causes of hearing impairment with social conditions, such as poverty and ill health, with a view to informing policies and practice. This section looks at prevalence and incidence, causes of deafness, early assessment and associated behaviour difficulties, and concludes with a critical evaluation of this approach to researching deafness in multiethnic societies.

Medically, hearing loss or impairment is described as a full or partial decrease in the ability to detect or understand sounds and is caused by a wide range of biological and environmental factors. There are two main types of hearing loss. Conductive hearing loss, due to obstruction in the outer or middle ear, may result in a mild or moderate loss and individuals are not usually classified as deaf or identify themselves as a member of the Deaf community. Language development may be affected by fluctuating hearing loss in young children, with possible consequences for developing literacy skills (see Chapter 4). Environmental causes are often linked to conductive hearing loss in minority ethnic groups.

Individuals with the other type of deafness, sensorineural hearing loss, are an important interest in this chapter because of their prevalence in some minority ethnic groups, particularly in the UK. Sensorineural hearing loss occurs when the inner ear or auditory nerve and nervous system is damaged, and loss whether it is mild, moderate or severe, including total deafness, is permanent. The main causes are infection and illness, medication, trauma, environmental noise and genetic, due to heritable dominant or recessive genes. Deafness can occur after speech and language have developed or before. Prelingual deafness is usually congenital, loss is stable, severe or profound, and the development of vocal/auditory language is severely or completely impaired. Children with this type of deafness and language development usually need special support in education. Yet, identity and self-perception of individuals who are deaf is not determined by clinical or legal criteria of deafness, but by identification with a community of Deaf people. Being Deaf has less to do with (in)ability to hear and more to do with membership of a community sharing similar cultural and linguistic (signing) experiences that follow from hearing differences from the rest of society.

There are almost 9 million deaf and hard of hearing people in the UK (RNID, 2004), although numbers are decreasing. About one in seven adults are deaf or hard of hearing. Between one and two people in a thousand of the general population are born Deaf or become deaf in early childhood in developed nations (ADSS *et al.*, 2002). The UK Deaf Community that uses sign language is thought to number between 50,000 and 75,000. A total of 90% of deaf children have hearing parents. The deafblind population is thought to number about 23,000. No figures are given for deaf people with minority ethnic, culturally and linguistically diverse backgrounds. Recently issued NHS guidance on ethnic monitoring in the UK also identifies the importance of ensuring appropriate communication methods are used when collecting information from people who are deaf or hard of hearing.

Biological causes

Congenital

Congenital and early onset deafness is the most common sensory disorder in children. In the USA, approximately one in every 1000 children has hearing loss sufficiently severe to interfere with normal speech development (Morton, 1991, cited in Fitzgerald *et al.*, 2004). There is concern for early identification of deafness to promote early intervention. Previously, the average age for identification of hearing loss using conventional audiometry was 14 months. Advocates of early identification argue that brain scanning techniques and genetic screening, that is DNA analysis, in newborn infants, can detect moderate/profound forms of hearing loss that may not be detectable for several months using standard audiometric techniques. Yet, when both techniques are used together, deafness can be identified prior to 6 months. Parents who know earlier about their child's deafness can, if they wish, engage their infants in early intervention programmes. Identification and intervention before 6 months shows that children had better language development than those identified later. This was the case for children with typical cognitive abilities across gender, ethnic group, socioeconomic background and degree of hearing loss (Yoshinaga-Itano *et al.*, 1998). A study conducted in New York (Fitzgerald *et al.*, 2004) showed that there was no significant effect of ethnicity across White, Hispanic, Asian and Black infants for particular genetic mutation, although one form of genetic mutation causing infant deafness was detected in Ashkenazi Jewish infants.

HIV/AIDS

There has been a rise in the incidence and prevalence of deafness and hearing impairment in countries with epidemic proportions of HIV/AIDS. HIV/AIDS affects the immune system to reduce resistance, and increase susceptibility, to infections, which affect auditory and hearing development. The unique population of HIV/AIDS-infected infants, particularly in populations of countries in sub-Saharan Africa, makes enormous demands on often limited medical and health care resources, usually to the exclusion of provision for deafness, including early screening (McPherson & Swart, 1997; Swanepoel *et al.*, 2006). There are implications for health and education provision within these countries for meeting the language needs of these children in contexts of economic stringency and CLD, as most countries in this region are multilingual. There are also implications for meeting language needs in the health and education provision for other countries as a result of migration.

Rubella

A mother's rubella infection (German measles) in pregnancy gives rise to a congenital syndrome in the baby, which includes deafness as well as other sensory, cognitive and physical difficulties. It is now rare in most countries with immunisation programmes in developed health care systems. Where it is still present, population movements between countries mean that rubella continues to be a cause of syndromal deafness. In some countries without immunisation programmes, such as in West Africa, where there is a 10–30% possibility of women being carriers, congenital rubella syndrome is still not reported. For example, a study in Ghana reported that infants with rubella syndrome are significantly associated with younger mothers from northern tribes (Lawn *et al.*, 2000). Findings like this can inform health campaigns.

Many young people with deafness caused by rubella go through mainstream school and into postsecondary education, while others may leave school for employment. Studies have shown that certain factors influence either going into further education or dropping out. In the USA, mainstreaming deaf children determines that they go into postsecondary education, and minority ethnic groups are less likely to go into further education and more likely to drop out of schooling and employment (Kasen *et al.*, 1990).

Interfamily marriage practices

In the UK, a main area of concern is the markedly higher rate of infant and childhood mortality in families from interfamily marriages, that is, the practice of consanguinity (Balarajan & Soni Raleigh, 1995). Consanguinity is a cultural practice among families from Pakistan, where close family members, such as first cousins, marry. The practice continues in transplanted Pakistani communities, such as in the UK and Norway (Stoltenberg *et al.*, 1997, 1998). In the UK, there is a higher incidence of children with severe and complex impairments due to genetic abnormalities and syndromes associated with consanguineous families, particularly deafness (Bullock & Khalid, 1995). Pakistani pupils are between 2.0 and 2.5 times more likely to have profound and multiple learning difficulties, visual impairment, hearing impairment or multi-sensory impairment than White British pupils, and Bangladeshi pupils are nearly twice as likely to be identified as having a hearing impairment than White British pupils (Lindsay *et al.*, 2006).

There are several critical reflections on these findings. Difficulties in consultation patterns and service conditions, such as the fact that health visitors' stereotyped views may lead to poorer maternity care and reduced access to it, tend not to be taken into account as part of the probable cause of both perinatal mortality and perceived higher incidence of congenital abnormalities (Ahmad, 1993). It is possible that risk of congenital abnormalities is increased by marriages within the transplanted Pakistani communities because of an overall decrease in the collective gene bank (Ahmad, 2000). These explanations might also interpret the findings for disability among certain other transplanted communities in the UK, such as from Bangladesh. For these reasons, consanguinity as a single explanation for severe disabilities in these minority ethnic communities has effectively been ruled out (Ahmad, 2000; Mir *et al.*, 2001: 10; Atkin, 2003).

Blaming cultural and linguistic practices potentially 'absolves the providers of responsibility for purchasing more imaginative and overtly equitable maternity and health care packages for this population' (Ahmad, 1993). It also ignores the social advantages of marriage within the extended family (Bullock & Khalid, 1995). The responsibility of health and education services is to remove barriers, such as negatively stereotyping cultural practices, and to improve access by engaging the existing social and cultural capital in minority communities.

Environmental causes

Otitis media is caused by chronic middle ear infection. Unilateral hearing loss often results from chronic middle ear infections associated with poor health and housing and it can have implications for academic achievement. Relating figures for prevalence with figures for poverty, housing and academic achievement in these children would be instructive. Studies of frequency of occurrence (prevalence) seek to support the notion of genetic predisposition in ethnic minority groups and link it to environmental factors. One purpose of health prevalence figures is to indicate where poor health can be improved. Findings need to be related to the impact of environmental factors, such as housing, nutrition, climate, in order to discern their social and educational importance and implications. Making this connection has been shown to be particularly important for understanding prevalence of deafness in CLD minority ethnic populations. Here are two examples of research with comparatively economically poor communities.

A large multiethnic prevalence study in the USA looked at population-based prevalence rates of unilateral hearing loss in school children. It compared students aged 6–19 years across five minority ethnic groups in the USA: African–American, Cuban–American, Mexican–American, Puerto Rican and non-Hispanic White. Cuban–Americans showed most prevalence of overall hearing loss and least prevalence of moderate to profound unilateral hearing loss. Puerto Ricans showed most prevalence of moderate to profound hearing loss. There were no significant changes due to age or gender. This study estimates that over a third of a million school-aged children in the USA have unilateral hearing loss (Lee *et al.*, 1998).

Another body of research compares prevalence of middle ear infections and resulting hearing loss between Inuit populations in Canada with their minority communities in other countries, such as in the USA. A recent study (Bowd, 2002, 2005) concluded that hearing impairment due to recurring middle ear infections (otitis media) is widespread among Inuit, First Nations and Metis children in Canada and may occur in some communities up to 40 times more frequently than in the urban south.

Implications

These findings have implications for policymakers and service providers, professionals and practitioners working with minority groups, concerning preventative work in school health. At the level of individual students, there are implications for preventing social and educational exclusion, such as by screening hearing in pupils, monitoring language development in both/all pupils' languages, as well as implications for teaching and learning with this group of children. At the same time, there are implications for action on a wider social scale, concerning the relationship between poverty/bad housing and ill health/hearing impairment that affects communities, like the Inuit and Puerto Rican illustrated in these studies, significantly more than their neighbouring communities.

There is an established link between socioeconomic deprivation, in terms of lower income, poorer housing, higher unemployment, a greater reliance on welfare benefit and the prevalence of mild or moderate learning difficulties. Overcrowding in housing and daycare facilities increases the risk of transmission of otitis media and upper respiratory infections (World Health Organisation, 2004). While the WHO report refers mainly to developing countries, in the UK, evidence indicates that many minority ethnic families live in poverty, where poor housing and chronic, poor nutrition leads to ill health particularly affecting children's hearing, and where families are more likely to have children with moderate and severe disability (see review by Mir *et al.*, 2001). Despite evidence of the influence of socioenvironmental factors, recent studies continue to attribute deafness and severe impairment in Bangladeshi and Pakistani families 'to a greater incidence of genetic factors related to consanguinity (parents are blood relations)' (Lindsey *et al.*, 2006).

Evidence concerning parents' and professionals' perspectives on consanguinity indicates that emphasising consanguinity as an explanation of deafness and/or other severe impairments engenders feelings of guilt in parents. This emphasis can also result in provision and professional practice that denies parents' equality of access to care entitlements, knowledge and information about reproductive decisions and their child's disability. Health provision for prospective consanguineous partners on genetic counselling is welcomed by the minority communities themselves (Ahmad *et al.*, 2000a).

One reading of a biological-genetic approach to researching deafness in particular, and disability in general, across ethnicity and cultures is that it constructs certain client groups as strange and 'Other', and distinct from a mainstream 'Us' who are providers of services and researchers. The purpose of this avenue of research is often to inform health or education policies. Research may also examine constructs that view cultural behaviour, such as consanguineous marriages, as aberrant moral practices, which are a cause of disease that weakens the nation physically and financially. One extreme response might be a set of proscriptive moral and educational recommendations to control and eradicate this epidemiological phenomenon. Alternative responses are advocated to develop provision and practice that enables 'professionals to become ... allies and facilitators to challenge both disablism and racism' (Ahmad *et al.*, 2000a: 44), as well as changing the social conditions of poverty that give rise to hearing impairment.

Assessment

Early detection and intervention of hearing loss and impairment in infants is widely established in countries with developed economies. There is increasing acceptance of the international benchmark of the Universal Newborn Hearing Screening (UNHS) programmes as part of an Early Detection and Hearing Intervention (EDHI) system. However, in countries with developing economies, early assessment may compete with other health priorities. Auditory research findings show that the bilingual experience may affect the outcome of auditory research, with implications for methods and improving descriptions of linguistically diverse research participants (Von Hapsburg & Peña, 2002). For example, assessments involving spoken word and sentence recognition (e.g. SCAN-C: Keith, 2000a, 2000b) have implications for bilingual and culturally diverse children. Dialect variations can influence scoring to such an extent as to place a small proportion of bilingual children on the 'borderline/disorder' category, so that caution should be used to interpret these scores and account taken of dialect variations (Woods *et al.*, 2004).

Cochlear implants

Research and professional practice on management and intervention with deafness has two perspectives. The 'hearing perspective' emphasises normalising, and promotes the use of various devices that may facilitate hearing, such as cochlear implants, as well as children's use of residual hearing, the acquisition of spoken language, speech and auditory training strategies and, based on the degree of hearing loss, the potential for academic achievement within particular educational settings. The 'Deaf perspective' emphasises Deafness and promotes the use of sign language in home and school, as well as the culture, heritage and resources of the Deaf community.

There is evidence of under-representation of minority ethnic deaf children accessing cochlear implant provision. A four-year study (Geers & Brenner, 2003) looked at 181 children from across the USA and Canada and documents characteristics of the children, families and education of children who were prelingually deaf and who received a cochlear implant by 5 years of age. The authors note that most families had normal hearing, were of majority (white) ethnicity and had more education and higher incomes than the general population. The families tended to be intact with both a mother and a father who involved their hearing-impaired child in family activities on a regular basis.

The study claims to be a large representative sample of this group of children. Yet, in a region with health statistics associating higher incidence of impairment with poverty and minority ethnicity, we could/would expect to see a sample with more representation of poorer and minority ethnic children. However, the authors also report that the sample is 'representative of those families seeking a cochlear implant for their child'. We could deduce that families from marginalised back-grounds, such as in poverty and from ethnic and linguistic minorities, do not seek cochlear implants for their deaf children. A different study (Steinberg *et al.*, 2003: 303) showed that this is indeed the case with Hispanic parents: 'Hispanic families are presented with fewer options such as cochlear implantation' by professionals.

Associated mental health needs

Behaviour and adjustment are important because they affect well-being in school, as well as in home and family relationships. They also indicate subjectivity and senses of self and identity. Yet, estimating prevalence of mental ill health in children with deafness is fraught with inconsistencies in the way data is collected and reported across studies. One review of research (Van Eldik *et al.*, 2004) presents prevalence estimates from the USA, UK and the Netherlands that range from 20 to 50%, and that prevalence can be between 1.5 and 2 times higher than for hearing populations, as well as studies reporting no difference in mental health between deaf and hearing students.

In the UK, the rates of referral for mental ill health and behavioural problems have decreased, probably due to improved general educational and environmental services for deaf people and better perinatal care (RNID, 2004). Nevertheless, deaf people seeking access to mental health care have to overcome considerable barriers to access services that meet their needs (NIMHE/DH, 2005). These barriers are constructed by lack of information and knowledge about deafness and its implications by service providers when assessing and treating mental health problems. The two recent reports that review research (Royal National Institute of the Deaf, RNID, 2004; Sign and Mental Health Foundation, 2006) make no mention of deaf people from CLD backgrounds who may have more complex communication needs that require different responses from service providers.

Mental ill health may also include behaviour difficulties, particularly in deaf children. A number of reasons are offered in the literature. Identifying associated behaviour difficulties may be due to professional practices of stereotyping personalities and behaviours in Deaf people that can obfuscate behaviours attributable to poorly expressed or received emotional expression that are also apparent in hearing people. Causes for difficulties in impulse control, such as aggression and anger, may be implicated specifically with deafness, such as due to brain damage associated with the cause of deafness, or it may be due to more pervasive deprivation concerning socioeconomic and educational environments which affect deaf and hearing children. Another possible explanation is that deafness, and in particular the communication difficulties that are associated with it, 'cause' these problems. Yet, few studies include minority ethnic or culturally and linguistically diverse communities, and where they are recorded in the cohort, ethnicity and CLD are not explored as a dimension of deaf family members with behaviour needs.

One study (Vostanis *et al.*, 1997) included culturally and linguistically diverse pupils and families in a primary and a secondary special school in the UK. The study was motivated by health provision entitlement, where deaf children might be under-represented, and consequently not receiving entitled support for psychosocial difficulties and mental health disorders, in comparison with their hearing peers. As practitioner-researchers in child and adolescent psychiatry, they were particularly interested in the interaction between methods of communication and ethnicity as a source of behavioural and emotional difficulties and sought to find a suitable measure of behaviour and emotional difficulties. The study used parent and child checklists, questionnaires and teacher/parent discussions to identify significantly more mental health problems in deaf children in comparison with the general hearing population. Vostanis *et al.* (1997: 233) claim that: 'behaviour and emotional problems were significantly higher in Asian children', and that there was a 'very high rate of social maladjustment of deaf children according to general population norms' (242). Yet, these claims are constrained by a narrow account of the impact of CLD on communication in deafness.

There seem to be assumptions made about the homogeneity of the deaf students, with little interrogation of the impact of ethnic diversity: 62% from an 'Asian' ethnic group, 34.5% White and 3.5% Black. It is widely acknowledged that the ethnicity category 'Asian', like 'Hispanic', indicates a range of language and cultural diversity rather than being 'relatively homogenous'. Even though students may identify with a deaf culture in school, the culturally and linguistic experiences that they engage with at home are likely to differ from each other and from school.

Different research methods yielded different knowledge about communication. It seems that the tensions in methods of communication between children and parents were not surfaced by the questionnaires, and the majority of parents indicated that they were following the policy promoted by the school by using sign language and speech. In contrast, the considerable anxiety-provoking behaviour of the children's emotional difficulties was signalled by the parents in the checklists and in discussions between teachers and parents.

Language practices across service needs-led provision and home offer insights into the relationship between deafness and behaviour difficulties. The school had a bilingual policy of using English in signed (BSL) and spoken forms. Asian children learnt to sign in English only and about half learnt to speak in English, and did not learn to sign or speak in their home language. While 'all parents have access to [BSL] tuition, although this is used in a varying degree' (Vostanis _et al._, 1997: 238), the result was that a quarter of the children had difficulty communicating with their parents and families. There are implications for researchers and providers to explore the variation and constraints in take-up and use of BSL, such as languages spoken at home, including English, cultural constraints on women (mothers, sisters) travelling on their own to school, expense of travelling to the school, competing priorities, in order to inform BSL provision for families.

The authors conclude that 'children of Asian origin were rated as having significantly more behavioural and emotional problems [than other children in the study and hearing children], at least in their family environment' because of the 'additional exposure to a third language at home' (Vostanis _et al._, 1997: 243). This explanation is a familiar one where nonschool languages in the home are interpreted as the cause, or exacerbating factor, of learning difficulties. An alternative reading would be that where Asian deaf children _lack a home language_ to communicate with parents, family and community friends, the situation is likely to be significant for their emotional and behavioural difficulties. Culturally and linguistically diverse parents and families admit to sadness and emotional loss when their deaf child cannot engage with the home language and cultural practices, particularly religion (Jones *et al.*, 2001; Steinberg *et al.*, 2003).

Thus, recent and relevant literature illustrates a continuum of critical approaches to deafness in CLD. Vostanis *et al.*'s study revealed examples of 'institutional racism' in at least two ways. There was reluctance by the school to engage with language and cultural needs specific to culturally and linguistically diverse families, which affected the education, communication and mental health of the deaf students. The research itself was an uncritical account of the practices, tools and analyses that did/could not embrace dimensions of CLD on deafness. Other research approaches engage with careful examination of the concerns of deaf Asian children and adolescents in the UK and reveals that they are engaged in negotiating complex identities across cultural, religious, ethnic and linguistic heritages with their families and communities, with their peers in school, and with the Deaf community (Ahmad *et al.*, 2002; Atkin *et al.*, 2002). While this group may need psychosocial support, they also require support in developing communication across all their communities.

Identity

In Chapter 1, I discuss identity as a fault line for exploring difference in the intersection of minority ethnicity and bilingualism in disability. I use this section to discuss issues emerging in research about developing identity across deafness and ethnicity, the role of languages and the demands of educational achievement. Identity research in Deafness studies has examined the extent to which individuals construct themselves primarily *either* as Deaf and members of the Deaf community albeit from minority families *or* as being members of a minority ethnic/ linguistic community who are also deaf. There is less research on how they construct themselves as being *both* Deaf *and* a member of the minority ethnic community. If identity is fluid and constructed *in situ* with the resources available, how do Deaf people with CLD backgrounds negotiate their identities across diverse groups? What are the implications for service providers?

Identity has become an important research site in social science study since the mid-1960s (Mead, 1967). One analysis is that research studies explore identity in four ways: personal, social, collective and 'the politics of' (Crossley, 2005: 144). A further analysis of multiple identities in culturally and linguistically diverse contexts is positioning theory. Pavlenko and Blackledge (2004) draw on positioning theory to analyse how minority ethnic individuals and communities develop identities that are either imposed on them, or which they assume because benefits accrue, and also flexible and fluid identities that they negotiate across majority and minority cultural and language sites, such as school and home. We may position ourselves and be positioned at personal, social, collective and political levels. Both analyses are used here to understand deaf people in Deaf communities in CLD contexts.

Our identity is the ways in which we make sense of ourselves. We make an account of ourselves according to who or what we are. We describe ourselves by categories that we place ourselves either in or out of. We identify ourselves by characteristics, and set boundaries that distinguish ourselves as much by being like the people in those categories as much as by being different from 'the other'. To have a conscious awareness of who we are, we need to be reflexive, and to look back, and in, on ourselves. Beyond self-perception we are aware of being agents of our personal identity and how and where we place ourselves in particular groups in society. Of interest is how people adopt identities and how they may change them over time and in different situations, together with the purposes for which they change and renegotiate their identity. The construction, purposes, and negotiation of identity by people who are deaf and with communication disabilities from culturally and linguistically diverse backgrounds should be of great interest to researchers, yet is under-researched.

Constructing identity is not always perceived by the individual as agentive and empowering. They may understand that they are positioned in social groups and awarded identities by more powerful others that they have not chosen or negotiated for themselves. Individuals may not be fully aware of their imposed identities. For example, people who are deaf may also be donated identities of learning difficulties, evidenced by low school achievement (Powers, 1998) and denied access to responsibility and employment opportunities. One response is that subordinated people may group together in opposition to imposed identities, to form new collective group identities. A good example of this is the emergence of the *Deaf* community, where 'deafness' as an identity marker of deficit and impairment has been reappropriated and transformed to identify a social group where deaf people seek to affirm their identity. As a group they have more power to negotiate their deaf identities. People with acquired deafness often do not regard themselves as part of the Deaf community (Ahmad *et al.*, 2000b). The collective Deaf community, like other social groups, is constructed with narratives of its members, deaf people. The impact and place of narratives of deaf Asian, Hispanic and other minority ethnic and linguistic people in the wider Deaf community is an important site for future research.

Recently, researchers of Deafness and the wider arena of disability have focused on identity and the way in which deaf people are perceived, categorised and positioned by society. At almost the same time, characteristics of race, ethnicity and language have become tools for people to work with to develop their personal and collective identity. They engage in 'the politics of identity' by articulating and engaging in a struggle against coercively imposed negative identity values for differences and diversity in race, language and ethnicity. The recognition of institutionalised racism (MacPherson, 1999), equality and human rights has contributed considerably to articulating this position.

Identity, Deafness and ethnicity

Deafness research is one of the few areas in disability studies that seriously engages with identity as an approach to understanding disability, ethnicity and linguistic diversity. Research in deafness and cultural and linguistic identity is relatively recent, both in the UK with young South Asian deaf people and their families (Ahmad *et al.*, 1998) and deafness in multicultural and multilingual families in the USA (Nuru, 1993, 1998; Steinberg *et al.*, 1997).

In work with South Asian deaf youngsters, reports of the same study (Ahmad *et al.*, 1998, 2002; Atkin *et al.*, 2002) examine the different identities that these young people construct. They argue that the young people negotiate and adopt identities that are complex, hybrid and situated in response to the demands of the different contexts they find themselves in, such as minority ethnicity in their families, religion in their families and neighbourhoods, and Deafness in schools, clubs, and friendships. Negotiating identity for young Asian people who are deaf presents tensions. They seek a community that reaffirms and respects their difference as deaf people. Deaf culture strengthens and includes them, yet at the same time denying and undermining their ethnic and religious differences. Parents and family members, particularly elder members, may see Deaf culture in opposition to their own heritage, language, values and beliefs. Deaf Asian young people must negotiate through these sites of support and contestation.

The reports (Ahmad *et al.*, 1998, 2002; Atkin *et al.*, 2002) give new interpretations to previous understandings. For example, in much research, age and gender have been found to be insignificant factors, yet in these reports, both have yielded crucial findings. The different ages of the deaf individuals has implications for the insight, reflexivity and experience brought to the research narrative. Gender in these studies has been crucial in revealing the different identities afforded to, and constructed by, Asian girls from that negotiated by and for Asian boys.

This study also throws light on a previously unreported area. It shows the importance that religion plays in the lives and 'performing identity' for the deaf young people and their families. Historically, in reportage of the 19th century, deafness was most often described as an affliction that isolated the individual from the Christian community (Bayton, 1996). Recently, religion is rarely if ever mentioned in the literature as an important dimension in the education and lives of deaf youngsters. This may be understandable from a perspective of researchers who may be members of a postreligious society. Nonetheless, this perspective obfuscates understanding the construction of identity in deaf Moslem, Sikh, Hindu and Christian young people. Steinberg and colleagues (2003) also note the 'great significance' of the religious beliefs of Hispanic Americans on their identity as parents through their care giving. They suggest that training programmes for practitioners working with Hispanic American families with deaf children should include a component on understanding religious values.

The importance of these studies and their findings is that they open up the complexity of the lives of young Asian and Hispanic American deaf people and their families to the view of professionals and researchers in the field. These young people and their families live with CLD and disability in contexts whose demands are far more complex than most of the professionals who work with them can begin to imagine. There are implications for professionals who are in positions to inform decision making and service delivery to these groups. There are implications for research approaches and professional practice to seek to understand and engage with the complexity of this situation and avoid simplification informed by monolingual and monocultural assumptions.

Bilingual professionals and researchers

The presence of deaf bilingual and culturally and linguistically diverse researchers in deafness studies is an important development. Several deafness studies note that bilingual sign/speech researchers, as well as bilingual minority ethnic researchers, were involved in the research process. In a very few cases is research conducted with multilingual deaf researchers, who are members of the same Deaf community as the deaf children and adults and their minority ethnic/linguistic and religious community. The advantages and benefits of working with bilingual researchers are noted in the reports. Researchers, such as Jones *et al.* (2001) and Steinberg *et al.* (2003), note the implications for service providers:

> The findings of this study underscore the need for a significantly greater presence of Hispanic professionals, educators, peer-to-peer support, parent liaisons and so on. (Steinberg *et al.*, 2003: 304)

Researchers and professionals who are members of the Deaf community are better positioned to reveal the perceptions, beliefs and values as community insiders. They are likely to be better positioned to interpret narratives of cohesion and dissonance across ethnic and linguistic families and communities and Deaf communities. Their reflections on the structures and processes of research and practice contribute to interrogating underlying assumptions of providers and users. Their liaisons with minority Deaf and culturally and linguistically diverse families support collaboration to develop co-designed services more informed by diverse communication practices.

Educational Implications

I use this section to discuss research on educational and environmental aspects, including oral/signing bilingualism for deaf youngsters in CLD contexts. Educational achievement is a focus of parent and professional concern for deaf children from majority and minority communities. Measuring educational achievement is more complex. It is usually considered along academic lines such as examination results, and reading ages, as well as nonacademic achievement, such as communicative competence, self-concept, social adjustment, mental health and social participation. Ultimately, parents and teachers are most concerned about the adult life outcomes, such as employment, financial security and long-term relationships (Powers, 1998).

A UK government report (Powers *et al.*, 1998) reviewed research literature (1980–1998) and identified a range of factors which influenced academic achievement: family socioeconomic status (SES), age of onset of deafness, additional difficulties, hearing status of parents, ethnicity, English as the home language, communication fluency at home, parental expectations and parental acceptance of the deaf child. The report found 'no clear evidence to demonstrate an overall significant advance in the education of deaf children' over that period (Powers *et al.*, 1998: 11). Indeed, there is a dearth of evidence, as the government does not provide regular comprehensive data on the educational achievements of deaf school leavers or any other comparable data.

Many deaf children have additional needs, as the case study illustrated. Overall, they are more likely to experience emotional, physical and sexual abuse than hearing children (Association of Directors of Social Services, ADSS *et al.*, 2002). They are vulnerable to delays in development, low academic achievement, behaviour difficulties and emotional distress as well as mental health problems. Of children with hearing loss, 10% have more than one disability, such as learning or communication disability, and a further 10% have additional clear neurological impairments, such as epilepsy or cerebral palsy (Hamblin & Kitson, 1992).

Deaf students leave school with a reading age well below their hearing peers and equivalent to primary school hearing children, across countries and languages. Studies do not seem to include deaf culturally and linguistically diverse students. In the UK, early studies show that 17-year-old deaf school leavers achieved average reading ages of about 9 years (Holt, 1993; Conrad, 1979). In the USA, a study conducted by Gallaudet University of children over a 30-year period found that half of the children with hearing loss graduated from high school with a 4th grade (9–10 years of age) reading level or less (Gallaudet Research Institute, 1996). A study in the Netherlands (Wauters *et al.*, 2006) of 500 deaf students aged 6–20 years showed that, on average, deaf students scored at a level equivalent to a hearing child in the first grade (6–7 years). Word identification scores of the deaf children, however, were almost equivalent to the scores of hearing children. More recent small-scale studies show that some deaf pupils can achieve similar to their hearing peers, and that there are individual deaf pupils who achieve very high levels of academic success at school and university. For example, the 10% of Deaf children who are born to Deaf parents do better academically, are more socially mature, and have more positive self-esteem than deaf children born to hearing parents (Health Advisory Service, 1995). Socioeconomic status and pupil intelligence are significant influences on school achievement. Other significant influences identified are ethnicity, languages other than English in the home, and parental acceptance of the deaf child. That is, White deaf pupils did better in school than non-White deaf pupils (Powers, 1998).

There were few studies on nonacademic outcomes; speech competence is influenced by the degree of hearing loss and a substantial minority have difficulties with speech. There is a lack of suitable measures for sign competence of deaf children (Powers *et al.*, 1998). In the past, service providers were often seen as privileging oralism. Although deaf clients may use sign language, the additional use of speech was promoted and understood to have a positive effect. Speech was seen as protecting deaf young people from social exclusion and from additional problems, such as emotional and behavioural difficulties (Vostanis *et al.*, 1997; Jones *et al.*, 2001). Deaf children's difficulties in speech and sign have influenced research methods with minority ethnic deaf youngsters (Ahmad *et al.*, 2002; Atkin *et al.*, 2002), driving researchers to find innovative visual tools and procedures to access the thoughts and feelings of these youngsters.

Environmental factors

Enhancing the hearing and listening environment is advantageous for hearing, L2 and hearing-impaired people. Children learning in their L2 appear to be at a distinct disadvantage when listening in rooms with typical noise and reverberation. Sound field amplification provides a way of teachers being heard in the full classroom without distortion and with full clarity by students. Nelson and colleagues (2005) compared native Spanish-speaking second graders learning English as their second language (L2) with English-only-speaking (EO) peers with and without sound field amplification. While no significant benefit was revealed with amplification on task performance in class, word recognition performance declined significantly for both L2 and EO groups in the noisy classroom and the impact was disproportionately greater for the L2 group.

In Canada, a recent study has explored implications for educating school-aged children with otitis media. A follow-up investigation (Bowd, 2008) on coping with otitis media in the north of Canada, including First Nations in Manitoba, had, as one of its aims, to explore adaptations for hearing loss in schools. The most significant innovation in meeting the needs of students with hearing loss, particularly the large numbers with minimal hearing loss who were not identified as hearing impaired, was the presence of classroom sound field amplification systems. The importance of this adaptation was emphasised in an earlier study for this region (Bowd, 2002). The current practice of installing amplification systems is a core support element for learning of all students. Observations that some teachers were initially resistant or felt uncomfortable using them were made by several participants. Recommendations included in-service training and support be made available to schools when new teachers are introduced to the amplification system, and when the system is first installed in schools.

Researchers in the USA (Muñoz-Baell & Ruiz, 2000) identify implications for improving work environments in education, health and elsewhere. Planning and design of an environment free from communication barriers should be one of the goals of any health care and education setting. They suggest this could be implemented by:

- Investing and equipping the setting with video-telephones, minicoms, faxes and the internet. This should always be accompanied by a previous consultation with organisations and representatives of deaf people.
- Installing emergency systems using visual/luminous means.
- Installing amplifying systems for hearing aid users.
- Presenting visual notices and important information on signs, panels or through the use of graphic symbols.

Further evidence for the need to reduce environmental communication barriers is identified in a recent report (RNID, 2004). Accessing health care reveals that for BSL users, who make up 30% of the total number of respondents, the communication barriers are significant. One third (33%) of BSL users were either unsure of the correct dosage of medication to take, or in fact had taken too much or too little medication, because of a communication problem with their health professional. Additionally, 70% of BSL users admitted to Accident and Emergency units, were not provided with a sign language interpreter, making an already stressful situation much worse. Recommendations called for by the RNID are similar to those of Bowd (2008). Simple and cost effective solutions through minor investment in simple technologies, such as visual alert displays and loop systems, would improve and encourage access to services, appointment letters written in clear English for BSL users, and deaf awareness training for all frontline health care staff, with specialist training in practical communication skills.

Most research discussed here evaluates improvements in workplace and school provision for first and second language English-speaking deaf people in the UK and Canada. The recommendations will improve the quality of life for many Deaf and deaf people. However, as Vostanis _et al._'s (1997) study revealed, there is likely to be a small but significant group of minority ethnic deaf young people who do not have any form of communication, including sign language. Considering facilities and support for them would need to be included in future investigations.

Deaf bilingualism: Sign language and oralism

In the UK and USA, Deaf culture and communities use BSL and ASL, respectively, as the Linguas franca, together with lip reading and spoken English. Limited evidence in the UK indicates that special schools for deaf children use bilingual BSL/oral programmes, although the case study that opens the chapter indicates that bi- and trilingual signing goes on in some provision in the British Isles. Recent policy initiatives in the UK have seen the closure of residential schools for the deaf and subsequent mainstreaming of deaf children. Some argue that this move will make it more difficult for deaf children to learn from the heritage language/culture of the Deaf community in education (Burch, 2000). Many mainstream schools are still developing bilingual sign/oral policies and programmes. Further, there is little evidence that schools' communicative practices encourage sign languages – other than BSL – in other minority languages.

In the USA, ASL is preferred in schools over other sign languages in the world, including Mexican Sign Language for Hispanic pupils (Allen, 2002). The rationale given is that:

> The underlying principle is the acquisition of a primary language that is accessible, that being ASL, the language of the deaf community in the United States ... an "accessible" and complete language is most critical in order to facilitate the child's linguistic, cultural, social and cognitive development needed for academic success. (Allen, 2002: 150)

Research evidence in the USA and in the UK is inconclusive about the significant effect on educational achievements of the type of language/ communication approach as well as the amount and type of preschool intervention. Powers and colleagues (1998) attribute this largely to methodological difficulties, such as gathering accurate information on exactly what communication methods are used. Nevertheless, they note that small-scale studies show that preschool sign language intervention can have measurable positive outcomes, although the long-term effects are largely unresearched.

Three studies are presented here from an oralism approach (so called hearing perspective) and a sign approach (Deaf perspective) in the early education of culturally and linguistically diverse children with hearing loss.

A study in the UK examines an oral approach from a hearing/normalisation perspective with deaf culturally and linguistically diverse learners. Evidence from this longitudinal study suggests that teachers of young Deaf children use interactional strategies similar to parents and caregivers of much younger hearing children, to develop first language as the language for learning in schools (Mahon, 2007). The study involved three teachers over two years working in oral schools with deaf children from culturally and linguistically diverse families and EO families. Parents' choice of an oral school for their deaf children requires that the spoken language of schooling, in this case English, is the main communication modality for social and curriculum learning. Teachers were aware that they interacted to develop both the deaf child's first language as well as the language of schooling. They tended to focus on developing the language of schooling as the main objective in the early years so that it became a tool for learning, socially and academically. They adapted their interactional strategies to facilitate spoken English, and perceived language-learning issues as being deafness-related developmental language difficulties rather than concerns of EAL pedagogy (Mahon, 2007: 9).

Another study looked at language practices in classrooms for secondary school Deaf learners with sign language as their first language, who were learning curriculum through their second language, spoken and written Swedish. The study took a Vygotskian approach through a classroom ethnography methodology to explore 'what life was like' in the bilingual (sign/spoken/literate) classroom. The researchers focused particularly on the way that everyday meanings of language are (re)constructed and learning is made possible in the context of the multilingual classroom. Cultural tools such as lesson plans and literacy tools (computers, internet, text-telephones) as well as different languages are used by teachers to shape language practices in the classroom to mediate learning (Bagga-Gupta & Domfors, 2003).

A third study in the USA (Allen, 2002) is taken from a Deaf perspective and offers an example of how researchers and practitioners examine practical, theoretical and ethnicity challenges when teaching deaf children from diverse cultural and linguistic backgrounds. The study contests the dominant discourse of the 'hearing perspective' that seeks to normalise deaf children in order to function in the hearing world. Instead, the study explores the affordances to parents of the 'Deaf perspective' that gives primacy to Deaf culture, communication through ASL, and support and identity in the Deaf community.

Theoretically, Allen draws on an ideological framework of societal resistance against recognising, respecting and implementing bi/multi-lingual programmes in the US education system either through Spanish or through ASL. She uses this framework to interpret the resistances of parents and teachers to the bilingual programme of ASL/English for deaf pupils. Allen (2002) takes an action research approach to investigate primarily parents' and families' perspectives of their children's deafness, communication and learning in a preschool intervention setting. Parents are hearing and deaf, and English speaking, Spanish speaking and ASL communicating. The study uses ethnographic and qualitative approaches to record the views of parents in interviews and exchanges between parents, researchers and teachers as they engage with their understandings and feelings about accepting their children's deafness, communication and learning.

As with the UK study (Ahmad *et al.*, 2002; Atkin *et al.*, 2002), the minority ethnolinguistic parents shared similar concerns as the EO majority ethnic parents, about achievement, friendships and communication of their deaf children. Moreover, Allen's study showed the additional difficulties that minority ethnolinguistic parents experienced, such as accessing resources and services, often exacerbated by low incomes and limited English. The study examined the structures and processes harnessed by parents to achieve their perceived learning goals.

The main findings indicate that parental difficulty was most acutely experienced in learning ASL and the concepts underlying it. Parents were supported in accepting their children's deafness through understanding the importance of ASL and Deaf culture. An important factor in this process was their interaction with their children's communication and learning through the bilingual ASL/English programme and being with deaf families and parents who used ASL; that is, through immersion. A negative finding was that there was little evidence to demonstrate inclusion, promotion or emphasis on Spanish language and culture of the Hispanic parents and families. Findings from studies in the UK (Ahmad, 2000) indicate similar tendencies. Minority culturally diverse children with hearing impairment learn only the dominant language and culture of English in school. The parents' perspectives on the outcomes of monolingual education reflect sadness and frustration that they are no longer able to communicate with their children who, in turn, are no longer able to communicate with them or the minority community.

Allen (2002: 165) recommends further research to address

> other linguistic minorities who have deaf and hard of hearing children within ASL-English bilingual settings in order to understand their perspectives about deafness, education and the specific needs of such linguistically diverse families.

Research studies like Allen's are located in both social and capability models of disability. They build on Vygotskian notions of intervention through learning, not only for the clients, but also for the clients' families and between providers and clients. Researcher-practitioner studies like Allen's offer strong models for generating further evidence in research sites, across provision, country, language, culture, to build new practices, skills and understanding for working with deaf children and their families from culturally and linguistically diverse backgrounds.

Conclusion

To what extent does research and practice in the field of deafness explore the intersection of CLD? Studies of the biological and genetic basis of deafness tend to continue to be uncritical of their position, their methods and assumptions at the intersection with CLD. Atkin notes that research in Deafness must take account of the social complexity of ethnicity:

> Identifying the genetic basis of disease is not a straightforward medical procedure but implicates the broader social, cultural and political context. Ethnicity represents an important part of this context, particularly given the confused and poorly informed debate about genetic differences among supposedly different "racial" populations. (Atkin, 2003: 91)

The extent to which causes of deafness and other disabilities are genetically linked to ethnicity and cultural practices, and the extent to which certain groups are treated differently because of their culture or perceived racial differences, is controversial. The studies discussed from this perspective tend to emphasise and oversimplify the causes of deafness in diverse ethnic groups associated with genetic predispositions and social practices such as consanguinity, and poverty. Furthermore, the main response to the increased incidence of deafness and other disabilities in culturally and linguistically diverse families are social and health initiatives focused on minority ethnic communities to prevent further incidence and lower prevalence; for example, genetic counselling, but not necessarily improvement in housing or economic support.

The case study illustrates the demands made by service provisions on deaf people and their families who migrate. It illustrates the implications for communicating and learning through sign languages that this group must engage with in migration and contexts of CLD. Lack of improvement in language and communication development is often attributed to noncompliance by minority groups, such as through varying degrees of engagement with learning the official sign language. Evidence, and critical interpretations of evidence, indicates that service provision in culturally and linguistically diverse contexts needs to become more responsive to deaf client needs. Developing alternative communication, such as sign language, with linguistic minority families needs to be sensitive to potential resistances, such as perceptions of abandoning the language of home, community and religion, and gendered cultural practices. Flexible approaches not only facilitate families to harness their own resources, but also support hearing impaired youngsters to develop personal, social, collective and political identities in the Deaf community and in wider society.

Chapter 7
Assessment Approaches: Comparison, Product and Process

Case Study

> In a preschool in a dominant English-speaking country, concern is raised by teachers about KP. KP is a boy aged 6;11 years and described as Taiwanese. Teachers are concerned because he is reluctant to participate in the classroom, has difficulty speaking, that is, others find him difficult to understand, and he has poor reading and writing in comparison with his age-peers. His parents are unclear both about their concerns for KP and what they want from intervention. The teacher has interviewed the boy's parents but these issues remain unresolved. His teachers report that KP has limited social skills in terms of reduced eye-contact and limited social interaction. He prefers self-directed activities and he has difficulty attending to unstructured and/or unfamiliar tasks. His parents report that he is difficult to control at home but his teachers report that he is quiet and cooperative at school. (Adapted from a case in *The ASHA Leader* (26 September 2006) publication of the American Speech-Language-Hearing Association)

Introduction

The next two chapters deal with aspects of bilingual language development and learning, namely assessment of, and intervention for, language disability. Both chapters draw on the notion of mediation, which is a central concept in Vygotsky's perception of learning (see Chapter 1). In this chapter, with reference to the literature, assessment of language disability is critically interrogated through the notion of mediation. To recap briefly, mediation is what Vygotsky argued to be the process by which external sociocultural knowledge is assimilated cognitively by individuals in order to (re)organise increasingly complex relationships with the external, through culturally constructed tools. Language is one of the most important cultural tools in mediating the relationship between externalisation and internalisation.

In this chapter, assessment of language disability is explored as a practice to examine language, both as a knowledge system of itself in terms of form and communicative function, as well as a tool for mediating meaning and learning. Reviewing the literature reveals three main purposes for assessment of language disability, namely research, clinical and educational. Studies researching the nature of specific language impairment (SLI) and speech, language and communication needs (SLCN) construct assessment tools through particular theoretical paradigms, resulting in a complex reflexive relationship such that assessment tools shape understanding of SLCN as well as practice and outcome. Previous chapters have indicated how research instruments can reveal something of the nature of language-related disabilities. This chapter is orientated mainly by clinical and educational considerations, which inform identification of difficulty and need, intervention and learning. Clinical purposes for assessing SLI and SLCN are mainly diagnostic, to identify deficit and to inform intervention. Assessment practices for educational purposes also include elements of identifying weaknesses and strengths and they inform teaching and learning approaches for intervention and development as well as to indicate allocation of provision.

Contexts of cultural and linguistic diversity (CLD) make specific demands on assessment practices of language disability because of the need to examine children's multilanguage knowledge systems as well as the social and cultural contexts that inform them. Some assessment approaches accommodate more easily these demands to examine how language knowledges are used by bilingual and culturally diverse children for building relationships (mediating) between themselves and the world. Approaches that privilege internal cognitive functions are likely to find it difficult to include CLD in assessment practices because they seek to minimise the influence of external factors, including even that of the 'examiner', by decontextualising the assessment from other social, cultural and linguistic learning. The case study highlights the purposes of assessing bilingual children's language needs at a particularly sensitive site, namely disentangling speech and language disabilities from additional learning needs and from additional language development (diagnostic and labelling purposes) and to inform educational management. The implications for the notion of a 'fair test' are discussed later.

In this chapter, practices of assessing the needs of bilingual children with speech and language difficulties are critically evaluated through the lens of mediation. Questions guide the discussion: to what extent does the assessment practice examine both the product and the process of the child's language learning? In what ways does it examine the child's mediation of social and cognitive tools for language learning? To what extent does the assessment practice take account of the tester's learning as well as the testee's?

The chapter is in four sections. I use the first section to revisit the remit for assessing bilingual children presenting difficulties in language development. The second and third sections deal with assessment of 'language learning as product' through normative comparison using standardised and criteria-referenced testing and language information processing approaches. The fourth section examines 'language learning as process' from sociocultural and ecological approaches to language development and multilingual language use, as well as dynamic assessment. Finally, I draw some conclusions.

Frameworks for Language Assessment

This section draws on research from provision-led approaches for assessment of bilingual children with alleged speech and language disability. This body of research literature reflects a concern that assessment practices for bilingual children with communication disabilities attend to both the individual and their context. The appraisal of the bilingual child's current learnt functioning and responsiveness to new language learning should be placed within a wider social context of families and provision, meeting the demands of bilingual communicative needs often in monolingual societies.

A provision-led approach to assessment of special educational need concerns:

(1) screening and identification of difficulty;
(2) classification of difficulty;
(3) profile of strengths and weaknesses;
(4) baseline to measure progress;
(5) allocation of resources and educational provision.
     (Cline & Frederickson, 1999; Peña & Valles, 1995)

Screening and early identification of students whose progress is causing concern, is often driven by a policy requirement for professionals, often teachers, to regularly evaluate students' learning and progress. While research and practice are increasingly focused on improving the efficacy and accuracy of assessment approaches for this group of students, students' needs may be misidentified when bilingual first language and second language development are confused with educational learning difficulties. The result for the learner is inappropriate educational management, possible underachievement and/or increasingly complex difficulties. Misidentification and under/over diagnosis of language-for-learning difficulties has happened in the past and continues to happen with bilingual students.

Language competencies

One focus for assessment is appraising knowledge of the language system itself in terms of form and communicative competence. Five aspects of language knowledge and communicative competencies are demonstrated by speakers when communicating effectively. They can be used to guide assessment to investigate the extent to which monolingual and bilingual children:

(1) know the forms of the language they use – how the words sound and how they go together (competence in phonology and syntax);
(2) are able to use those forms to convey meaning and can understand what others mean when they use them (competence in semantics);
(3) understand the social conventions that determine how people use language to each other, so that they can appreciate another speakers' intentions in speaking and can communicate their own intentions to a listener (pragmatic competence);
(4) can vary their style of communication and the language they use to suit the needs of different listeners in a conversation (conversational competence);
(5) understand how language use and language conventions vary with the social and cultural context (sociolinguistic competence).
(Frederickson & Cline, 2002: 266)

These competencies focus on formal aspects and social use of language. A further competence that can be investigated is *language competence for academic learning* (Cummins, 1984). Policies advocate that language knowledge and competencies of both (all) languages and cultures of culturally and linguistically diverse children with alleged difficulties are assessed (DfEE, 2001a).

A strong tendency in the assessment of language competencies is to draw on a container metaphor, suggesting that these competencies can be located and measured in the individual and measured 'in much the same way as one would measure liquid in a container' (Kovarsky *et al.*, 1999: 18). However, the container metaphor fails to account for the situatedness of individuals in contexts, particularly of social, cultural and historical diversity among children and between children and adult testers.

Multiple perspectives, professional cultures

Assessment practices for allocation of provision for children with SLCN in culturally and linguistically diverse contexts are multiprofessional, in contrast with research assessment practices, which focus on exploring one aspect of difficulty/need. Multiprofessional practices are premised on specialist knowledge and responsibilities, which are shaped and informed by historical and social factors and professional cultures. Simply put, assessment practices within medical/psychological paradigms leads to diagnosis, and making judgments about development and difficulty to inform intervention. By contrast, and often complimentary, assessment practices are framed by social and capability paradigms and are concerned to inform teaching and learning for immediate and life-long needs. Dimensions of power around diagnosis tend to privilege certain professionals over others and over the client and families. The implications for culturally and linguistically diverse children and families with language-based needs are fragmentation and 'underlapping' knowledges. There may be limitations in professional education, with an unpreparedness for CLD demands. There may be a reliance on tacit knowledge of monolingual/cultural assessment practices for language difficulties, which relies on 'reaching for old tools'.

In addition, parents and the young people themselves are likely to have opinions about the difficulty. Diagnosis and disclosure of difficulties is a key identity marker for clients, parents and families (Kovarsky *et al.*, 1999). With the availability of information on the internet, many parents and young people can become knowledgeable about their difficulty, particularly issues around hearing impairment, dyslexia and Asperger's syndrome. The increasingly common scenario of informed and knowledgeable parents and clients and shared knowledge across professional groups has implications for the professional–client relationship and collaborative interprofessional working (see Chapters 9 and 10). The manner in which different professional groups and parents and clients come together to discuss assessment information, has become an important part of the assessment process.

Increasingly, researchers and practitioners seek to develop tools – conceptual and procedural – for the assessment of bilingual children, which minimise sources of bias. One approach advocates adopting a cyclical, consultative and multipractitioner process, involving problem definition, hypothesis generation, data collection and analysis, which inform intervention planning and implementation, evaluation of outcomes and problem redefinition (Cline & Frederickson, 1999; Hall *et al.*, 2001). This approach is revisited later in the chapter.

Many researchers and practitioners see beyond the technical issues involved in assessment practices. They are concerned for social justice and equality of opportunity for this group of learners, which becomes a further reason that drives research and practice for effective assessment to inform educational management. Notions of a 'fair test' of the child's abilities and difficulties underpin perspectives of equality and are themselves orientated by theoretical perspectives. For example, issues in constructing 'fair' assessment practices from a cognitive psychology perspective may privilege assessing only one of a bilingual child's language repertoires, exploring language in decontextualised modes and making comparisons with monolingual norms. There are concerns about privileging 'tests' that are standardised and decontextualised over assessment practices that are situated and interpretative. Many current tools and approaches for assessment practices are likely to be unfair to bilingual and bidialectal children.

This discussion surfaces several implications. One implication is for collaborative interprofessional working which brings together specialist technical knowledge about language difficulties with specific knowledge of the implications for CLD for the client and family. Another implication concerns expanding professional development to include assessment practices in contexts of CLD. There are implications for research on assessment of language difficulties to include CLD dimensions. Finally, there are implications for assessment practices with clients and families to be embedded in their CLD context, to support identity and decisions for language and cultural choices. These issues point to developing joined-up practices among professionals for assessment in CLD contexts, orientated by a theory that 'joins up' social, cultural and linguistic aspects of families and children's lives, that links assessment and pedagogy, and embraces a perspective for social justice (see Chapter 9).

Assessing Product: Comparative Performance

A frequently used approach in assessment is comparison with typically developing children through normative testing and developmental stages. This approach does not engage mediation. It explores the product of prior learning and can provide a baseline of knowledge and performance for planning intervention and support. In this section, I review the problematic of norm-referenced tests and apparently nonbiased assessment for language information processing, and in the next section I review criteria-referenced comparisons for bilingual children across speech and language development.

Norm-referenced testing approaches

A large proportion of speech and language assessment tools are norm-referenced tests, standardised on monolingual and monocultural populations. There are widely acknowledged problems with standardised L1 monolingual tests for bilingual/second language acquisition (SLA) children with alleged language difficulties. Most of this advice also holds for avoiding IQ or other cognitive tests that are linguistically and culturally embedded. The most familiar problems concern tester bias, content bias, linguistic bias and disproportionate representation in normative samples (Wheldall *et al.*, 1987; Duncan, 1989; Cole & Taylor, 1990; Laing & Kahmi, 2003; Genesee *et al.*, 2004).

Tester bias

The effect of practitioner bias has been identified as a powerful influence in the misidentification, both over- and under-identification, in testing procedures with culturally and linguistically diverse pupils. Researcher-teachers identify language impairment and dyslexia in children with English as an additional language (EAL), even when these needs are *not* identified as a cause for concern (Valdes & Figueroa, 1994; Lock & Layton, 2002). Further evidence of tester bias comes from studies demonstrating statistically significant disparities in inter-rater reliability for test performances. Most reliability (100%) was shown by highly trained raters and lowest reliability among least trained raters (Pray, 2005).

Content bias

Content bias addresses the validity of tests. Test items and procedures, which assume that all children have similar experiences, concepts and vocabulary, demonstrate bias in their content. Children from CLD backgrounds may perform more poorly on standardised measures relative to dominant (mainstream) language and culture because of variations in life experience, socialisation practices and early literacy experiences (Stockman, 2000). For example, pointing to and labelling objects or actions may not be a typical communicative experience for Hispanic children (Anderson, 2002; Peña *et al.*, 1992). Items usually draw on concepts and vocabulary from white, middle-class schools settings, such that children from CLD backgrounds perform poorly on widely used language tests for some or all of these reasons (Laing & Kahmi, 2003).

Vocabulary testing is particularly problematic not only because many procedures demonstrate content biases, but also because they adopt a reductive conceptualisation of vocabulary, that is, single word recognition. Some tests assess a range of semantic knowledge, such as associations, categorisation, functions, linguistic concepts and similarities and differences, across a range of languages, with comparable but not directly translated items (Peña *et al.*, 2003). Nevertheless, Peña *et al.* (2003) note that content bias may still be evident as an intrinsic aspect of drawing on learnt language performance (language as product). Other assessments of vocabulary and language for conceptual meaning (Woodcock & Muñoz-Sandoval, 2001a, 2001b; Muñoz-Sandoval *et al.*, 1998) run into problems distinguishing language knowledge from academic learnt knowledge (MacSwan & Rolstad, 2003).

Even first language speakers may not do well on these tests. Widely used language tests have been shown to designate first language speakers as nonspeakers of the language. Comparison with their performance in language sampling shows some errors (e.g. MacSwan *et al.* [2002] for Spanish speakers, Pray [2005] for English speakers).

Linguistic bias

Linguistic bias affects test reliability. In standardised tests, this is exemplified when there is a disparity between the child's language and that of the assessor, or a mismatch between the language/dialect used by the child and the language used/expected in responses in the test. The outcome is a recorded poor performance by the child, which can be interpreted in two ways. Assessors identify language difficulties when there are actually language differences (over-identify) (Cole & Taylor, 1990). Or, assessors over-compensate for this mismatch and attribute poor performance (i.e. different responses) to dialect or language differences and ignore real difficulties (under-identify). Assessments claim that they are culturally fair when they try to reduce linguistic bias by attending to language and dialect differences in the way responses are elicited (Craig & Washington, 2002). In the case study, the language(s) that KP hears and engages with in his home, e.g. a dialect of Mandarin, has implications for the language of assessment.

Yet a further source of linguistic bias is when tests are translated. The translation from the language of the test to another language disrupts the original aims of the test in a variety of ways. As the grammar, morphology, vocabulary and phonology of the translated language may not address the original test's assessment aims and may not be age-appropriate in the child's first language, no comparison can be drawn. The standardised information cannot be referred to.

Judgment is needed about the appropriateness of the language match between the normed population and the bilingual children being assessed. Using tests standardised on similar speech groups has been advocated for some time (Romaine, 1995). Languages in contact generate codeswitching which can result in code change. Minority languages are more likely to take on features of the dominant/majority language, in vocabulary borrowing and loan words as well as in grammar, such as word order and morphology changes (Myers-Scotton, 2006; Martin *et al.*, 2003; Pert & Letts, 2003). Consequently, over time, such as 10 or 20 years, the L1 code of linguistic minority groups may change considerably. Thus, L1 normative performance on assessments standardised on a population over 10 years ago may no longer correspond to the normative performance of present populations. There may be substantially more evidence in the minority L1 or majority L2 vocabulary, grammar and morphology, so that language patterns previously thought of as indicators of problematic development in children (such as word order changes) may now be more widely used and not considered odd (Martin *et al.*, 2003).

Disproportionate representation in normative samples

Children with CLD and EAL backgrounds are disadvantageously compared on tests standardised on monolingual normative populations, whether for their first or additional language. Although standardised tests have not usually included culturally and linguistically diverse populations in their normative samples, increasingly they are attempting to have more diverse normative populations (see review, Laing & Kamhi, 2003). However, if standardised tests only extend their normative populations, they only lower the arithmetic bands of 'normal' without presenting qualitative markers for evidence of difference or difficulty in language performance. For example, while performance by a group of at-risk African American preschoolers suggests that the Peabody Picture Vocabulary Test-III (Dunn & Dunn, 1997) is more culturally fair than the older version, Peabody Picture Vocabulary Test – revised (Dunn & Dunn, 1981), the African American children's scores were below those of the standardisation sample, although there was a normal distribution of scores (Washington & Craig, 1999).

Summary

There are implications for critical awareness of biases in language assessment for the allocation of educational resources to culturally and linguistically diverse students on the bases of performance on tests. As we saw in previous chapters, assessment tools, practices and knowledge may be inadequate for the educational needs of these children. Their language and educational needs may go unrecognised or their abilities underestimated, and their educational opportunities in comparison with their peers may be restricted and without additional support.

Despite these considerable caveats about using standardised tests with bilingual children, there are assessments that claim to be culturally and linguistically sensitive in terms of appropriate linguistic items and responses, presentation and procedures, as well as generating norms from appropriate linguistic populations (e.g. Carter *et al.*, 2005). Content and linguistic bias can be addressed to some extent by developing assessments with multicultural and multilingual colleagues. Content bias may decrease for older students who are familiar with the culture and testing behaviour through years of schooling (e.g. labelling, pointing, performing to speed) and with decontextualised nature of language use (Cummins, 2000; Kohnert, 2002). Linguistic bias is minimised by accepting responses in either language, allowing students to access their shared bilingual lexicon and language resources (Cummins, 2000; Peña *et al.*, 2003).

Language-processing measures

Language-processing measures have been assumed to be nonbiased alternatives to traditional experience-dependent measures and offer promise for identifying language difficulties in culturally and linguistically diverse learners (Campbell *et al.*, 1997). While advocates of language-processing measures purport they do not assess 'products of learning', they may do; these measures seem to assess products of learning processing language information. The frame of reference of assessment remains normative, standardised and task-specific, and prey to the linguistic, cultural and representational biases discussed earlier. Moreover, this approach does not assess mediation and new learning.

A core characteristic of children with SLI and dyslexia is difficulty in storing, accessing, retrieving and manipulating word level language knowledge; that is, memory knowledge of phonological information. Nonword repetition (NWR) tasks probe language-based processing (in)abilities for learning new phonological sequences for new words. They focus on processing and manipulating language-specific phonological information. The task appraises skills in language processing when there is no support from semantic knowledge or prior rote learning of the word (Kamhi, 1998; Gathercole & Baddeley, 1996). The task uses either equally familiar (high frequency) words or equally unfamiliar (nonsense) words which follow the permissible phonological (phonotactic) patterns of the language.

Studies have shown that NWR is an effective procedure for detecting SLI across languages and ages (Botting & Conti-Ramsden, 2001; Girbau & Schwartz, 2007). A meta-analysis of NWR studies across children with and without SLI found that children with SLI showed very large impairments in nonword repetition, with difficulty repeating even short nonwords, with greater difficulty for long nonwords, and performing an average (across 23 studies) of 1.27 standard deviations below typically developing children. They also found that there was no association between effect size and the age of children with SLI, although effect sizes meant that NWR measures were not interchangeable (Graf Estes *et al.*, 2007).

There are few cross-linguistic studies of NWR. However, one cross-linguistic study with Cantonese children found that sentence repetition tasks, but not NWR, discriminate between children with SLI and their age-matched and younger typically developing peers, although the authors felt more cross-linguistic study of processing strategies was needed (Stokes *et al.*, 2006).

Claims are made that language-processing measures are less biased than experience-dependent measures, yet cultural vocabulary knowledge is evident in assessment material for processing sentence information. The Competing Language Processing Task (CLPT, Gaulin & Campbell, 1994) looks at memory knowledge in sentences, in particular functional working memory (in English, Gaulin & Campbell [1994], Dollaghan & Campbell [1998], and in Spanish, Gutierrez-Clellen *et al.* [2004]). Children are asked to recall linguistic information (repeat last words in an increasing number of sentences) after responding to the truth of each sentence (e.g. 'pumpkins are purple'); that is yes/no judgments and word recall. Items are high-frequency words in simple sentences. Children are required to perform two operations simultaneously: to store increasing numbers of lexical items at the same time as they process incoming information. The task emphasises storing rather than processing (Montgomery, 2002). Further to the case of bias in standardised testing, NWR procedures are claimed to be a 'culturally nonbiased measure of language processing' (Ellis Weismer *et al.*, 2000: 865); while the CLPT is also assumed to be, some sentences seem to depend on cultural knowledge. The example sentence cited about 'pumpkins' has cultural weighting.

The claim that processing-dependent measures hold considerable promise for distinguishing between children with language disorders, whose poor language performance reflects fundamental psycholinguistic deficits, and children with language differences attributable to differing experiential backgrounds (Campbell *et al.*, 1997) has since been contested and found wanting (Kohnert *et al.*, 2006). The potential value of CLPT and NWR as nonbiased assessment measures to distinguish between bilingual/EAL learners and learners with language difficulties was investigated. In an experimental design, 100 school-aged children (7–13 years) participated in three groups, typical monolingual English, typical bilingual Spanish–English and monolingual English with SLI. The children were initially assessed on English and Spanish where necessary on the CELF-3 (Semel *et al.*, 1995, 1997). The groups achieved from highest to lowest: English only, bilingual, and the language difficulties group.

It seems that 'these tasks did not provide compelling diagnostic power for separating typically developing bilinguals from monolinguals with language difficulties' (Kohnert *et al.*, 2006: 19). The authors also note that 'these results suggest that performance on language based processing measures are not independent from previous language experience and cannot, without further refinement, be considered nonbiased assessment measures when used with bilingual children' (Kohnert *et al.*, 2006: 27). Kohnert and colleagues conclude that the anticipated promise of these tasks is not realised.

There are neuropsychological limitations on a language information processing approach. The assumption that the link between brain, cognitive processes and behaviour is uninterrupted and can achieve decontextualised, culture-free assessments has been questioned (Perez-Arce, 1999). Moreover, from a sociocultural perspective, while the tasks are not based (entirely) on directly learnt language experience, they are based on memory 'capacity', which is culturally and linguistically learnt memory knowledge (Claxton, 2002). Assessment practices for culturally and linguistically diverse children reliant on normative task-specific testing of products of language knowledge and language-processing knowledge are constrained by a range of procedural biases as well as theoretical limitations. The tools offered by research studies are unable to distinguish, for clinical and educational purposes, between children developing EAL typically and those with language disabilities.

Criteria-Referencing Language Development in Bilingual Contexts

In this section, the problems and potential of criteria-referenced measures to identify language difficulties are discussed. Core areas of difficulty learning language knowledge, specifically morphology and verb grammar and phonology, are examined, with reference to relevant studies of criteria-referenced measures, such as development stage information and standard language descriptions.

Criteria-referenced measures compare a child's performance on a specific skill, grammatical structure or linguistic concept to independently predetermined criteria (Laing & Kamhi, 2003: 46). They can be sensitive to the child's social, cultural and communicative context and reduce the biases evident in normative testing. They include language sampling, probing techniques and other informal techniques for sampling interactions. Claims are made that they are usually more accurate than norm-referenced measures for identifying a child's SLI and indicating a focus for intervention (Battle, 2002).

Criteria-referenced measures for language assessment largely depend on developmental data or language descriptions. As difficulties with morphology are a core feature of SLI, developmental information about morphology in bilingual children is an important tool for identifying language difficulties. However, the profiles of morphology development across languages are unlikely to be the same (see Chapter 4). For example, English-speaking children have particular difficulty in English, marking tense on verbs (Rice & Wexler, 1996), while French-speaking children omit French object pronouns in the middle of sentences (Paradis *et al.*, 2003a). There is an increasing body of research on early development of grammar and morphology across a range of languages (see Pienemann [2005] for German, Swedish, Japanese, Arabic, Chinese, and Thoradottir [2005] for French), which could inform analysis of language sampling in first languages. Further research on assessment practices using language sampling and comparative analysis might identify qualitative indicators of morpheme 'error type' that might contribute to distinguishing EAL learners from those with specific language learning needs.

A recent study (Paradis, 2005) used comparative criteria based on the morphology development across EAL learners and L1 English learners with language disability. Paradis set out to specifically investigate whether the expressive language characteristics of typically developing EAL children are similar to the characteristics of English spoken by monolingual children with SLI, and the impact of these similarities on 'errors of judgment' in the assessment of EAL learners as having SLI. The main finding of this study for assessment practices is that early morpheme development in additional English of bilingual learners with less than a year's EAL development can look like SLI patterns. This is further evidence that tests of early grammar standardised on typically developing monolingual children are not necessarily helpful for diagnostic purposes for EAL learners.

In families with linguistic diversity through regional variation and dialect, comparing the speech and language patterns of children with their parents from culturally and linguistically diverse families may be insightful (Terrell & Terrell, 1993). The parents' language offers a model to compare and contrast the child's dialect in typical and atypical development. A drawback of this approach is that the anticipated model of the parents' language may be different from the child's, for reasons of code change, frequency of use of structures, vocabulary (Martin *et al.*, 2003; Washington, 1996).

I use the rest of the section to examine other aspects of speech and language development, which present as potential sites for criteria-referenced differentiation between developmental and problematic patterns of learning languages.

Slow or late talking

An important feature of later language difficulties is a history of late talking. In monolingual studies, young children between 2 and 3 years who show delay in talking are known as 'late talkers'. Late talkers are identified when they have less than 50 words/lexical referents in their expressive vocabulary and/or show no word combinations. Monolingual studies show an important wider picture for this group of children. There are several significant risk factors, including a family history of speech/language delay. While a high proportion of children who are late talkers spontaneously improve (e.g. Rescorla *et al.*, 1997), most demonstrate, whether or not language improves, substantial subsequent problems, particularly in literacy skills (Law *et al.*, 2000a), education achievement and behaviour (Caulfield *et al.*, 1989).

In a bilingual context, late talking in the first/home language will be an important indicator in case history taking, of difficulty in the child's other languages (Genesee *et al.*, 2004). A Swedish study found different patterns in speed of bilingual language development. Typically, developing bilingual first language children show a higher level of language development in at least one language, while children with language difficulties tend to have a balanced low level of language development in both languages (Håkansson *et al.*, 2003). Evidence for monolingual slow talkers indicates that intervention is recommended whether by working with parents or directly with toddlers, rather than a 'watchful waiting' approach (see a review of evidence by Eadie, 2004a). There are clear implications for work with minority linguistic families.

Speech difficulties

The child in the case study, KP, has difficulty making himself understood by others. Unintelligibility is a frequent early indicator of later speech difficulties. Speech development and difficulties in bilingual children can be assessed using criteria-referenced measures of development. Speech has two components: phonology which is language-specific, and articulation which is a motor function, and they are differentiated in assessment with bilingual children. Phonological development, similar to morphology and grammar, is language-specific with a developmental sequence within maturational constraints. Transfer across languages is unlikely and phonological profiles across languages are likely to be different (Zhu & Dodd, 2006a; Salameh, 2003).

One analysis of typical and atypical phonological development draws on phonological simplification processes (Stampe, 1979). Phonological processes simplify syllabic information (e.g. reducing clusters, deleting final consonants) and simplify segmental speech sound information (Grunwell, 1987; Ingram, 1989; Stampe, 1979). Assessment of phonological difficulties in bilingual children must be language-specific (Holm & Dodd, 1999) and reliant on language-specific information about developmental phonological processes (Zhu & Dodd, 2006a). Using a criteria-referenced approach, an analysis of phonological processes could inform a comparison of the child's emerging phonological system in each language with the adult system. Comparisons of typical and atypical phonological development of first and additional languages are emerging and informing intervention (Zhu & Dodd, 2006a).

By contrast, motor difficulties in articulation of speech sounds and sequences are not at a level of linguistic meaning. Thorough motor assessment of speech movements is likely to reveal organic/maturational/neurological-related speech motor difficulties, which affect articulation of speech sounds in both languages. An assessment tool used by speech and language therapists to reveal neurological difficulties is diadochokinetic rate (DDK), which measures how quickly an individual can accurately produce a series of rapid, alternating sounds. The rate is calculated and compared to published norms. There are two considerations for culturally and linguistically diverse people with speech difficulties. Studies show that DDK rates for articulation in other languages differ from those reported for English-speaking children and vary across languages rather than being a universal comparator (Prathanee *et al.*, 2003). Although in clinical practice DDK is generally measured perceptually, without support from instrumental methods that display the acoustic waveform, no standard measurement procedures are employed and studies on inter- and intra-rater reliability are lacking (Gadesmann & Miller, 2008).

Literacy difficulties: Dyslexia and bilingualism

In the case study, KP was observed as having difficulties with reading and writing in comparison with his peers. While these difficulties may be developmental, nevertheless they deserve to be explored, particularly in the light of his possible speech difficulties. Within a language-processing model, speech-processing difficulties are closely related to dyslexia. (Assessment of dyslexia is discussed in Chapter 5.) For KP, it would be important to explore the literacy systems and practices used in KP's home and the extent to which KP was included in them. Again, researchers and practitioners are urged to look for means, other than normative or comparative, for assessing and identifying bilingual students like KP as either typical but slow progress or with language learning difficulties.

A Sociocultural Approach

So far, the chapter has explored evidence about assessing the psychological knowledge of language in the child. Yet, Vygotsky asserts that what individuals do and how they learn cannot be predicted on the basis of their psychological attributes alone, because as Claxton (2002: 25) notes 'these are selected, customized and instantiated, in unpredictable ways on the basis of shifting context'. This section looks at assessment practices that examine the interaction between social and cultural settings and their communicative demands with bilingual learners' cognitive language learning and socialisation. Mediation is directly addressed in discussions about dynamic assessment.

An ecological approach

Ecological approaches to assessment are based on the assumption that every individual is 'an inseparable part of a social system' and that one's 'behaviour cannot be understood without considering its context' (McCormick, 1997: 227). Ecological approaches stress the importance of:

> Sampling communication in a variety of differing contexts and environments, including classroom, community and home,
> Obtaining information concerning the communication expectations of adults who are part of a child's natural environment, and
> Considering the contexts in which a child's learning occurs before drawing conclusions about his/her communicative abilities. (Wyatt, 1999: 199)

Furthermore, ecological assessment approaches can inform culturally relevant intervention and planning.

For example, in play contexts for language socialisation, observations of peer reactions, such as engagement or puzzlement to talk with a culturally and linguistically diverse child, like KP who has raised teachers' concerns, can provide data for analysing inclusion/exclusion and contribute to distinguishing between typical and atypical language development and dialect. The considerations identified by Wyatt are important when communicative expectations differ from those valued in the dominant culture of professionals and schooling. She emphasises, for example, that practitioners need to know that in the first three years of life, children who are speakers of nonstandard English (NSE) dialect have the same language skills as those who speak a standard dialect (standard American English [SAE] or received pronunciation [RP] in the UK) if they are typically developing. Children follow a broadly similar path in phonological, grammatical and communicative functions development, albeit at different paces (Wyatt, 2002). Dialect differences in grammar usually begin to emerge only at around preschool age, with differences becoming more noticeable as children become older (Craig *et al.*, 2003; Craig & Washington, 2004).

One of the most influential models for conceptualising influences on a child's environment has been Bronfenbrenner's (1979) ecosystems approach. His model depicts the child at the centre of a multisystem society, represented as concentric circles, like onion rings or 'a set of nested structures, each contained inside the next like a set of Russian dolls' (Bronfenbrenner, 1979: 3). There are four main subsystems: a microsystem (e.g. family), a mesosystem (e.g. school), an exosystem (e.g. education policy) and a macrosystem (e.g. migration), which impact on the child's development. The relationship between the subsystems is based on the individual's ability to use accessible resources to achieve goals that meet needs. Bronfenbrenner's model is relevant in analysing factors such as poverty, discrimination and immigration on the psychosocial development of children and young people from minority cultural groups. In cases of recent migrants and refugees, the model affords examination and analysis of the different sets of values and norms which children are exposed to in different settings and the potential areas of conflict this can give rise to (Gibbs & Huang, 1989, cited in Frederickson & Cline, 2002: 110). However, it is not a framework that draws on learning and learning theories to explain or interpret development, growth and change.

Spolsky (1989) developed an ecological approach to understand bilingual learners' needs, based on second language research. Spolsky's model of the relationship of the environment to the learner posits that there are two major clusters of conditions that affect bilingual and second language development. One cluster is external to the learner and related to the social context in which language learning is taking place.

(1) *Motivation* to engage with languages that is encouraged through teaching/learning.
(2) *Opportunity* to be exposed to and engage with languages, particularly that of schooling.

The second cluster is internal and related to the learner as she/he is engaged in the language-learning process.

(3) *Knowledge* about both (all) languages known to the learner.
(4) *Ability* of the learner to learn and develop language.

At the centre of Spolsky's model is the interplay between the potential of the language learner and the opportunities provided for language learning that determines the outcomes. Spolsky asserts that when learning outcomes have not been achieved in school, the learning environment in the school needs to be evaluated: teacher expertise, curriculum and quantity and quality of teaching and support given, as well as aspects of the student and their learning, and the features of the interface between the school and the student.

An important aspect of the ecological approach is the relationship between assessment, planning and intervention. In many cases, the practitioners who assess are not the practitioners who implement educational management of the child, with implications for the information obtained in the assessment process informing teaching and support (Cloud, 1994).

Spolsky's model offers a theoretical frame and rationale to specifically address the individual and environmental needs of bilingual children with SLI. Using Spolsky's model, we can reinterpret the general guidelines for an ecological approach to SLI for the purposes of bilingual assessment. We can ask: what are the purposes of data collection for understanding bilingual children's language knowledge, ability, motivation and opportunities for learning both languages? While Spolsky's model fits well with a Vygotskian approach, it does not focus on mediation and learning.

The RIOT procedure

The RIOT procedure is a set of generic guidelines for practice that take an ecological approach to assessing SLCN in learners. It orientates practitioners towards methods of collecting information, which provide a historical, social and cultural story about the family and child with language concerns. The main actions of the RIOT procedure are Review, Interview, Observe, Test.

> Review all pertinent documents and background information
> Interview teachers, peers, friends, family members and other informants
> Observe student in multiple contexts with a variety of people engaging in both (all) student's languages
> Test both school and home languages

The guidance can be amended and extended to orientate practitioners to identify the language difficulties and needs of bilingual children (Isaac, 2002). From a critical perspective, there are important implications for the RIOT procedure. It is a procedure that is broadly applicable to all children whose language development is causing concern and here it is modified for bilingual and culturally and linguistically diverse children.

(1)   Minority bilingual children and their families live as a microsystem within the larger social system. Critically evaluating the interaction of these systems offers valuable insights on the language practices and expectations of the family for the emerging bilingual child.

(2)   Access to minority communities may need to be negotiated by practitioners from the majority communities, who may also need to work with trained bilingual personnel.

(3)   Judicious use of formal language testing is seen as an important although small part of ecological approaches to assess the intrinsic needs of the child. Testing may not always be appropriate for bilingual children.

(4)   Assessment concerns not only language learning as product, such as language knowledge and abilities of the child, but also the motivation and opportunities afforded by contexts. Continual assessment tracks children's developing language to distinguish between difficulties and needs that are intrinsic to the child or a function of the environment.

Multiple realities of language socialisation

Studies of bilingual language development indicate that bilingual children are socialised by person/domain/place of language use (Fantini, 1985). A complex interplay of languages may be performed by bilingual families in codeswitching, as well as complementary language use by person and specific context (domain), such as a geographical place or a subject of conversation (e.g. shopping, hobby, place of worship).

There are multiple communicative realities for researchers and practitioners to investigate around bilingual children's language development. A record of reported parental/caregiver perceptions of bilingual language socialisation practices offers perspectives of a family's 'map' of language choice. Further perspectives are afforded by practitioner observation, bearing in mind the affect of the presence of the professional, who may be a stranger and not share the family's languages and cultural practices. For sequential bilinguals, enquiry needs to explore the amount and kind of exposure and engagement with the L2 that the child has. Drawing a map of language use entails information about who speaks what language, to whom, when and where, and how frequently and about what, and usually takes place over time. While practicable for researchers, practitioners may have logistical and financial constraints.

More subtle socialisation practices around children with language needs can be recorded and analysed by detailed observation of speech events developed in sociolinguistic research (SPEAKING in Hymes,

1972; Gee, 2005). Hymes' approach takes account of a range of details which interpret meaning-making in an exchange: the setting, participants, purpose, sequence/organisation of the exchange, the manner, linguistic code(s), social and cultural rules, and the type of event. Comparison of a series of speech events with children with needs yields detailed language socialisation evidence to support assessment. Other sources for observations include schedules, diary data and questionnaires for language socialisation (Mattes & Omark, 1984; Westby, 1990; Langdon, 1992; Baker, 2001).

Appraising risks and resilience

Risk and resilience factors for language disability arise from historical, social and cultural experiences as well as bio/medical and psychological reasons. Common risk factors in families with children with language difficulties include a family history of speech, language or literacy difficulties, poverty or low socioeconomic circumstances, low level of maternal education and negative attitudes towards disability. African American children and mothers with low education levels are at risk of being unfairly identified in formal assessment procedures as presenting with potential language 'disorder' (Restrepo *et al.*, 2006). Minority and migrant families may present additional risk factors, such as traumatic migration histories, few local supportive networks and limited majority language and literacy skills. An important risk factor is ineffective communication between practitioners and parents, which may not be due to language differences. Assessing family circumstances on Maslow's hierarchy helps practitioners to understand a family's priorities, such as housing is likely to be perceived as more urgent than EAL classes. Resilience factors that enable families to cope with adversity are evidenced in a family's and children's positive approach to these issues, such as a sense of wellbeing, coping strategies, resourcefulness and (re)sources of community networks and support. Part of the assessment process entails identifying resources to ensure assessment in the child's languages and that each party understands the nature of the child's communication difficulties and needs, and their role, responsibilities and rights concerning the child (Shah *et al.*, 2004; Lozano-Rodriguez & Castellano, 1999).

Practitioner knowledge

Practitioners assessing culturally and linguistically diverse learners may identify their own impoverished resources in terms of their multicultural knowledge. In multilingual and multicultural classrooms which seem like a 'mini-United Nations', teachers, therapists and other professionals may not have sufficient current knowledge about the variety of languages of their students to allow them to engage with the family, for example, in case history taking. This situation can be approached by using electronic tools such as search machines on the web. The case study described KP as Taiwanese. A few minutes on *GoogleScholar*, with the search term, 'Taiwanese languages' yielded the following peer reviewed information.

> (i) From 1945 until 1987, the KMT (Nationalist) government enforced its strict Mandarin Language Policy in schools throughout Taiwan, and students were forbidden to speak local languages or dialects. Recent reversal of this policy allows schools to teach these formerly forbidden varieties. Despite some attention from scholars, it remains to explore the impact of these policies on successive generations of bilingual speakers. This study explores the perceptions of parents, grandparents, and young adults. The data show that school-based policies have an impact on family-based speaking practices. They also demonstrate the complex interplay between public and private histories in the development of linguistic ideologies and language as capital. (Sandel, 2003)

> (ii) Taiwan's political climate, which has been the single most important influence in the development of the island's local languages, has changed dramatically since the mid-1980s. One of most important consequences of Taiwan's democratisation is the Tai-yü language movement, which aims to revive this major local language and which symbolizes the recent, rapid growth of local identity awareness. The promoters of the movement reject the official definition of Tai-yü as a "dialect". For them, bilingual education and the establishment of a Tai-yü pronunciation and writing system are crucial to the rebirth of the language. The movement has posed a threat to the status of Mandarin as the national language and the symbol of Chinese identity and political dominance of the ruling Nationalist Party. This paper analyses the official language policy, which had exalted Mandarin and suppressed other local languages, and the efforts to revive Tai-yü. The paper points out that the Tai-yü language movement shares with the official policy a language ideology which is based on the nation-state idea. The dynamics of the Tai-yü language movement reveals a pressing problem facing

Taiwan: how to balance national cohesion with multilingualism and multiculturalism? (A-chin Hsiau, 1997)

The information given in these two abstracts from academic papers informs practice in several ways. It could inform and sensitise professionals with background information for interviews with parents and students about language use in the home and across the family as well as recruit, if necessary, a language/culture-appropriate interpreter or co-worker. It could inform approaches to home language assessment. Printed information relating to language and culture could be kept with the student's records for purposes of multidisciplinary professional collaboration, and to inform further assessment and educational management. In addition, the information could inform local policies of school and support services for educational management, in its widest sense, of students 'described as Taiwanese'.

Approaches to assessing social knowledge

The social competence of KP is a feature of his communicative (in)competence in the case study at the beginning of the chapter. Children's social competence in managing social entry into friendships and managing disagreement and conflict plays an important part in social acceptance by peers and teachers. Children's social knowledge is played out in their behaviour. Similar paradigms are reflected in assessment practices for social knowledge as for language. Traditional approaches to assessing social competence compare children usually through task-specific nomination rating scales and experimental approaches. Studies with children with language and/or learning difficulties reveal three findings, which reflect the biases discussed earlier for CLD. Children have trouble performing tasks designed to measure social competence; teachers rate them as less socially competent than their peers; and peers rate them and low achieving peers as less popular than their schoolmates (for a review see Saenz *et al.*, 1999; 112–113). Monolingual children with difficulties with social competence may be identified as having pragmatic language impairment or difficulties on the autistic spectrum.

Alternative approaches to evaluating social competence include comparative cross-cultural study looking at specific social interactions and how commonly occurring behaviours are interpreted by different groups. For example, in a study by Chen *et al.* (1992) low income African American and European American children were found to value verbal assertiveness and witty verbal play in others. Canadian and Chinese children were found to differ in their interpretations of shyness and sensitivity in others. These traits were negatively correlated in Canadian children, but positively correlated in Chinese children. The implications of these findings for the case study concern interpreting the child's different behaviour across nursery and home. Might KP be transferring assertive social behaviour favoured in the nursery to home where it might be less accepted? Or are there other explanations?

Ethnographic studies that look at specific social interactions between children with and without speech and language disabilities reveal the complexity of social interaction as it is enacted during a specific activity. Language difficulties may or may not impact on a child's success in entering play. Successful entry into play depends on whether the child uses nonverbal behaviour compatible with the ongoing play activity (Craig & Washington, 1993). A later study (Saenz *et al.*, 1999) of two preschool Latino boys with SLI, studied their social knowledge and competence managing their 'ownership in play' of toys. One boy without verbal language managed to obtain objects that were in the other child's possession irrespective of the other's verbal protests. The microstudy showed that while both children behaved with limited social competence, the teachers demonstrated different notions of appropriate social competence in the boys' play, and that overall they favoured competence which showed peer cooperation rather than territorial play. Saenz *et al.* (1999) conclude that social (in)competence and 'social problems' should not be evaluated as intrinsic (dis)abilities of the individual. Rather, social competence is a complex of social constructions that are based on the interpretations of those making the evaluations of competency as much as those who are being evaluated. The implications for KP are that professionals need to notice not only how KP constructs his social (in)competence in specific activities at home and school, but also how others evaluate it. There are implications for practitioners and parents sharing their views in order to assess KP's social cognitions, as well as for intervention approaches.

Dynamic assessment

Dynamic assessment engages Vygotsky's notion of mediation, as the child builds relationships between her/his private internal world and the external social, cultural world. It focuses on the moment when children interact with unfamiliar material in social and cultural settings and they become 'person-plus' (Perkins, 1993). Their zone of proximal development (ZPD) is expanded and their cognition distributed. In any such instant, the 'person acting with mediational means' is the irreducible unit of analysis and of intelligence (Wertsch, 2000; Claxton, 2002: 25). As a result of a succession of such instants, both person and culture are changed. Dynamic assessment explores the process of language learning through these moments of co-construction of mutual understanding and learning; '. . . it includes deliberate and planned mediational teaching and the assessment of the effects of that teaching on subsequent performance' (Hayward & Tzuriel, 2002: 40).

With dynamic assessment, the practitioner can determine not only the child's current level of functioning, but also the best means to facilitate further learning. The primary focus of dynamic assessment is the engagement between adult (practitioner, parent) and child with language needs and how they both engage in negotiation of meaning and learning. It focuses on how the adult scaffolds the child's language learning, through temporary, graduated assistance. In dynamic assessment, assessment and teaching/learning co-occur. For children with language-learning needs, language becomes not only the object of learning (e.g. new vocabulary, morphology), but also the tool for teaching/learning the child's language or conceptual learning needs.

Dynamic assessment is yet to become a routine part of evaluations of language of children who have speech and language needs. Its process is similar to analytic teaching, diagnostic teaching and microteaching, because of its focus on examining the moments of children's learning and nonlearning and the negotiation of teaching. Peña and Gillam (2000) note that there is increasing use of dynamic assessment for differentiating language difference from language difficulties and needs, and for informing practice. They have contributed to developing dynamic assessment procedures for these purposes.

In the literature, there seem to be three main approaches to using dynamic assessment with bilingual and culturally and linguistically diverse children: test-teach-test, task/stimulus variability, graduated prompting (Laing & Kamhi, 2003). Some of these approaches are less successful at engaging with mediation than others.

Test-teach-(re)test

A familiar approach to dynamic assessment is test-mediate-(re)test;

> the modifiability of a child by examining changes between baseline testing and re-testing and by careful observing learning behaviours exhibited during mediation (teaching) sessions. (Peña & Gillam, 2000: 543–544)

This conceptual slant privileges measurement of progress and outcome of mediated intervention. It focuses on the *'stimulability'* of the learner, that is, how the learner responds to the number and type of exchanges with the practitioner in order to complete the task. One interpretation could be that this test-teach-(re)test approach seems very like teaching for the test. Several sources report that children's scores go up after mediated learning experiences (MLE) (Lidz & Peña, 1996; Ukrainetz *et al.*, 2000).

Three important findings emerge from MLE research for diverse learners. First, this way of using dynamic assessment differentiates strong from weak language learners among culturally and linguistically diverse children. The MLE process claims to distinguish language-learning potential between individual bilingual and culturally and linguistically diverse children who start with similar scores on a standardised assessment of vocabulary (Lidz & Peña, 1996; Peña & Gillam, 2000; Gutierrez-Clellan & Peña, 2001). Furthermore, identifying prompts, cues and negotiation strategies that the teacher uses and the child responds to in the MLE informs subsequent planning and intervention. Thus, dynamic assessment bridges assessment and intervention.

However, the notion of post-testing is arguably unnecessary. Determining that a child has learnt the object of learning in a MLE is demonstrated by the child doing unaided what she/he could not previously do, either in the mediated session or in a subsequent session, or in observation in wider contexts. Test performance is not necessarily a more robust context. It also emphasises the product of learning rather than the process.

Task/stimulus variability

Another form of dynamic assessment modifies and adapts standardised tests to overcome content and linguistic biases and to meet the child's CLD. So, tests seem to become scaffolds for the practitioner to support the student's learning. Adapting tests for use in contextualised learning, such as thematic activities, results in more differentiated performance among the culturally and linguistically diverse children (Fagundes *et al.*, 1998). Researchers and practitioners conclude that children whose performance does not improve after this scaffolding and contextualising are most at risk for linguistic and/or academic learning difficulties.

Graduated prompting

Practitioners use graduated prompting techniques to determine children's stimulability and responsiveness to teaching/learning language. From a range of verbal cues embedded in general statements, they identify which are least supportive models to direct language learning and which are most supportive. Standardised tests are also modified and adapted in this approach. Intervention overlaps with assessment across all levels of language, phonology, vocabulary, morphology and reading. Scoring children's responsiveness appears to be a shortcoming of this approach because it transforms a dynamic learning process into a static number. An important critique of aberrations of dynamic assessment comes from Valdes and Figueroa (1994). They note that when dynamic assessment becomes prescriptive and controlled by the examiner, it becomes more like normative testing through specific tasks and less like co-constructed learning, negotiating for meaning, through graduated assistance working within a child's ZPD.

Dynamic assessment offers a theoretically informed, sensitive and flexible approach that contributes to distinguishing between CLD students of different language-learning potential. It can also inform planning and intervention. Yet, there are important shortcomings in the ways that it is developed in the literature, such as ensuring reliability of assessment across different testers, issues of validity and developing a reliable metric for measuring graduated learning. Practitioner knowledge is problematic. Professionals need to have the knowledge and trained skills to engage effectively in dynamic assessment for language learning, yet it is not usually included in professional training programmes or recommended as the preferred choice of assessment practice (Hayward & Tzuriel, 2002: 59). Similarly, bilingual co-workers require training to do dynamic assessment in languages that the practitioner does not speak.

Conclusion

The case study that opened the chapter highlighted major concerns for researchers and practitioners assessing bilingual learners. Approaches to assessment are needed that distinguish between SLCN and slow development of additional languages. It is crucial to go beyond assessing language already learnt and to examine how new language for learning is learnt in interaction. Assessment of language must include wider notions of social cognitions. The case study prompts self-reflection by practitioners on their assumptions about language and cultural practices.

This chapter has discussed disadvantages of using standardised tests with monolingual norms with bilingual or SLA children. While we can draw on developmental cross-linguistic language information to inform professional judgment, we do not yet have unique markers that distinguish between learners who have typical bilingual and EAL development and SLCN development. The promise of a language information processing approach was explored and found wanting.

From a sociocultural perspective, two further approaches were examined, which foreground assessing language-learning potential as well as social, cultural and linguistic influences shaping children's language learning. Dynamic assessment investigates the process of language learning in interaction and seems to be able to throw some light on differentiating between bilingual SLCN and EAL groups of learners. An ethnographic approach, using methods, such as case history, interviewing parents and family members and observation, holds an important place in distinguishing between EAL progress and SLCN. However, the efficacy of all these approaches hinges on sufficient professional knowledge to reduce practitioner bias and inform practice with bilingual/EAL learners. Working with multidisciplinary colleagues, particularly with bilingual practitioners, can ensure preferred practices in assessment based on adopting a cyclical, consultative and multi-practitioner process. Interprofessional working and learning is explored in Chapter 9.

This chapter takes the notion of mediation, that is, how people build relationships between their internal knowledge and the process of appropriating new external knowledge, as a central plank for under-standing difficulties in language learning. Assessment of language development needs to examine sites of mediation to appraise how bilingual children draw on their knowledge of language and cultures to accomplish new language learning. The concept of mediation as central to language learning is taken up in Chapter 8 on intervention.

Chapter 8
Learning, Teaching and Intervention

Case Study

> J is Spanish-speaking girl, about 11 years of age. She has recently been reunited, from being in a Spanish-speaking country, with her mother in the USA. She has a record of interrupted school attendance due to childhood illnesses. She has started to attend school in the USA with a mainstream teacher and a bilingual special educator. Notes from the language support teacher read:
>
> "J is making progress and completing more work in class and at home. I make sure that directions are understood, translating them [from English] into Spanish when needed, circling the key words, giving physical cues, and writing the homework directions in Spanish. In math we use cooperative learning. I frequently modeled for them how to interact with each other during discussions and how to take turns. During math I helped J work on vocabulary definitions. Her homework assignment for that day involved understanding the word 'congruent'. I explained the word and concept to her in Spanish and she understood and was able to complete her homework assignment". (From Highbeam Research, Salend *et al.* (1997), *Remedial and Special Education*)

Introduction

In this chapter, the focus is maintained on mediation as a central feature in a Vygotskian orientation on teaching, learning and intervention in language disability in cultural and linguistic diversity (CLD) contexts.

Mediation is central to learning as it is the process by which external social, cultural and linguistic knowledge is assimilated cognitively by individuals in order to (re)organise increasingly complex relationships with the external, through culturally constructed tools. An important feature of this chapter is the emphasis on the important Other who usually guides the process, working in the zone of proximal development and negotiating with shared tools. Language is the most important cultural tool in mediating the relationship between internalisation and externalisation (see Chapter 1).

The absence of studies of intervention with bilingual/English as an additional language (EAL) children with language disability in three major UK publications of evidence-based practice (Enderby & Emerson, 1995; Law *et al.*, 1998; Reilly, 2004) suggests that the area is under-researched. Yet, there is an emerging body of qualitative research in the field of intervention in bilingual language disability, particularly case studies detailing the efficacy of intervention in response to specific individual needs, such as speech/phonological intervention (Zhu & Dodd, 2006a). Therapeutic intervention and pedagogy requires the interaction of theory and practice. Theory can inform practice by informing the relevant dimensions of speech, language and literacy intervention. Practice can inform theory by providing a critical test of the implications of a theory or approach (Dockrell & McShane, 1993: 206). The trajectory of researching complex phenomena usually has foundations in descriptive model building to enable later more complex, comparative research designs.

The case study presents an inclusive classroom scenario to illustrate several points that are addressed in the chapter. The language support teacher, while offering one-to-one learning support with the learner, includes other learners in cooperative learning. She is responsive to the learner's needs for language and for curriculum learning. She draws on the student's first language, Spanish, to support learning both EAL and mathematics. Yet, the case study does not tell us about the involvement of the curriculum class teacher or whether J has further language learning needs, such as language disabilities. The main issues for this chapter are the role of both the learner's main (first) language and the language of instruction for academic learning where language learning is both the focus of learning and a tool for academic learning, and the pedagogy of intervention to meet the learner's needs – linguistically, academically and socially.

This chapter on language learning and intervention draws on Halliday's (1975, 1979) theories of language and learning, and Cummins' (1984) hypotheses on the relationship between languages in learning for bilinguals. The first section examines key concepts about teaching and learning, including therapeutic intervention and specialist pedagogy for special needs. The second section focuses on evidence to support developing first/home languages with culturally and linguistically diverse children who have speech and language delay and disability. In the third, fourth and fifth sections, I draw on Halliday's frame of language learning, namely language learning, learning about language and language for learning, to interpret evidence and to explore the implications of this approach for intervention for speech, language and communication needs (SLCN) in bilingual learners. Finally I draw some conclusions.

Inclusion and continuum of need

Implementation of inclusion policies means that, increasingly, learners with language-related disabilities are supported in mainstream classrooms for curriculum learning. Practitioners in mainstream classrooms deal with competing priorities: while they may be well disposed to the diversity of learners across culture, language and ability, they are also held accountable for teaching a national curriculum and achieving a set of standard outcomes. Alexander's (2004: 11) definition that pedagogy

> is what one needs to know, and the skills one needs to command, in order to make and justify the many different kinds of decisions of which teaching is constituted ... [including]
>
> - *children*: their characteristics, development and upbringing
> - *learning*: how it can best be motivated, achieved, identified, assessed and built upon
> - *teaching*: its planning, execution and evaluation, and
> - *curriculum*: the various ways of knowing, understanding, doing, creating, investigating and making sense which it is desirable for children to encounter, and how these are most appropriately translated and structured for teaching.

It is not the differences among children, their characteristics or upbringing that is problematic, but it is when the magnitude of these differences exceeds what schools can accommodate that children are considered to have special educational needs (SEN; Davis & Florian, 2004). With respect to culturally and linguistically diverse learners with language disability, this chapter considers, what Cummins (2000) calls, 'pedagogic disability'.

I argue here that there is a continuum of educational language learning need across culturally and linguistically diverse learners, from those with substantial intrinsic language 'impairment' to others who fail to thrive in classroom learning contexts. This group of learners is at risk of being pedagogically disabled to varying degrees (Cummins, 2000), and pedagogic attention needs to be focused on pedagogic knowledge of language learning needs for learners who are CLD and/or with language disability. It is difficult to distinguish between these groups of learners through testing, even after a year's exposure to the school language (Paradis, 2005); only over time do substantial individual needs become obvious which affect achievement. They constitute a continuum of language learning need. Do learners with SEN require a special education, a special pedagogy? The evidence so far in several reviews suggests a qualified 'no' (e.g. Lewis & Norwich, 2000, 2005). Lewis' and Norwich's analysis indicates that specific strategies, techniques and materials are usually employed to mediate learning with unique common or individual need. Evidence suggests that pedagogic practices based on the same research are taken up by mainstream and special needs, suggesting that sound teaching and learning practices benefit all learners, not only those with additional educational needs. For example, phonological awareness in national literacy programmes, cooperative learning with learners with SEN, and pedagogic strategies for EAL language learning, such as language task analysis and language-focused curriculum work are also effective with SLCN language learners. This chapter builds on this conceptualisation of pedagogy, and draws on evidence from studies and analyses of language learning needs in mainstream classrooms to explore pedagogy for language disability in CLD contexts.

Pedagogic and Therapeutic Practice: Key Concepts

In this section, the relationship between therapy, intervention and pedagogy are explored along a continuum of types of pedagogy (more often known as teaching and learning) in the context of language disability and CLD. The focus is on inclusive pedagogic practice. Most reviews of literature of SEN pedagogy reveal evidence that supports a move away from segregation models and towards inclusive pedagogic practices (e.g. Davis & Florian, 2004). This section examines key concepts: pedagogy, scaffolding and generalisation.

A biomedical approach to therapy and intervention

Therapy is a term from a biomedical frame of reference. It usually signifies an attempted remediation of a health problem, following diagnosis. In the medical field, therapy is synonymous with 'treatment'.

Professional groups with histories of working in biomedical paradigms, such as special educationists and speech/language pathologists/therapists, describe intervention as 'therapy', adminstered in 'packages of care' and 'treatment programmes', including to children in educational contexts (Law *et al.*, 1998). There is a persistent belief in aptitude-treatment interaction (ATI) models of meeting special educational needs, where intervention is understood as 'person-fixing rather than context-changing' (Norwich, 1990; Linton, 1998).

Therapeutic intervention is usually a personalised programme of work that a practitioner, such as a speech and language therapist or specialist teacher, plans and implements to improve a child's speech, language and literacy skills informed by the assessment process. Mediation practices usually involve correcting, reducing or preventing the nontarget behaviour, and while the approach is based on cognitive learning processes, it has different goals from therapy, such as non-curative, rehabilitative therapies. Specialist teaching on the other hand is often constructed as restorative.

Pedagogy

Therapy and intervention can be analysed as models of pedagogy. Transmission models emphasise the transfer of knowledge and transmission of skills. The teacher's/practitioner's role is 'teller'/giver of knowledge and the learner is 'listener and answerer/repeater'. Knowledge is clearly not co-constructed between teacher and learner or learner and learner, as knowledge is already known by the practitioner and the learner must respond culturally and linguistically appropriately (Tharp & Gallimore, 1988; Cummins, 2000). So-called progressive pedagogic approaches are usually based on a Piagetian understanding of development, where learning is a child-centred notion of discovery learning and active exploration. The practitioner is the facilitator of the stimulating and culturally relevant environment. Both these models are visible in traditional therapeutic intervention. Traditional intervention may also recruit behaviourist models and techniques, such as drills, as well as exploratory approaches with facilitative techniques.

Pedagogy, from a sociocultural perspective, entails constructing a responsive relationship between practitioner and learners, involving joint knowledge building that takes account of the cultures and identities of learners. It draws primarily on Vygotsky's and Bruner's ideas of learning as social and then cognitive through the key concept of mediation. There are three central ideas about all teaching and learning: that cognitive processes are understood in terms of their origins and the mechanisms by which they change; that the development of all higher order psychological processes have their origins in interaction with individuals; and that it is through communication using signs and symbols that individuals can eventually come to regulate their own behaviour (Bruner, 1986). As children make meaning and interpret their environments through socialising with others, so they learn, particularly about both curriculum knowledge and language in school settings.

Vygotsky (1978) also postulated a specific relationship between teacher and learner, or the individual, family and society. They co-exist in an interdependent relationship, each shaping and being shaped by the other. These interactions take place in contexts of purposeful activities that are determined by the larger historical, cultural and linguistic framework in which the teaching and learning occur. Teaching and learning is social and interactive (Lantolf, 2000; Mayer *et al.*, 2002). The key tool in these interactions is language. It is through language that children learn to make sense of the world(s) around them, and in particular, language practices such as conversation and dialogue.

Children, including those with disabilities, in school bring knowledge from their culturally and linguistically diverse homes. They have already learnt, to varying degrees, to mediate through communicative practices including language, between sociocultural external contexts and their internal sense making, and to transform their everyday experiences into higher order thinking. An important challenge for practitioners is to draw on children's diverse cultural and linguistic resources to develop language and content of schooling. For culturally and linguistically diverse children and those with language-related disabilities, language is both the tool and the focus for learning to address problematic aspects of communication.

Thus, pedagogy is a social and interactive enterprise where adult and learners co-construct meaning together. The co-constructed meaning and knowledge takes place through language and other signs and symbols in purposeful activities. The interaction is dependent on the ability of the adult to work in a 'contingently responsive manner' with the learner.

Scaffolding language learning

There is an increasing body of evidence that developing knowledge about language and how it works in one language scaffolds the development of additional languages (Cummins, 1984, 2000). The phenomenon of languages scaffolding learning in and of another language is discussed in the Language Interdependency Hypothesis (Cummins, 1984). Working through an established language can be used to scaffold cognitive understanding across both languages in bilingual learners. Cummins explains this by drawing on the notion of Common Underlying Proficiency, that is cognitive resources are accessed and developed by both/all languages (Cummins, 1981). Research in bilingualism (e.g. Cummins, 1977, 1981, 1984, 1994, 2000) supports the necessary relationship between a well-developed home (first) language and the development of a second/additional language of schooling and academic learning. Cummins hypothesises that a degree of language proficiency, a threshold, may need to be achieved in one language for scaffolding development of other languages, and for language to be a tool for conceptual and curriculum learning: the Language Threshold Hypothesis (Cummins, 1977).

Research with young Portuguese students shows that their awareness of morphemes and grammar in their first language is a predictor of how well they perform in learning a second language, English. They received the same teaching from the same teacher for a year, and although they started the year with a better awareness of morphology and grammar in their first language, they learned the second language better than those who had lower levels of awareness. Children can scaffold their awareness of grammar and morphology in the second language they learn, from their awareness in their first language (Castro *et al.*, 2004, cited in Nunes & Bryant, 2006). Comparisons between Italian/English bilingual and monolingual English preschoolers showed that bilingual children had increased metalinguistic awareness of manipulating speech sounds in words (phonological awareness) (Campbell & Sais, 1995).

Bruner's notion of scaffolding (see Chapter 1) in developing generalisation of language learning is referred to in research with bilingual learners for language knowledge, literacy knowledge and academic knowledge. Children and adults who are additional language learners use their knowledge of first language to scaffold language learning with a positive effect on learning in and of other languages. Further evidence of scaffolding language-related knowledge is shown in studies of literacy skills, where similar results across languages were found for achievement in reading (Cobo-Lewis *et al.*, 2002; Genesee *et al.*, 2004; Gutierrez-Clellan, 1999). Reading studies indicate the need to take account of levels of proficiency in the home/first language and its effect on phonological awareness, which is important preknowledge for reading and literacy skills (Lopez & Greenfield, 2004). There is evidence of scaffolding language knowledge for academic learning. Typically developing bilingual children who are instructed in maths through their home language for a year performed in the end of year assessment through L2 English as well as and better than their L2 peers who had been taught through English only (Fitzpatrick, 1987). There is also evidence of increased academic achievement for immigrant children in the USA who become proficient speakers of home and community languages (Feliciano, 2001; Portes & Hao, 2002 in Kohnert, 2005).

Generalisation

Generalisation describes the process when a child learns a new skill and applies it to instances that are similar to the examples used in the original learning. A conceptual frustration in transmission pedagogies, such as therapy approaches, is that although a child may produce appropriate and accurate speech and language in linguistically highly controlled situations, this does not *generalise* to other contexts such as their everyday speech (Grundy, 1989: 264). The underlying concern is how learning becomes conceptual rather than remaining tied to specific instances. An assumption in sociocultural approaches is that learning is situated, and skills are not learnt as autonomous and independent of context. Generalisation is explained in Vygotskian terms when everyday actions across a range of contexts are transformed by higher order thinking into an abstract concept that can be applied across contexts.

Nunes and Bryant (2006: 90) describe generalisation as the learning of *principles* in contrast to learning *specific facts*. They identify two crucial ways to ensure that children learn principles: one is through teaching strategies to develop categorisation (e.g. encourage children to see the similarities between specific instances and to form the principle or concept) and the other is through learning strategies, to promote learners' engagement in different operations of thought in solving problems (e.g. making analogies, focusing on grammatical categories, analysing novel words). These two ways involve a metacognitive approach to learning language.

There is evidence to indicate caution in anticipating scaffolding and generalisation of learning in young bilingual children with language learning delay or difficulties. Children with learning and language learning difficulties need more support than their typically developing peers to learn principles or concepts (Dockrell & McShane, 1993; Grundy, 1989). According to these authors, in addition to metacognitive and metalinguistic strategies, practitioners need to attend to the type of learning task and how they present it to the child, as well as manipulating the context of the learning, e.g. different words and sentences, books and talk partners. Owens (1995, 1999) offers a 10-step plan to develop generalisation of skills for children with speech and language difficulties.

Although there is evidence that older bilingual learners and adults scaffold knowledge between their languages, for young bilingual children cross-linguistic scaffolding may be restricted by their different levels of cognitive and linguistic development and metalinguistic knowledge (van Tuijl *et al.*, 2001; Kohnert *et al.*, 2005). Learners with SLCN have difficulties developing, learning and managing implicit knowledge about language and processing. The knowledge that is required to manipulate language in metacognitive and metalinguistic approaches is unlikely to be available to these learners in the way it is available to their peers. (These approaches are discussed later in the chapter.) Bilingual learners with SLCN need additional support and intervention that explicitly addresses knowledge and skills about language knowledge that their peers develop implicitly, in order to scaffold knowledge from the first/ home language into the second language and vice-versa, as well as 'generalising' the language knowledge learnt in one context to another.

Language of Intervention for Bilinguals with Language Needs

I use this section to examine early interventions of service provision with bilingual children with SLCN for language delay which are largely indirect, that is mediated by people other than professionals. Issues are surfaced concerning potential dilemmas in the interdependence between provider and client because of CLD.

Early years intervention

In early years intervention, providers are aware that the 'client' is both the child with needs and their parents and family. For children who have difficulties and delay developing early speech and language, intervention and support are recommended, evidence-based practice rather than a 'wait and see' approach (Eadie, 2004a). There is a great deal of evidence to support parent–child language intervention and many programmes for this purpose (e.g. Hanen programme: Watson, 1995). Language of intervention with very young children is not controversial when child, family, professional and school share the same language. Yet, the issue can appear problematic when the family language is not shared by service providers or the wider society. The decision to select a language for intervention and academic learning is unique for bilingual families. Genesee *et al.* (2004) examine likely social and educational scenarios for bilingual families and children faced with this choice. They discuss the issues that parents, children and professionals are likely to have to consider in order to agree about language(s) for therapeutic and educational intervention. They argue that the choice of language for support and intervention is determined by several factors: the communicative demands on the child and family, the nature and severity of the child's difficulties and the demands of academic learning in each language for the child both in the short term and in the long term. Parents and child need to be responsible for the choice (see Chapter 2).

Using several languages and mixed codes across languages are bilingual home scenarios for children with language difficulties that seem to have little research-based evidence to support professional guidance. Families that are second or third generation members of transplanted communities may speak a home language which is not a standard variation of the minority language, and/or there may be codeswitching and code change in the home language. These variations need not pose a problem for children developing language or with difficulties learning language. Like regional variations, code change and codeswitching have predictable and learnable patterns as they are sociolinguistic phenomena. Families who speak two or more languages regularly in the home/family provide children with a bilingual first language. Fantini (1985) recorded that his preschool child spoke French, Spanish and Italian to family members. Interestingly, Fantini also reported that his trilingual son was referred to the speech-language pathologist shortly after entering school because he was not speaking English, and was an example of misidentification of SLCN for EAL.

Misleading advice

There is a belief that variations in home language, such as bilingual first language and codeswitching across languages, make children vulnerable to language learning difficulties. This mistaken belief can lead practitioners to advise parents and families to use a monolingual code, which is misguided for several reasons.

There is no evidence to support the belief that using diverse languages at home is a cause of language learning difficulties. In fact, most culturally and linguistically diverse children grow up without language difficulties. Yet, in certain circumstances, advice to give up the home language may make children vulnerable to language difficulties. For example, rather than find this advice easy to follow, culturally and linguistically diverse families find it very difficult to follow, as code-switching is often their communication code. Where families use two or more languages regularly in the home, it is likely to be communicatively impossible for them to follow advice to use one language only. Studies show that suppressing one language in bilinguals is more effortful, in terms of inhibiting processing, than alternating between languages (Hernandez & Kohnert, 1999).

Furthermore, not speaking the language of the home is likely to disrupt cultural learning and the emergent identities of the child, with longer term implications. Electing not to develop the home language would entail rejecting evidence of the reciprocal relationship between social, emotional and cultural factors and language development in first and second languages (Okamura-Bichard, 1985). In addition, being advised to abandon the home language may bring a degree of distress to parents and older family members. Distress in parents that is caused by environmental factors increases stress in children with a negative impact on children's wellbeing (Belsky *et al.*, 1995, 1996).

There are three bodies of evidence that positively support bilingual development in language disability. Apart from the evidence in our everyday lives, there is evidence that children with speech and language difficulties can grow up bilingually (Paradis *et al.*, 2003b). Much earlier, Bruck (1984) in discussing assessment and intervention considerations for linguistic minority children with language disabilities notes that

> in addition to psychological and pedagogical factors, one must also consider the sociolinguistic and cultural background of the child and attempt to place him or her in a situation where the mother tongue will not be replaced by the second language, and where pride in his own culture can be fostered. (Bruck, 1984: 125)

Second, does learning through both languages confuse linguistic minority and culturally and linguistically diverse children who have language difficulties? The evidence would suggest not. Rather than confusing bilingual children with language disabilities, it seems that offering more ways of accessing meaningful communication encourages language learning. In a study with bilingual students who had classroom anxiety and learning difficulties, their needs 'were exacerbated by use of low-redundancy structurally based methods allowing little place for hypothesis testing and other processes thought to underlie unconscious second language learning' (D'Anglejan & Renaud, 1985: 13).

Third, being bilingual supports early literacy skills (Campbell & Sais, 1995). Further, a substantial review of research on preschool inclusion in the USA (Odom *et al.*, 2004) found 'only two recent studies have investigated the influence of cultural and language diversity on inclusive preschool experiences' (Hanson *et al.*, 1997, 1998). They found that Individual Education Plans (IEPs) lacked goals related to language for second language learners, that language differences were sometimes barriers to children's friendships and social relationships, and that there were complex interactions between disabling conditions and language differences (Hanson *et al.*, 1997; Odom *et al.*, 2004: 38). Three themes emerged relating to successful experiences for children: children's belonging and membership within their peer culture, teachers' practices and philosophies supporting diversity in classroom culture, and families' perspectives on the meaning of disability (Hanson *et al.*, 1998).

To summarise this section, where client/learner needs are culturally and linguistically diverse and service/education provision is monolingual, language choice becomes a main issue around intervention. Evidence supports home language intervention for children who show signs of early language delay and difficulty in development. Advice to give up interacting with children in home language is likely to have negative effects on communication development. Home language development is not at the expense of learning the language of schooling, and intervention for language difficulties can support both languages. Language development in all languages underpins reading readiness and literacy development. Maintaining the language spoken between parents, siblings and children with delayed language development is likely to strengthen the sociocultural context for language and dialogic interaction which is fundamental to children's language learning.

Language Learning

I use this section to examine evidence of therapy interventions for difficulties with language form, that is, speech and grammar, as well as language use and learning narrative language. It is a comparatively under-researched area, with little research on bilingual children, although intervention on speech difficulties in bilinguals seems to be more researched than other areas of SLCN/specific language impairment (SLI). I draw on Halliday's ideas of language and learning. One of Halliday's three inter-related language knowledges is *language learning*. This particular knowledge is problematic in children identified with

SLCN or SLI. Learning language knowledge is emphasised in therapeutic and remedial interventions to develop language skills and proficiency.

Like Vygotsky, Halliday perceived an intimate relationship between meaning, language forms and learning. In his work on child language, Halliday (1975, 1979, 1993) identified three inter-related language knowledges in children's development: learning *language*, learning *through language*, learning *about language*. Studies of typically developing monolingual children demonstrate the emergence of these three knowledges (e.g. Painter, 2007). Painter's work reveals how children learn language knowledge of language features and functions from a series of context-embedded interactions to the abstract conceptualisation of the feature 'rule'. At the same time, children use language as a tool to access other knowledge and thinking skills, such as matching and categorisation. Her study also shows that children show metalinguistic awareness by learning 'a language to talk about language'.

Bilingual children and children with SLCN may have difficulty with learning one or all three language knowledges. *Learning language* knowledge is emphasised in therapeutic and remedial interventions, to develop language skills and proficiency. Yet, there is evidence to show that *learning about language*, that is metalinguistic knowledge, facilitates learning the other two language knowledges. Metrics to evaluate research on successful intervention include the extent to which these three inter-related language knowledges are drawn on and the extent to which intervention is dialogic and that there is information given about social interaction.

Speech difficulties

Dodd (1995) claims that the type of speech difficulty determines the type of intervention that is appropriate. Working within the framework that phonological-based knowledge is language-specific and articulatory knowledge is language-general, recommendations about protocols for language choices for intervention is informed by the child's communication needs (see Chapter 4).

The research literature gives clear guidance for management of provision for speech difficulties in bilingual children. The literature indicates that bilingual children develop separate and differentiated phonological systems, although each system may not develop in the same way as in monolinguals (Zhu Hua & Dodd, 2006a: 3–14). Thus, intervention for phonological difficulties in bilingual children needs to be language-specific, and need not follow a monolingual developmental sequence. Studies indicate that familiar therapeutic approaches can be used successfully to intervene with language-specific phonological difficulties in bilingual children, which work on phonological processes, language processing and metalinguistic skills (Holm *et al.*, 1997). Moreover, therapy with bilingual children may precipitate complex intraphonological generalisation as well as interlanguage generalisation. A study of a Welsh/English child showed transfer across phonological systems as well as within each system, and loss of contrastive phonemes as well as gains (Ball *et al.*, 2006).

Usually, intervention for motor speech (articulation) difficulties in one language of a bilingual child scaffolds articulation learning in the other language; that is, improved motor skills are likely to show across languages (Holm *et al.*, 1997). For bilingual children who present with articulation difficulties, a conventional programme of articulation therapy in the language of schooling is likely to improve not only the articulation of speech in that language, but also in the child's other language(s).

Intervention with bilingual children with verbal dyspraxia is an under-researched area. Children with verbal dyspraxia have inconsistent speech patterns due to difficulties in learning control and development of motor patterns in speech sound sequences in (new) words, which in turn may affect the linguistic and processing knowledge of speech. The implications of theoretically informed intervention approaches for bilingual speech difficulties are that choice of language for intervention is not only a matter of client preference and provision resources, but is also informed by the type of speech needs of the child. Furthermore, the language of intervention may only be possible in the language/literacy of schooling.

There are likely to be further implications for intervention/support in schooling. Children with verbal dyspraxia may develop social, emotional and behaviour difficulties as a result of frustration with their communication difficulties. Children with dyspraxia usually require additional support programmes for speech, language and literacy, which need to be included as far as possible in the child's Individual Education Plans and curriculum planning. For bilingual children with verbal dyspraxia, language of intervention may only be possible in one language/literacy of schooling. Educational management of children with dyspraxia requires collaborative work between teachers, speech and language therapists and possibly occupational therapists. An example from multilingual Singapore illustrates that children with motor neurone disorders that affect their speech and/or feeding/swallowing, and most of them have sensory/proprioceptive issues, many of them need an

Alternative and Augmentative Communication (AAC) device to help them communicate effectively in the classroom. They may need adaptations to their AAC device for communicating in English in school and other languages at home.

Examining the literature on intervention for speech difficulties, the focus is on theoretically informed outcomes, and the product of teaching and learning in the intervention. There is little information given in the research reports on the process of pedagogy, of teaching and learning and the responsiveness in interaction. As I note in Chapter 4, descriptions of psycholinguistic processes are often agent-less. Terms describing language learning in bilingual learners, such as 'transfer' and 'normal interference between languages' (e.g. Holm & Dodd, 1999) are underspecified regarding how this new learning has come about. There is a need to examine further the process of teaching and learning in therapeutic intervention research with all children, and particularly with bilingual children.

Auditory perception and classroom noise

Many children have difficulties with auditory perception (Roeser & Downs, 2004), which is exacerbated in noisy classrooms with poor acoustics and makes learning difficult. Studies with bilingual Spanish/ English children show that they have difficulties distinguishing words that are minimally phonologically different, such as pin/pen, boat/vote (Nelson *et al.*, 2005). Snow and Brinton (2001) discuss implications for curriculum learning of auditory perception and discrimination difficulties in EAL learners. They give examples where EAL students may have difficulties distinguishing key vocabulary: in maths teaching, 'thirteen/ thirty', and in history, 'a state dinner'/'a steak dinner', particularly when frequency and familiarity of vocabulary is influential. Children with moderate hearing difficulties and auditory perception difficulties are shown to benefit measurably from learning in classrooms with auditory loop systems (Berg *et al.*, 1996).

Intervention with difficulties in grammar

There are few studies on intervention with grammar with bilingual children. We are thrown back to examining intervention with monolingual children with SLCN and extrapolating from them to bilingual children. Most children, monolingual and bilingual, with language difficulties, although they may have significant difficulties in other aspects, have difficulties with grammar and morphology. Fey and colleagues review the literature on intervention with monolinguals to set out 'ten principles' for facilitating grammar development for three purposes (Fey *et al.*, 2003). Practitioners can offer direct or indirect intervention. Educational planning may be informed by these principles and place a special emphasis directly on the development of grammar to meet the needs of students with SLCN. While Fey and colleagues focus on first language English speakers, they suggest that the principles are sufficiently broad to cut across many linguistic and cultural boundaries. The 10 principles are based on evidence-based practice.

---

(1) The *basic goal* of all grammatical interventions should be to help the child to achieve greater facility in the comprehension and use of grammar and morphology in the service of conversation, narration, exposition and other textual genres in both written and oral modalities

(2) grammatical form should rarely, if ever, be the *only* aspect of language and communication that is targeted in a language intervention programme

(3) there should be intermediate goals

(4) there should be specific goals

(5) manipulate context to create opportunities for grammar targets (forced contrasts)

(6) exploit different textual genres for contexts for intervention targets (obligatory context contrasts)

(7) manipulate discourse to make targeted features more salient (emphasis, forced contrasts)

(8) systematically contrast child forms with adult forms (immediate and frequent corrective recasts); can be used by parents and support workers who are trained

(9) avoid telegraphic speech, present grammatical models in well-formed phrases and sentences (modelling and expansion)

(10) more controversially, use contrastive elicited imitation to make target forms more salient, and to give child practice with phonological patterns that are more difficult to access or produce; to be consistent with recasts (principle 7).

Fey *et al.* (2003)

These principles suggest that they may be used for both L1 and L2 intervention in bilingual children. The first four principles are relatively uncontroversial, although for L1 intervention they depend on sufficient assessment information of the home language for planning intervention. The subsequent principles depend on necessary detailed grammar and phonological knowledge of other languages, in order to work with bilingual children and/or trained home language speakers. Studies show that parents can be as effective as trained staff (Law *et al.*, 1998). Intervening to develop emerging, delayed and atypical language development can be effective when certain well-researched interaction techniques are used; for example, recasting and modelling children's utterances to include the mature form (e.g. Saxton, 1997, 2005). *Recasts* maintain the meaning of children's utterances while modifying their structure. *Modelling* mature utterances for children with language learning difficulties, as noted in the opening case study, offers cues for grammatical relationships that the child may not yet use although may understand (Maratsos, 1982), and *expansions* develop semantic as well as grammatical knowledge. Thus, a further principle might be that intervention should develop knowledge of grammar in the home language to scaffold knowledge of learning grammatical knowledge in L2.

In 'real life', parents in child interactions recast articles and copulas 0.25 times per minute on average in comparison with clinicians who recast 0.8 times per minute. Tallal (2000: 180) notes that to have a significant impact on children with SLI, it appears not to be enough just to recast the children's utterances at rates found in their environment. Instead, successful intervention efforts involving recasts have increased the rates by approximately two to four times those observed in naturalistic contexts. The study concluded that elicited imitation and modelling approaches were insufficient and limited to teaching contexts and underestimated the complexity of what the children had to learn (Tallal, 2000: 187). When intervention with clinicians ends, learning does not generalise to typical communicative contexts.

Salience and meaning making are emphasised when focusing on form with bilingual children with SLCN, and contexts, discourse and textual genres need to be manipulated to achieve this. Fey and colleagues (2003) argue that it should be feasible to incorporate these techniques in classroom dialogue where the teacher and support staff maintain the emphasis on form to intervene with the child. Planning inclusive intervention in classroom contexts, where it may only be possible to intervene in the additional language, is discussed later.

A recent study demonstrates effective intervention on grammar with monolingual English students with persistent complex difficulties with grammar who are 11–13 years in specialist educational provision (Ebbels, 2007; Ebbels & van der Lely, 2001). The intervention programme in one-to-one therapy draws on a specially devised visual aid for coding sentential thematic role and argument structure, using shapes, arrows and colour. In addition, an effective group intervention on past tense morphology is reported with a class of nine children. The results are statistically significant although the numbers are small, and it is noted that there are students whose needs in learning grammatical forms are not met by the intervention. The efficacy of the intervention approach is contrasted with a less successful approach using computer-mediated therapy (Bishop *et al.*, 2006).

An explanation from a Vygotskian and Hallidayan perspective suggests that the intervention allows therapist and student to engage in dialogic interaction around the material tool and language, within the student's zone of proximal language development. A computer-mediated approach may not afford these dialogic opportunities. Furthermore, from a Vygotskian perspective, approaches to intervention such as Ebbels', use the notion of 'double stimulation' (Vygotsky, 1978), that is the learner is presented with both the problem and the means (tools) to resolve the problem. Ebbels presents the learners with an aspect of grammar that is problematic for them and becomes the focus for learning. She also presents them with visual aids that can resolve the problem by mapping the grammatical relationship and word sequence. This approach has implications for researching intervention in different languages with minority language and bilingual children.

To sum up, these studies have illustrated one of Halliday's language knowledges, language learning. They focus on teaching aspects of language for structural skills and proficiency. An important criticism of these studies of intervention with children with SLCN is that intervention is not explicitly embedded in a theory of learning. They focus on the product of learning rather than on giving an account of co-constructing language knowledge and responsive interaction. Studies that focus on 'generalisation' of newly acquired language skills may be better orientated by sociocultural theories of learning.

Learning about Language

The language knowledge of learning about language is evident when learners develop metalinguistic knowledge through cognitive resources to suspend using language for communication in order to learn about language. There are only a few approaches that take a metalinguistic perspective to intervene for language learning for children with SLCN. The approach directly and explicitly presents the aspect of language difficulty as a focus for learning, which requires learners to reflect and talk about the language feature in specific terms. There are metalinguistic approaches for speech intervention such as Metaphon (Howell & Dean, 1991), which is a commercial programme for speech difficulties. These approaches seek to promote learning strategies that can be drawn on by the learner beyond the context of the intervention.

Metalinguistic approaches seek to make language learning visible in the classroom. They encourage learners to develop *learning strategies*. Learning strategies are employed by learners and shaped by learners' psychological and social resources to scaffold their own learning, such as strategies for repetition due to short-term memory or processing needs, motivation to learn. Practitioners can encourage learning strategies (Palinscar & Brown, 1984) that usually depend on developing materials and social rules to encourage talk to develop language for learning language (McGuinness, 1999). For example, phonological awareness develops metalinguistic knowledge.

A growing body of research supports the explicit teaching of phonological awareness in young children to prepare them for successful learning of literacy skills (e.g. Nunes *et al.*, 2003). The metalinguistic knowledge of literacy skills, mainly reading and spelling, is often built into literacy curricula, as in the UK and USA. Part of a 10-year study on improving literacy skills, focusing on a metacognitive approach to teaching morphological knowledge to primary school children, showed that literacy skills improved significantly in children with this teaching approach over children who experienced typical noninterventionist teaching (Nunes & Bryant, 2006). Not only children who had a good awareness of morphology improved significantly, but also 'low achieving' children who did not have good awareness of morphology and grammar. Nevertheless, even after the direct teaching intervention there was still a substantial gap between the higher and lower achieving groups. The research did not identify EAL learners specifically, although it is noted that one teacher of EAL children reported that the students benefited from explicit teaching of morphology and grammar (Nunes & Bryant, 2006: 151). A similar recommendation came from an earlier study of children with SLCN who had word-finding difficulties. The study found that they had difficulties accessing words whose form had changed due to irregular morphology in past tense and plurals (swim/swam, tooth/teeth). The authors suggest that intervention should be targeted at supporting lexical comprehension and the development of strategic responses possibly through explicit teaching about morphology (Murphy *et al.*, 2003: 23).

A study with adolescent bilingual learners by Goldfus (2001) drew on a metacognitive and metalinguistic approach to learning strategies. Her study investigated how teenage bilingual learners with language-related learning needs engaged with direct explicit teaching about the language in textbooks, and the discourse of expository texts. The study was classroom-based, where the teacher followed a structured programme drawing on a metalinguistic approach. The students were taught how to make conceptual, inferential and implicit links in simple, and then increasingly demanding, discourse texts in English, their second language, which was the language of schooling. After two months, the students showed substantial progress in personal reports and on testing, although improvement did not reach statistical significance. There was evidence of sustained improvement after a year.

Intervention for difficulties in language use

Although children with difficulties in the domain of language use (pragmatics) are increasing demographically, there is little systematic evidence that demonstrates either the benefits or efficacy of speech and language intervention with these children, or measurability of changes in pragmatic behaviour resulting from the intervention (Adams *et al.*, 2006). There are some studies on L1 English-speaking students which show that specific intervention focused on social cognition and skills has positive outcomes (e.g. Rinaldi, 2000; Adams *et al.*, 2005). However, these studies, while located in school, are outside academic classroom learning. They do not offer specific evaluation of the impact of intervention on language demands and use in instructional and regulatory classroom contexts. These contexts are particularly important for bilingual learners (Wong-Fillmore, 1982: 3), namely for academic curriculum learning, social cognition in classroom behaviour or long-term effects (e.g. one year) of intervention. Researchers identify methodological challenges embedded in this research field, such as measurability of change in language and social knowledges in communication. Investigating bilingual children with these difficulties remains substantially under-researched.

Intervention with narratives for bilingual children with SLCN

Interventions using narrative and story telling are often linked with preparing children for learning literacy skills, and studies tend to focus on preschool children. Narrative intervention is usually measured by development of identified 'story elements', that constitute the sequential development of 'story' through story grammar, and the nature of characters. Intervention usually supports recall and generation of stories. Older learners develop subjective concepts of perceptual action, psychological action and private states, as well as personal narration skills indicated by the development of propositions across explicitness, implicature and inference (Mainess *et al.*, 2002). Furthermore, narrative and story telling is culturally and contextually specific (Gutierrez-Clellen & Quinn, 1993). Claims are made of the close association between narrative language and academic skills (Hughes *et al.*, 1997). However, narrative is different from language used in curriculum learning, which is largely expository and explanatory. The relationship between learning narrative and learning expository language is not clear in terms of the generalisation of language knowledge between them and the efficacy of similar intervention strategies.

Little is known of the narrative skills of bilingual children who are in the process of becoming bilingual. Sequential bilinguals may show differences in the language of narration, but may not always show differentiated skills across language, in aspects of grammar complexity (Gutierrez-Clellen, 2002; Westby *et al.*, 2002; Silliman *et al.*, 2002). Narrative interventions with typically developing primary age bilinguals to enhance communicative competence show that first language narrative skills develop more than second language skills (Schoenbrodt *et al.*, 2003). Narrative is a popular intervention tool, but is under-researched and there are implications for researching its use with bilingual learners with language disability.

This section has dealt with research on learning about language, that is, interventions sought to develop language knowledge by developing metalinguistic knowledge. Evidence suggests that this approach helps many children improve *language learning* knowledge, although possibly to a lesser extent those with substantial difficulties in language knowledge and processing. More important, there is very little research evidence for bilingual children with SLCN. The next section examines the literature on intervention approaches to culturally and linguistically diverse children with SLCN who are in school learning contexts, with language demands on social learning and academic curriculum learning.

Learning Through Language

This section deals with the third of Halliday's language knowledges, *learning through language*, as it applies to culturally and linguistically diverse students with speech- and language-related difficulties in school. The issues here mainly concern pedagogy of inclusion of learners with language-related educational needs in mainstream classrooms. Specifically, how do bilingual learners with SLCN learn new language and conceptual material when the main tool for curriculum learning, language, is developmentally emergent and/or problematic? I review the evidence through three theoretical orientations: Cummins' work on language and learning in bilingual children; Bernstein's theory of language for learning; and sociocultural approaches to dialogue and joint meaning making. I draw on evidence of pedagogic practice in classrooms with L1 English, pedagogic intervention in classroom learning with bilingual learners and, to a lesser extent because there is less evidence, with bilingual children with SLCN. I also look at the evidence for peer mediation and pedagogy of affect for learners with language and behaviour needs.

A theoretical framework developed by Cummins (1984), based on educational research with EAL learners, constructs a relationship between language proficiency and academic language for learning. He identified an important fault line in developing second language distinguishing language for social and for academic purposes. In academic teaching and learning, language proficiency is used for conceptual development and higher-order thinking (e.g. inferring, predicting, hypothesising, analysing, evaluating) (cognitive academic language performance; CALP). Research studies show that bilingual children and young adolescents learn conversational skills in the newly acquired language relatively quickly, typically within two years (basic interpersonal communication skills; BICS). However, it takes between five and seven years, or longer, for bilingual learners to use the second/ additional language for learning language for academic purposes in a similar way as monolingual peers (e.g. Thomas & Collier, 1997). In later work, Cummins (e.g. 2000) argues that failure in academic achievement can be attributed less to individual bilingual learner 'deficit' in language skills, and more to inappropriate pedagogies and teaching strategies for language for academic learning.

Cummins' early ideas about the distinction between language for social and academic purposes have been contested, for example, by pointing out that conversational skills are necessary for both social and academic learning (Martin-Jones & Romaine, 1986). A shift of emphasis was able to take more account of the complexity of language and learning, leading to more sociolinguistic and socialisation perspectives of language for learning. The notion that language is a tool for thinking remains central.

Approaching learning *through language* from a socialisation perspective is important in inclusive classrooms and inclusive pedagogy. Bernstein's work (e.g. 1999), influenced by Vygotsky's ideas, identifies the importance of language as a tool for higher order thinking. He is concerned with how children learn to move from the 'common-sense' talk of understanding their everyday lives (horizontal discourse) to the scientific concepts of curriculum subject domains (vertical discourse), and how this occurs in the socialisation of classroom learning. Learning the language of a curriculum subject allows the learner to join in the learning activity and practice of that subject (Lemke, 1988; Daniels & Anghileri, 1995: 101). When learners access the language of the domain, they make meaning and knowledge in that domain and use the symbolic language of the domain to reason with. That is, children learn the social languages of maths or geography as they talk and read about the subject discourses, so that they can talk and write like 'mini mathematicians' or 'mini geographers'. This analysis of the social use of academic language has implications for pedagogies with children learning the language of instruction and children with language disabilities.

Curriculum subject domains have different discourses that bring different and unique language learning demands. Christie and Martin (2007) draw on Halliday's and Bernstein's work to examine these demands. Studies working in this paradigm explore a variety of aspects. For example, the learning demand of geometry in maths not only concerns learning specialist vocabulary (e.g. *angle, rhomboid, acute* and *obtuse angles*) and polysemy across disciplines (e.g. *degrees*: angles versus temperature), but also the semantic taxonomy of concepts by developing webs and frameworks of meaning through synonomy, antonomy and subordination. Understanding and using metaphor is another challenge. The grammatical metaphor in the nominalisation of verbs (explode-explosion, he departed–his departure) leads to further abstraction from the specific context (Unsworth, 2000: 246; Painter, 2007). Semantic metaphors such as 'heart as a pump' may be inaccessible when the understanding of a pump no longer matches the action of the heart (Cameron, 2003). Literal interpretations of idioms, such as 'skating on thin ice', obscure the socialisation meaning.

One of the drivers for moving from horizontal to vertical discourses is that horizontal discourse, which is context bound and specific, has limitations for accessing new knowledge. Moving to vertical discourses that are self-contextualised, enables talking about the topic within its own discourse and without reference to a tangible contextualised specific (Painter, 2007). Pupils can talk about geometry using the language of geometry, rather than an everyday language of shapes.

There are implications for teaching specialist/technical domain language to students with different languages and cognitive and language ability. Lack of pedagogic differentiation across language and concepts makes learning inaccessible for students with delay or difficulties learning the language of schooling. Similarly, simplifying curriculum language for learners with language needs, limits them moving from common sense discourse to more scientific discourse. There seems to be little research evidence of the development, implementation and impact of differentiation to meet the language-related learning needs of monolingual or bilingual children with SLCN, from this perspective.

Here are two examples of a language-focused approach to curriculum pedagogy with EAL learners. 'Rich scripting' (McWilliam, 1998) is an approach for EAL learners. It is based on a metalinguistic approach and in addition emphasises a sociocultural pedagogy of dialogic learning in groups, collective remembering and problem solving. Learners are encouraged to suspend using language for learning, and to make language an object of learning in itself in order to examine the meanings and forms of the language, e.g. cognate lexis, suffixes, meaning and semantic webs, polysemy and irregularities. One of the purposes is to empower learners in their use of language as a tool for learning through understanding the social and cultural dynamics of its construction and use. It also seems to have a positive effect on learners' conceptual learning and literacy skills, although the 'rich scripting' approach has not been evaluated with EAL learners, and it has yet to be researched for children with SLCN.

A second approach presented by Gibbons (1993, 2002) is orientated by a Vygotskian perspective to learning through a language-focused curriculum. It addresses all three language knowledges. Gibbons recruits a functional model of language (Halliday & Hasan, 1985) and a sociocultural theory of learning (Mercer, 2000) to inform teaching strategies. Activities in curriculum contexts are language focused and promote joint meaning making. A language-focused curriculum engages teachers in explicitly planning for language learning in curriculum learning so that children can learn language through academic learning.

Professionals can personalise planning for individuals and it is likely that further accommodation for language learning would be needed for monolingual and bilingual learners with SLCN. There is no published evaluation of this approach.

These approaches support inclusive education. Studies show that teachers can learn to change their interaction with learners from a domain-specific to an integrated (language and curriculum) perspective of knowledge (Stoddart et al., 2002). An integrated approach to language learning supports monolingual and additional language learners who have communication difficulties that although may not be severe enough to be immediately noticeable, nevertheless interrupt and constrain learning. However, withdrawal practices are often justified by lack of distributed professional expertise and organisational constraints for planning and implementing language-focused teaching. Learners with SLCN may be vulnerable to other social threats, particularly culturally and linguistically diverse children, which may impact on communication and learning.

Affect Pedagogy

A proportion of children with language disability have difficulties learning social cognition, knowledge and skills, which makes them vulnerable to being regular targets for victimisation and who grow up to live isolated lives often with mental health problems (Botting & Conti-Ramsden, 2000; Knox & Conti-Ramsden, 2003; Conti- Ramsden & Botting, 2004). Students with these difficulties often have social, emotional and behavioural difficulties, as well as isolation and attachment needs. Some groups of culturally and linguistically diverse children may be particularly at risk, such as EAL learners with language disability, refugees and 'late arrivals' in school, displaced and highly mobile/ transient children who have had distressing, traumatic or unsettled earlier experiences. In this description, language with behaviour difficulties are attributed to intrinsic needs in individual pupils as well as environmental reasons. Yet, culturally and linguistically diverse children may be the recipients of antisocial behaviour. Black and minority ethnic pupils in mainly white schools are especially vulnerable to bullying (Cline et al., 2002). Schools often have an exclusive focus on negatively perceived misbehaviour and the response may be school exclusion (Stirling, 1992; Parsons & Howlett, 1996; Fletcher-Campbell, 2001). Studies in the UK show that the highest proportion of pupils excluded from schools is black (Osler, 1997). Yet, intervention approaches to behaviour needs tend to remain blind to colour, culture and language diversity (Hallam *et al.*, 2006).

An essential aspect of intervention and support for children with communication needs is a focus on social and emotional learning with language learning. Studies indicate that there are two main approaches; one concerns direct support to students and the other is support to practitioners. Direct intervention may include developing social language skills groups through social stories (Rinaldi, 2000) as well as nurture groups (e.g. O'Connor & Colwell, 2002) and therapeutic teaching skills (Morris, 1991), such as 'Circle Time' and 'Circles of Friends' (Newton & Wilson, 1999). These interventions offer opportunities to ensure inclusion of individuals who face the greatest risk of rejection or isolation from the class, school and wider community where they live, and they may need to be specifically orientated for culturally and linguistically diverse learners' needs.

Three approaches to supporting practitioners and other adults and parents through school-based approaches to professional development are offered here. They have been designed primarily for learners with identified SEN and are adaptable to culturally and linguistically diverse learners: whole school culture, dialogic pedagogy and teacher support groups. An inclusive school culture enhances all children's personal experiences. Cooper *et al.* (2000) suggest developing experiences of being valued as a person, belonging and being involved, feelings of personal satisfaction and achievement, congruence between personal and institutional values, and personal meaningfulness in the teaching/learning tasks. Affective, cognitive and social dimensions can be included in pedagogic practice in curriculum interaction. A 'joint systems approach' (Dowling & Osborne, 1994) shows practitioners how to understand and sharpen their recognition of learners' difficulties in order to engage in dialogue and joint problem solving with them. Practitioner support groups, and Teacher Support Teams, are recognised as being effective mechanisms for professional development through problem sharing and solving (Creese *et al.*, 1997; Baca & Cervantes, 1998).

Conclusion

For historical and professional reasons, teaching/learning and therapy have been understood as different. In this chapter, I have demonstrated with reference to the literature that pedagogy and therapeutic intervention with children who have language disabilities with culturally and linguistically diverse backgrounds can be informed by similar concepts of learning, in particular mediation in interaction.

Children scaffold additional language learning from their first language. The case study illustrated how teachers can use students' first language to learn the new language. Most typically developing minority linguistic bilingual children develop the additional language of schooling within 2 to 7 years, with subsequent advantages for literacy skills. As with monolingual children, early difficulties that do not resolve quickly indicate serious needs that require professional responses. Delays or difficulties in early language development are not caused by bilingual environments. Culturally and linguistically diverse children with SLCN can become bilingual and a family's decision to give up the home language needs to be an informed decision.

Children learn language in contexts that are meaningful to them. They develop from context-specific language to language for learning and conceptualisation. Teaching or intervention for language learning on its own may not lead to wider language use in other contexts without graduated support. Other approaches to language learning develop psychological resources and strategies in learners that enable them to learn *about* language. Teaching metalinguistic knowledge is illustrated in the case study by the support teacher instructing not only the bilingual learner with additional needs, but also her peer group, about ground rules for discussion and interaction in class.

The case study also illustrates how the teacher performs language teaching and learning through other teaching and learning, particularly academic learning. That is, learning language as a tool for understanding and examining concepts, particularly in curriculum subjects. It usually takes several years for learners to become capable of using language in this way. Additional language learners and learners with SLCN often take longer and require language-focused pedagogic approaches, teaching strategies and materials. Mainstream and specialist professionals could effectively share their knowledge to meet the needs of these learners.

Culturally and linguistically diverse learners with language disabilities appear to present numerous challenges to monolingual services and provisions. The challenges do not usually lie within the children or their families, but in the responsiveness to their needs by monolingual services and provisions. Responsiveness draws on a range of knowledges and skills, across cultures and languages as well as application of specialist technical knowledge about speech and language needs and learning. The next chapter explores these challenges further.

Chapter 9
Collaboration as Interprofessional Learning

Examples of Multiagency Work

A Royal National Institute of the Blind survey (1992) revealed that 27 different professionals were involved with a group of 45 children with multiple disabilities. These professionals included some who came from a variety of medical disciplines from paediatrics, orthoptics and orthopaedic surgery to speech and language therapy, physiotherapy and dietetics. There were several different educationists involved including peripatetic teachers for the visually impaired, educational audiologists and Portage workers. There were also a group of professionals with semi-medical roles, for example an aromatherapist, a music therapist and a chiropodist. Social services were represented by a residential social worker, and the voluntary sector through the Barnardos fostering team. The Community Mental Handicap Team was also involved and they are themselves a multidisciplinary body. (Lacey, 2000: 158)

[for refugee and asylum seekers] Targeted services (which offered extensive focused support) ... cover a range of issues: EAL support, after school activities, access into mainstream curriculum, special provisions for post 16, or early years, supporting refugee communities through supplementary schools, psychological support, pastoral support, raising awareness through citizenship education, liaison with other agencies, home-school liaison.

(Findings from a survey of school districts, from Arnot & Pinson, 2005: 38).

Introduction

This chapter and the next, present collaboration as learning: *learning to work together* and *working to learn together*, for children with substantial communication needs and their culturally and linguistically diverse families. Collaboration around cultural and linguistic diversity (CLD) has the necessary feature of working between monolingual and bilingual colleagues across languages and cultures, particularly where agencies, practitioners and the child/family do not share a language. Attention to learning highlights that, as practitioners and researchers, we are continuing to develop expertise in this area. I draw on learning theories to interpret inter- and intraprofessional learning in service provisions.

This chapter offers a frame for understanding and transforming the phenomena of overlapping, 'underlapping' and fragmentation in professional work around children and their families with substantial complex needs. The literature on professional collaboration for language disabilities in CLD contexts is orientated by a Vygotskian approach to organisational learning, using sociocultural historical activity theory. The chapter has four sections. With reference to the literature, I set out the context, terms and theoretical approach, Activity Theory, to understanding collaboration for culturally and linguistically diverse children with additional communication difficulties. The second and third sections critically examine collaborative interprofessional working through Activity Theory. The fourth section presents an analysis of demands and implications of intraprofessional learning between professionals and bilingual paraprofessionals, and the chapter ends with some conclusions.

Context, Terms and Theory

Internationally, the wider context of this discussion is the current policy initiatives in the UK, North America, Australia and other countries that require agencies to develop 'joined up' responses to the needs of those children and families identified as being at risk of social exclusion. Educational inclusion policies orientate agencies, which previously provided separate services, to work together (UNESCO, 1994). More locally, in the UK, the Education Act (1981), the Code of Practice for the Identification and Assessment of special educational need (SEN) (DfEE, 2001) and the policy Every Child Matters (2003) provide the impetus for agencies to collaborate to support children at risk and with educational difficulties.

Schools in many countries are assigned a key role in recruiting and coordinating specialist services as well as providing support and monitoring progress. The two surveys cited at the beginning of the chapter present the possible range of agencies and professional groups that can be involved with children with multiple needs, and with culturally and linguistically diverse children and families. These examples underscore the imperative for a 'joined up' response to prevent vulnerable children from 'falling through the net' (Roaf, 2002: 3). Uniting the various agencies working with children's needs is not a new idea (e.g. Bronfenbrenner, 1970), but it has yet to be achieved, particularly for culturally and linguistically diverse children with language-related disabilities.

Specialist provision for bilingual children with speech, language and communication needs (SLCN) in the UK is largely under-served and under-reported (Law *et al.*, 2000b). Speech and language practitioners and educational specialist professional groups (such as English as an additional language (EAL) teachers) maintain professional discreetness, while sharing a common goal of wanting to meet culturally and linguistically diverse children's educational and communication needs. One study of specialist language provision (language units) with bilingual children showed that about 11% of children (27 of 247) in language units were bilingual, which was a similar proportion to the national figure (Crutchley, 1999). Crutchley noted that bilingual children's CLD was better served in provision that was part of a school with experience of diversity. She also found that there was no contribution from EAL staff or collaboration between EAL staff and speech and language therapists (SLT) staff for bilingual children in language units.

Terms

Agencies refer to the systems of health, education and social services comprising the statutory and voluntary bodies that offer universal and targeted services. Roaf (2002: 36) describes 'agency purpose as consisting of a core of responsibilities, translated in a range of services decreed by government and tradition'. The nature of these responsibilities is evolving, sometimes arbitrary and overlapping, and can be interpreted, negotiated and disputed across agency boundaries. For example, education in mainstream schools is a universal service, while EAL support and speech and language provision offer targeted services. In the UK, tradition determines that speech and language provision is a health service that is requisitioned by education.

*Inter*agency work refers to collaboration across the major service systems, which for culturally and linguistically diverse children, refugees, asylum seekers and travellers usually includes education, health, social services, police, law and housing. In the USA, a similar range of agencies and professionals are involved (Baca & Cervantes, 1998: 299). Interagency collaboration across targeted services often shares a focus to meet individual children's and families' needs. Those involved with disability and/or with CLD may have distinct conceptualisations of how inclusion can be realised. *Intra*-agency work refers to collaboration within a single agency between practitioner and professional groups; for example educational psychologists, teachers and other educationists planning a cross-school referral system for students with SEN.

Interprofessional collaboration refers to learning to work together across professions or discipline groups, such as between classroom teachers and SEN teachers and SLTs, or EAL teachers and subject teachers. This particular example has been researched as 'partnership teaching' (Bourne & McPake, 1991). *Intraprofessional* learning refers to learning to collaborate within a single profession, either across specialisms or hierarchies, such as between a teacher and a support assistant, or between a SLT and a bilingual therapy assistant. Bilingual paraprofessionals are also known as bilingual assistants and co-workers and usually have roles and responsibilities including and beyond interpreters and translators (Mattes & Omark, 1984).

The two surveys at the beginning of the chapter give examples that multiple agencies are involved at any one time for children with complex educational needs. Are agencies and professional groups learning to work together and working to learn together to overcome overlapping, underlapping and fragmentation of services? The rest of the chapter presents a Vygotskian-based approach to interpret organisational learning for the language needs of culturally and linguistically diverse children with SLCN. I start by offering a rationale for this choice.

Theory

There are several theoretical approaches to understanding organisational learning. In the USA, a major cross-State initiative to pull together the various stakeholders involved in special education draws on the approach known as 'communities of practice' (Lave & Wenger, 1991; Wenger, 1998) as offering a new approach to solving complex educational problems. The authors of the evaluation report that:

> The [Individuals with Disabilities Education Act] IDEA Partnership's Communities of Practice approach offers a promising strategy to support positive change. It is our hope that, together, we can discover what it will take to engage state agency personnel, policymakers and

stakeholders as partners in a way that truly improves the system – to effectively translate policy and research into practice to ensure successful outcomes for students with disabilities and their families. (Cashman *et al.*, 2007: 38)

The term 'communities of practice', although appropriated by Lave and Wenger, is used with a similar meaning by other approaches to organisational learning. They accept that learning is situated and reproductive, in that newcomers acquire competence and status through engagement in activities in the community, with specialist language, skills and cultural (professional) knowledge. However, there are important distinctions in conceptualising learning between 'communities of practice' and 'learning communities' (Eraut, 2002). A substantial criticism of Lave and Wenger's notion is that while this approach focuses on reproducing commonalities of knowledge rather than diversity and agency, it offers no explanation for how communities transform themselves. Yet, this is the principle challenge facing providers, stakeholders and clients in service provision for disability in culturally and linguistically diverse contexts. An alternative approach is a post-Vygotskian perspective, which offers conceptualisations of transformative, self-conscious learning to communities of learners (Engeström, 1999), particularly intraprofessional learning for language disability in contexts of CLD (Martin, 2005) and interprofessional learning in schools (Martin, 2008).

Sociocultural Activity Theory (SCAT)

Traditionally, from a psychological view, learning is understood as individual-, cognitive- and content-based; that is: learning-as-product and evidenced in outcomes. An alternative conceptualisation prioritises the *process* of learning, that is, learning as practice which is collective and constructed through historical, social and cultural contexts; learning-as-process (Vygotsky, 1978). Mediation between the external-social and the internal-cognitive brings about internalisation of new knowledge, meaning making and learning. Vygotsky called the set of interactions in this learning space the zone of proximal development (ZPD) (Vygotsky, 1978). Human *activity* (not actions) is *learning* that results in being able to think or do something that was previously beyond one's capability and to do this *practice* in a historical, cultural, social context with another or others (Vygotsky, 1987).

Vygotsky believed that human activity happens in a relationship where those whose actions are the focus of analysis (subjects) resolve a shared problem which is their 'focus of learning' (Object) by using 'mediating means' (tools) to achieve a goal. Practitioners are familiar with the notion of mediation and 'scaffolding' in their work with children. Successful teaching/learning is embedded in aligning the appropriate tools with what is being worked on. Tools are the fundamental elements of human activity, as they shape the learning for which they are used. Tools may be conceptual, material or organisational, and the primary tool is language. Activity Systems are the unit of analysis for organisational learning. Human activity systems engage in purposeful, motivated, goal-directed learning, which produces outcomes. These relationships are diagrammatically represented in Figure 9.1. This basic learning relationship depicts the Activity System in teacher–SLT or other dyadic/small group collaboration and emphasises individual learning.

Engeström (1999), a Finnish academic, has taken the basic triangle of relationships for human activity and expanded the model for the purposes of organisational analysis, which includes historical and contextual factors that shape current collaborative work. A further lower part of the triangle incorporates institutional level components: the community of others who are involved in the problem, the rules, routines and professional conduct that support and constrain participants in solving the problem, and the way the participants share their work and responsibilities, division of labour in resolving the problem. The components and their interactive relationship are represented in Figure 9.2. Engestrom emphasises the importance of the interactions between the different components in the expanded Activity System for understanding and analysing learning at organisational level. Tensions and dilemmas, or *contradictions* (not to be confused with problems or conflicts), which arise from the structures and processes within and between components in the Activity System, for historical and cultural reasons, become the Object of

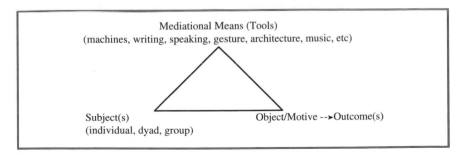

Figure 9.1 The principle relationships in an activity system

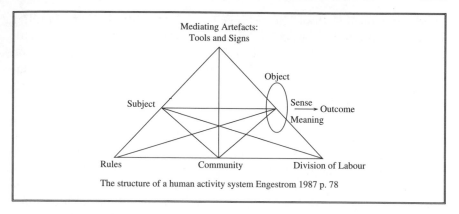

The structure of a human activity system Engestrom 1987 p. 78

Figure 9.2 Second generation Activity Theory model

collaborative learning. There is an iterative cycle as contradictions are resolved and new ones are brought to the surface.

Activity Theory focuses on instability and contradictions that are a 'motive force of change and development' (Engeström, 1999: 9). The purpose of an Activity System is to resolve contradictions as they evolve towards the desired outcome, so that subjects and their environment change and are transformed through activity. It is more accurate to think of a large and complex organisation like a secondary school or a SLT service not as one activity system, but as a network of activity systems. Individuals can be in several activity systems within a service or school, wherever they work on common contradictions to achieve a common goal.

Activity systems can be differentiated from 'teams'. Teams that are designated, such as single service professionals grouped for administrative purposes, or multiprofessional teams working around a child, performing roles and responsibilities according to recognised professional 'scripts', may work in parallel or in liaison without addressing issues that prevent better collaborative working (Engeström, 1995). Researchers using Activity Theory are interested in the process of transformation, when groups become Activity Systems.

To understand the complexities of two interacting activity systems, Engeström formulated a third generation activity theory model (Engeström, 1999) (see Figure 9.3). Every activity system is a community of multiple points of view and perspectives. Within them, people have different positionings, with distinct traditions and multiple layers and strands of histories, which multiply the multivoicedness in interacting activity systems (Daniels, 2001: 94). This model is particularly relevant

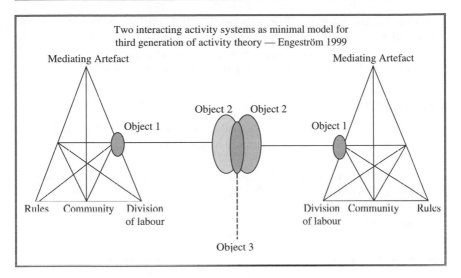

Two interacting activity systems as minimal model for
third generation of activity theory — Engeström 1999

Figure 9.3 Third generation of Activity Theory. A minimal model for two interacting activity systems

for analysing the integration of Speech and Language (SL) provision into schools, where an aspect of the SLT service with its historical and cultural factors must engage with an activity system of the school. Within secondary schools, there is a similar scenario when staff in the SEN department engages with curriculum subject departments.

Interprofessional Learning

This section discusses the application of Engeström's interpretation of Activity Theory to models of interprofessional collaborative working for culturally and linguistically diverse children with additional educational language needs. Engeström *et al.* (1997) developed a three-level analysis of forms of knowledge that are learnt in systemic collaboration: co-ordination, cooperation and communication. These terms pepper the literature on collaboration, most frequently to refer to models of practice, but Engeström *et al.* use them in a specific theorised way that was developed in a study of collaborative practice in the legal system. They refer to knowledge of collaborative work that practitioners learn about relationships between practitioners, the problems they think they are resolving and the learning they believe they are accomplishing to achieve goals for the child (Daniels, 2001: 141). This analysis can be applied to examine learning for multiprofessional collaboration in historical, cultural and social contexts of key practitioners who work with culturally and linguistically diverse children with communication needs, and inform the beliefs and values that influence how they work.

Coordination level

The first level of knowledge of collaborative working is coordination (Figure 9.4). It represents how professionals/practitioners from different disciplines (*actors*) work within their discrete professional roles on aspects of the child's needs to achieve successful performance of assigned actions (*the object*). They use existing decision rules already established to work collaboratively in their shared task environment (Rogers & Whetton, 1982, cited in Daniels *et al.*, 2000). They share a set of assumed rules and traditions about their work (*a shared script*) which 'co-ordinates the participants' actions as if from behind their backs without being questioned or discussed' (Engeström *et al.*, 1997: 372). The overarching goals of the child's long-term wellbeing are assumed and, together with the script that operates behind the actors, remain habitual, unconscious and unquestioned (Engeström *et al.*, 1997). 'The co-ordination actors follow their scripted roles pursuing different goals' (Daniels, 2001: 141). Work in services and agencies that is role-focused, maps on to the coordination activity system of interprofessional work (Figure 9.4).

Coordination most accurately represents knowledge reflected in traditional models of professional collaboration. It indicates the potential

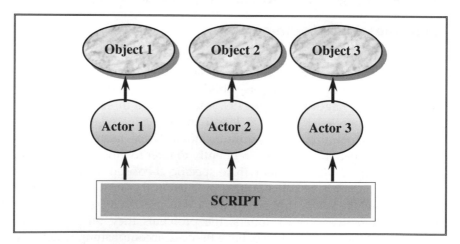

Figure 9.4 Coordination

for overlap between provision as well as the more likely 'underlapping' and fragmenting of provisions meeting children's needs. In Chapter 3, we noted that disability and SEN are more often constructed categorically, that is by children's specified difficulties. Writing about California, Mitchell and Scott (1994: 89) note that:

> The single most potent threat to successful interagency collaboration lies in the historical division of client needs in to distinctive "problems" ... Once service agencies have been assigned unique responsibility for dealing with particular sets of client problems, the stage is set for systemic failure ... As a result client needs come to be defined in terms of an agency's capacity to respond.

Two forces tend to maintain the status quo: inertia and resistance in historical professional cultures and systemic structures.

Professional cultures

Agencies involved with learners with SEN and EAL/CLD have operated discreetly, as the opening case examples show. This is partly explained historically, by their piecemeal, idiosyncratic development as agencies, defined and distinguished by distinct roles and functions in respect to children's needs (Lacey, 2000, 2001). Another explanation is a privileging of *vertical knowledge*, that is expertise derived from distinct bodies of cognate knowledge and skilled practices which gave professional groups distinct identities and specialist status. These groups have developed strong notions of professional autonomy, responsibility, self-reliance, which shape their approach to organisation of work, decision making about children and recording their practice (Nias, 1993; Miller, 1996). For example, specialist learning support teachers develop nuanced sensitivities of their distinctiveness from classroom and subject teachers. Similarly, professionals specialising in the area of language, such as EAL teachers, advisory language teachers, educational psychologists and SLTs, may have finely nuanced sensitivities leading to hyperdistinguished work. Ideologically, services and professionals involved with the learning needs of culturally and linguistically diverse learners have been keen to distinguish their work from the bio/medico/psychological needs of learners with SEN (Tomlinson. 1982). Rivalries and misconceptions of professional role, knowledge and practice can maintain coordinated level work.

Nevertheless, potential for collaborating lies in considerable overlap of knowledge, skills and values across professional disciplines, for assessment, intervention and support for culturally and linguistically diverse children with SEN. For example, health professionals in education, such as SLTs in the UK, bring values derived from health/medical cultures, such as 'duties of care', diagnosis, intervention and meeting individual children's needs. Teachers in special education often bring similar values, derived from a historical medical paradigm of SEN, to work with children in education, as well as an 'ideology of child need' and 'protectiveness' to meet the severest needs of children (Croll & Moses, 2000; Troyna & Vincent, 1996).

Systemic structures and personal attributes

Successful collaboration requires both systemic (structural) and personal attributes. Structural differences between agencies and services present barriers at operational levels for learning to work together. They can be mitigated by appropriate strategic collaboration, signs of which are beginning to emerge in local agreements between health and education agencies for speech and language provision in the UK (Law *et al.*, 2000b). Evidence indicates that the necessary characteristics of successful collaborative work are an agreed assigned time and place to share interprofessional information, knowledge, understanding and skills (e.g. Wright, 1996; Roulstone *et al.*, 2005). From an individual perspective, some studies cite personal attributes as important in collaboration, such as being friendly, having a sense of humour and having friendships with colleagues (Roulstone *et al.*, 2005; Creese, 2005). An important characteristic is practitioners' disposition to learn (Carr, 2002). Practitioners need to be professionally knowledgeable, motivated and willing to learn new practices by working with colleagues from different professional, cultural and linguistic backgrounds for the needs of bilingual children with communication difficulties. The extent to which individual and systemic characteristics integrate remains under-researched.

Professional learning, in order to change from a co-ordinated level of work for children with communication needs, can present challenges for working together. On the one hand, collaboration between teachers and SLTs for children with speech and language difficulties can be a rewarding experience, which can achieve improvement in children's speech and language needs (Roulstone *et al.*, 2005). By contrast, it can provoke a mixed response from practitioners in terms of positive feelings of extended knowledge and improved skills, but also negative feelings (Miller, 1996; Wright, 1996). Negative feelings and misgivings have been associated with loss of specialist knowledge status and loss/fudging of professional identity (Robinson *et al.*, 2004).

Studies of the micropolitics of professional work find negative approaches to changing from a coordinated level of working, namely resistance to collaborate to meet the particular needs of children with learning disability if constructed as outside the professional's remit (Benjamin, 2002). This can lead to professionals working in the same classroom with different pupil groups and individual pupils. For example, EAL teachers and class/subject teachers may work in parallel within the same class session focusing on different teaching/learning objectives (Creese, 2005); EAL teachers and SLTs may work separately with bilingual children with SLCN and EAL needs (Crutchley, 1999). This approach can lead to fragmentation and 'underlapping' of services to culturally and linguistically diverse students with multiple learning and language needs. It can also lead to high levels of inefficiency (overlapping). More important, it can confuse pupils and parents.

Where collaboration is organised as coordinated, provision of multi-disciplinary support to children is maintained as separate programmes and even through pull out/withdrawal. Liaison is maintained through official and legitimated channels, such as professional letters, case meetings, home-school notebooks, school reports. Historically, in many countries, there has been little interagency collaboration between educational EAL services or health based SLT provision, or between either of them and schools. The drive for inclusive education is changing these practices.

Work between professional and interpreter is a further example of coordinated role/agency collaboration. Participants coordinate their actions according to accepted pre-existing roles and rules, in order to meet bilingual children's and family's needs. The role and expectations of the interpreter may not go beyond accurate rendering of the exchange between client and provider, for example to contribute to diagnosis. Working within a coordinated approach may explore but rarely challenges the accepted scripts (e.g. Isaac, 2002). The evolution of the role of bilingual co-worker/paraprofessional (Mattes & Omark, 1984) goes some way towards disrupting a role/agency-orientated approach to collaboration between therapist and bilingual co-worker.

In the absence of coordination and further learning across professional groups and services, practice can be ineffective. Research reveals characteristics of unsatisfactory professional practice, which should be avoided in the best interests of client, family and practitioner. For example, where clients and professionals do not share a language or culture heritage, consultations are unprepared between practitioners and interpreters and/or family and friends are recruited as interpreters (Mills, 1994; Pöchhacker & Kadric, 1999; Isaac, 2002; Hale, 2007).

The importance of one-to-one, specialist professional-to-child model of provision is that it has facilitated the development of expertise, that is, specialist 'craft' knowledge among professionals. As expertise becomes routinised, it can become mass customised through commercial programmes, be offered to more children with needs by a range of practitioners. Expertise in developing routinised skills, practices and knowledge with bilingual children with language-related disabilities is largely under-researched and under-reported. However, a body of evidence-based specialist practice is emerging for work with bilingual children in speech and language assessment and intervention across both languages (Duncan, 1989; Kayser, 1995; Holm & Dodd, 1999; Battle, 2002; Pert & Letts, 2003; Mahon *et al.*, 2003; Martin *et al.*, 2003; Zhu & Dodd, 2006a).

Traditional one-to-one work practices between professionals and children are not the only method of generating high levels of routinised expert knowledge and skills in working with bilingual children with communication needs. Parents and professionals can learn 'craft' through dyadic or small group work and through informal and formal learning practices (Duncan, 1989). Specialist knowledge, skills and understanding, are required for working with bilingual children with communicative needs, particularly in a specialist professional capacity. While an aspect of this level of learning is dyadic between specialist and novice professionals in apprenticeship models usually through the first generation models of learning, there are implications for organisational learning at later stages.

Roaf (2002) argues that the fundamental importance of interagency and intraagency work is to prevent children whose life chances are at risk from 'falling through the net' of provision so that they become 'difficult to place'. That is, to prevent underlapping provisions. For the focus of this book, 'underlapping' service provision for culturally and linguistically diverse children with speech and language difficulties poses several threats. For example, where there is little interagency collaboration, single agency and single profession approaches are likely to threaten the quality of assessment and planning intervention and support. It becomes easier to confuse and conflate EAL needs with speech and language difficulties/needs in linguistic minority children. It is more likely that minority linguistic children will be placed with either EAL support or SLCN support, but not both as may be needed. As a result, achievement and attainment outcomes are likely to be threatened. This predicament may be construed by agencies or researchers as a failure of single professional competence to manage the perceived excessive complexity of the placement and resource needs of culturally and linguistically diverse children with additional language-related needs (Lindsay *et al.*, 2006).

In summary, the coordination level of collaboration based on role/ agency is historically the most familiar model for practitioners. It is also the one that is the most likely to have to change in order for agencies and services to engage with implementing policy initiatives and imperatives for 'joined up' service responses to bilingual children with complex needs.

Cooperation level

The second level of knowledge of collaborative work is cooperation. Cooperation involves different professionals in their joint work focusing on a shared issue concerning a culturally and linguistically diverse child (object of learning) to reconceptualise or solve a problem. They are not so concerned with performing set assigned roles or presenting themselves. There is a given script, but while not questioning or reconceptualising it, the actors may go beyond it. The main focus of attention is the shared object of learning (Daniels, 2001; Engeström *et al.*, 1997). For example, in the UK, at an operational level, subject teacher, EAL teacher, SLT, bilingual home-school liaison and the Special Educational Needs Coordinator (SENCo) may focus on developing a programme to include minority ethnic/linguistic parents in supporting the special learning needs of their children. Another example would be subject teacher, EAL teacher and the SLT working together online on a bilingual child's individual educational plan (IEP) and focused on developing targets and activities to support particular children's vocabulary learning, drawing on their distinct and overlapping professional knowledges to create repositories of new knowledge (Figure 9.5).

Knowledge of collaboration as cooperation can effect organisational learning strategically to change provision. Demands on limited bilingual resources within single provisions can precipitate discussion around best use, such as sharing trained bilingual staff across services. Cooperative learning is evidenced when specialist services, schools and funding authorities renegotiate their relationship to meet the needs of culturally and linguistically diverse learners with additional needs, to create joint funding, new work routines, distribution of work and decision-making

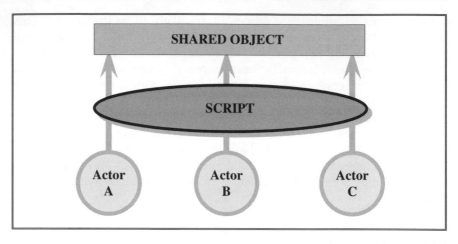

Figure 9.5 Cooperation

policies for work in schools and services. However, there is little evidence of this due to the inflexibilities of funding practices (Law *et al.*, 2000b).

Studies of cooperative learning show that strategic and operational staff create and respond to opportunities for information and knowledge exchange. They respond formally through shared staff meetings, training courses and shared professional work, such as shared cases, assessments and joint report writing or with less formal discussion through staffroom and corridor chats (Robinson *et al.*, 2004). Provisions in school, where practitioners work through cooperative learning, show improvement in aspects of service delivery, such as procedures for referral, assessment and review (Roulstone *et al.*, 2005; Daniels *et al.*, 2000). Lindsay *et al.* (2005) found that in specialist and mainstream speech and language provision, educationists preferred needs-led work practices and SLTs preferred procedures-led work. Roulstone *et al.* (2005) concluded that needs-led flexible work by practitioners was crucial for meeting children's needs, so long as it was within pre-agreed approaches. These studies also report the importance that practitioners place on clarifying roles, responsibilities and expectations.

The role of bilingual specialist paraprofessionals is emerging as a needs-led flexible approach to working with professionals. Collaboration is focused on bilingual children's and families' needs, where professionals and bilingual practitioners are willing to go beyond teacher/therapist and interpreter roles to develop new forms of practice (Barnett, 1989). However, professionals and bilingual support practitioners do not critically attend to *all* aspects of their work and bilingual co-workers, advocates and assistants usually work within a defined script, role and responsibility.

Studies in language teaching support in mainstream schools shows the complexity of joint construction of role and responsibility between expert practitioners working to meet individual children's needs (Creese, 2005). In EAL provision

> Co-operative teaching is where a language support teacher and class or subject teacher plan together curriculum and teaching strategies which will take into account the learning needs of all pupils in the class, trying to adjust the learning situation to fit the pupils. (Bourne, 1997: 82)

Creese (2005) gives accounts of partnership teaching where subject teachers and EAL teachers are 'joint experts' in curriculum teaching. She focuses on their interactions and the discursive construction of joint responsibility as they teach in classrooms. While engaging in a co-operative level of interprofessional learning, the practitioners remain grounded in their professional roots. This research approach into collaborative work has implications for exploring aspects of practitioner support for bilingual children with educational needs in mainstream.

Structural models of skill-mix teams organised to meet multiple needs of culturally and linguistically diverse children, tend to work through co-operative learning. Baca and Cervantes (1998: 298–307) describe a whole school approach to bilingual children's linguistic and cultural needs in learning, in schools in the USA. The initiative is the Teacher Assistance Child Intervention Team (TACIT). TACIT is a collaborative team assembled to identify and support bilingual students whose language, learning and behaviour needs are not being met within mainstream and special language classes. TACIT is a small, selected, loosely configured school-wide team with a wide skills mix, including languages, learning, cultural diversity, counselling and special educational needs, that meets weekly to discuss issues concerning supporting individual children's needs through intensive in-class support. Team members work with class teachers and other agencies and may recommend pupils for further specialist support. The TACIT team works through a staged-process for each pupil and records and evaluates its efficacy. Baca and Cervantes (1998: 299) claim that research has shown that TACIT achieves high levels of responsiveness from children during the two-month intervention period, but the source is not given. The account given of TACIT reports cooperative learning and offers models of good collaborative practice for culturally and linguistically diverse children with educational needs.

Flexible structures exemplified in team teaching models and TACIT, and also in Sure Start (UK) and Head Start (USA) initiatives, afford opportunities for practitioners to embrace more fluid positions, extend their roles and knowledge, engage with new responsibilities and construct new identities. Professionals' responses to working in these types of teams are diverse. There seems to be a tension between embracing the changes, and fears of losing specialist knowledge and specialist status, with implications for their position and identity in the team as well as for career progression within their 'home' professions (Robinson *et al.*, 2004). It is possible that less powerful members, such as bilingual assistants, may fear losing autonomy and status afforded by specialist services. Robinson *et al.* (2004) recommend that teams move to overcome or prevent these fears by developing cultures and management that accords value to practitioner knowledge rather than to professional position.

To sum up, studies reviewed here of interprofessional collaboration show how practitioners are sharing information, problem solving and working closely together, that they are performing within a cooperating learning system. Practitioners engage in identifying, reconceptualising and resolving tensions and dilemmas in shared work while leaving unchallenged their acceptance of professional or service boundaries. They do not seem to reconceptualise the script of their professional or service heritages.

Communication level

Communication, or 'reflective communication', is a way that practitioners work together when they critically attend to all aspects of their joint work (Engeström *et al.*, 1997). That is, when they address both the hidden script, the unquestioned professional roles and rules that govern their actions and work practices, as well as new shared dilemmas and tensions (objects of learning) (Figure 9.6). Learning through reflective communication describes interactions between practitioners when they focus on reconceptualising their own services and communication systems in relation to their shared object of learning. Everything is subject to discussion and reconceptualisation. This transition to reflective communication is rare in the 'ongoing flow of everyday actions' (Engeström *et al.*, 1997: 373). Moreover, reflection *during* an action is more difficult to accomplish than reflection *after* an action and, furthermore, is particularly difficult to recall and report (Eraut, 1995).

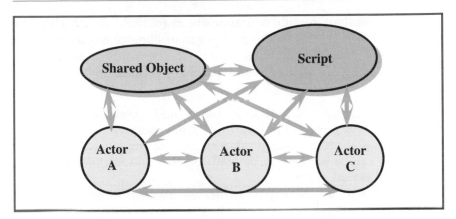

Figure 9.6 Communication

Systemic communicative learning is evidenced in responsive, flexible and reflective work practices that go beyond professional structures and heritages. Good service delivery through flexible work practices helps create positive work climates (Glisson & Hemmelgarn, 1998). The study found that practitioners are motivated to work to achieve the best results for children's needs and do whatever it takes to get the best result for the children in working environments that support risk taking and rule bending in professional practice. It seems that this approach contrasts with colleagues in similar departments who follow prescribed procedures and practices of service delivery in work environments that are more heavily monitored. Glisson and Hemmelgarn (1998) argue that research needs to focus more on how effective learning environments are constructed, rather than on role/agency organisation.

Communicative collaboration, with its characteristic of professionals reconceptualising their professional boundaries and statutory work practices, could be seen as risky business. Change is not only of role and responsibility, but also of working context. Nevertheless, learning how to create effective joined up service provision requires this kind of new learning. Two examples from the literature on interprofessional learning to collaborate for bilingual children or children with special needs, critically engage with role/agency-based work and present ways to create more reflective communicative activity systems: Partnership Teaching (Bourne & McPake, 1991) and Teaching Support Teams (TST; Creese *et al.*, 1997, 2000; Daniels, 2001).

Partnership Teaching (Bourne & McPake, 1991) is a programme developed from research with local education authorities (LEAs) and extensive consultation with educationists in the field in the UK. The researchers intended this model to apply to meeting *all* pupils' needs. It aims to build on and fit into whole school development planning phases and to become part of the cyclical planning process: the Partnership Teaching Cycle:

(1) Reviewing national and local policy and observing practice in classes, year groups and departments and identifying areas of need.
(2) Setting realistic goals that address these specific needs of pupils, which can be worked on by staff together and evaluated after an agreed period of time.
(3) Experimenting with ways to achieve these goals (action research).
(4) Evaluating the achievement of the goals and setting new goals.
(5) Disseminating ideas, strategies, techniques and materials that have been developed through the partnership to colleagues within and beyond the school through partnership networks. (Bourne, 1997: 82)

Bourne is keen to emphasise that Partnership Teaching while building on the concept of joint teaching by linking the work of two teachers, concerns a whole departmental team or other partners, with plans for curriculum development and staff development across the school (Bourne, 1997: 82). She emphasises the importance of understanding that Partnership Teaching is an approach rather than a method, that is intended to operate within the whole school, encouraging a learning community among the staff, facilitating, nurturing and creating new responses to teaching and learning challenges (Bourne, 1997: 85). The planned aspect of 'action research' is a potential tool to allow reflective communication about traditional professional boundaries in order to create new contexts, conceptualisations and practice with culturally and linguistically diverse learners and those with additional needs.

A further example in the literature is a study that seeks to change the context of work for professional participation to a communicative environment is the creation and development of collaborative problem-solving groups in schools in England (Creese *et al.*, 1997, 2000; Daniels, 2001). The context of work concerns learners with social, emotional and behaviour difficulties in schools. The aim of the study was a form of intervention to change the sociocultural context of schooling through the development of a culture of collaborative professional peer problem solving. The Teacher Support Teams (TSTs) comprised a small group of teachers who took referrals from individual teachers on a voluntary basis. The referring teacher brought concerns about classes, groups or individuals to discuss and problem-solve with peers, where expertise was shared.

There are apparent similarities between TSTs and TACITs, yet they are differentiated by the activity systems of collective learning that they develop. The focus for TACIT's work is the development of the learner, while TSTs aim to develop both learners and teachers. The expertise of specialist staff in TACIT was self-maintained and possibly shared, while the aim of TSTs was to distribute teacher expertise, and in this way engage whole school improvement. The child-focus and professional role orientation of TACIT may prevent it from engaging in questioning and changing the school environment to become more communicatively collaborative. The TSTs' purpose was to engage in dilemmas and tensions which referring teachers experienced in the social worlds that they inhabited with the learners (Daniels, 2001: 144). The underlying differences in the focus of activity constructs TACITs as learning at a cooperative level and TSTs seeking to learn to work at a communicative level.

To sum up, interprofessional learning to collaborate through reflective communication is not widely reported in the literature, which may indicate that it is not widely practiced. The examples from the literature reflect Glisson and Hemmelgarn's (1998) argument that research should focus more on how effective learning environments are constructed, rather than on role/agency organisation. They illustrate how a measure of effective learning environments is the extent to which reflective communicative collaboration develops and informs practice, which goes beyond role/agency organisation in order to make effective work around culturally and linguistically diverse children with additional and special needs.

I turn now to examine the literature concerning how professionals and bilingual paraprofessionals learn to work together to meet the needs of culturally and linguistically diverse children with language-related disabilities and their families.

Intraprofessional Learning

In this section, I explore, with reference to the literature, essential questions in professional collaborative learning: what is being learned, how is it being learned, and what are the factors that influence the level and directions of the learning effort? The context is professionals and bilingual paraprofessionals working with culturally and linguistically diverse learners with language disabilities and their families, where professionals and clients do not share language or culture sufficient for managing their needs. I give a brief description of the role and expectations of bilingual co-workers, before moving on to questions about collaborative learning: what is the focus of learning? What is being learned and how is it being learned, and the influential factors that orientate level and direction of learning? The therapist, co-worker and client and their family constitute an activity system that interlaces and networks with other activity systems. These activity systems tend to be multiple, loosely connected, emergent, abstract and contested (Blacker *et al.*, 2000).

Bilingual paraprofessionals

Many professions and service providers in the UK, USA, Canada and Australia have become multiprofessional by recruiting assistants/aids to support various aspects of professionals' work and service provision. They are referred to in the literature as co-workers, assistants and advocates and paraprofessionals (Mattes & Omark, 1984). Bilingual support workers from bilingual client communities are recruited as funds of linguistic and cultural knowledge as a 'tool' to enhance and enable monolingual provision for culturally and linguistically diverse communities and clients. Some terms/phrases, such as 'to *use* an interpreter or bilingual assistant', emphasise the instrumentality of bilingual human resources with nuances of power asymmetries. By contrast, other discourses refer to 'bilingual co-workers and paraprofessionals' to emphasise distributed cognitions and expertise with more egalitarian status. Bilingual assistants are typically less qualified practitioners working within services, alongside professionals, and receiving in-service training from colleagues, the profession and their employers. They are 'invariably low-status staff ... with few paths of professional development open to them' (Martin-Jones, 1993: 26). They are a disparate group, although mainly female, with a range of language, oracy and literacy skills and educational backgrounds (Mills, 1994).

The responsibilities of bilingual co-workers for SLCN are more extensive than interpreters and translators. Expectations of their role also usually go beyond those of monolingual SLCN assistants. They are expected to interpret and facilitate case history taking by offering cultural information about child rearing and communication practices. They assist and may take a lead in assessing clients' home language, and support professionals to identify areas of difficulty or delay. They are expected to progress to working independently in some areas, such as developing intervention materials, running intervention programmes in both languages, and counselling parents. They are also usually involved in administrative support of the bilingual caseload. Their work is supervised through the professional responsibility of therapists (Mattes & Omark, 1984; Barnett, 1989; Isaac, 2002; Martin, 2005) and they work within the same codes of ethical conduct.

What is the focus of learning?

The focus of learning is determined by the participants of an activity system working on the dilemmas and tensions that they identify as preventing them achieving their overall goal. While the long term goal of specialist professionals and bilingual co-workers working together is to meet the needs of bilingual children with language-related disabilities in one or both of their languages, the focus, or object of learning will change continually as the professional and bilingual co-worker move through a needs-led 'curriculum' of learning knowledge, skills and work practices This 'curriculum' has two main aspects of learning tools. Monolingual specialist professionals need to learn about the language and cultural practices of clients from the bilingual/bicultural co-workers. Co-workers need to learn not only specialist knowledge about language-related disabilities, but also specific practices and conduct of being a paraprofessional, as well as organisation and distribution of work, 'who does what', and who is accountable to whom. 'Knowing what', 'knowing how' and 'knowing who' are necessary characteristics of learning for both groups of practitioners in a reflective communication activity system. Actors reflect on their shared script, questioning and reconceptualising it as they develop collaborative work practices around bilingual children.

What is being learned?

There are two approaches to answering this question about new learning and knowledge in provision for culturally and linguistically diverse children with language disabilities and their families. One approach looks at learning of new knowledge in the interpersonal mediation between professionals and bilingual co-workers. There are three main types of learning and knowledge being learned in the activity systems around monolingual professionals and bilingual co-workers: explicit learning, tacit learning, and the relationship between them.

(1) Explicit learning is learning knowledge that can be explained, such as through formal and informal training, discussion with knowledgeable others and by reading texts. In the context here, SLCN professionals can

learn explicitly about the cultural and language practices of culturally and linguistically diverse communities of their clients. Professional training to develop cultural competencies has been urged as a foundation for professional practice in this field (Cheng *et al.*, 2001; Isaac, 2002). Professionals with personal motivation attend language learning courses, cultural training and read about culturally and linguistically diverse communities (Martin, 2005), as well as learning in discussion with bilingual colleagues and paraprofessionals. Bilingual co-workers learn interpretation and translation skills explicitly through formal training courses. There are few formal training courses and accredited pro- grammes for co-workers and monolingual assistants. They usually learn more informally through discussion, videos, and reading about knowl- edge of SLCN and knowledge and conduct of paraprofessionals, e.g. confidentiality and departmental procedures (Martin, 2005).

Explicit learning is also described as 'deliberative learning'

> where there is a definite learning goal and time set aside for acquiring new knowledge and engagement in deliberative activities such as planning and problem solving for which there is a clear work-based goal with learning as a probable by-product. (Eraut, 2004: 4)

In a case study of a bilingual co-worker learning to work in a SLT department (Martin, 2005), deliberative learning is evidenced in several ways. Specialist practitioners and bilingual paraprofessionals engage in deliberative teaching/learning about professional knowledge for plan- ning case history taking, assessment and intervention, such as child development, particular speech, language and communication difficul- ties, speech and language analysis, counselling, using assessment and teaching materials. They also engage in deliberative learning to solve work-based problems both authentic and reconstructed, and they rehearse future events, such as decision-making scenarios and giving advice to parents and other professionals. Monolingual and bilingual professionals can lead these learning events.

'Shadowing' is another example, where a co-worker observes experi- enced colleagues in their work without being expected to engage in the work (Martin, 2005).

> *Bilingual therapist*: Part of the induction when they [bilingual co-workers] come in is they are not just inducted in the clinical specialisms and go to the specialist to have a chat to them but I will get them to shadow one of the more experienced co-workers so that

they can look at the work relationship and look very carefully at how the person writes down the information. (Martin, 2005: 150)

Later, the experienced practitioner discusses the events and processes in the 'shadowing' and makes explicit any learning that the new co-worker will have experienced.

(2) Tacit knowing is best described as 'know-how', knowing by doing, such as riding a bike, baking bread. Acquiring this kind of knowledge is usually not done through discussion and reading. Tacit knowing is difficult to articulate so that reading or talking about riding a bike, bears little relation to actually knowing how to do it. For example, anyone can develop tacit knowing by engaging with organised cultural activities with culturally and linguistically diverse communities, hanging out with families, and visiting, living and working in heritage countries.

When learning from experience takes place and without a conscious awareness, this learning is referred to as implicit learning, that is,

the acquisition of knowledge independently of conscious attempts to learn and in the absence of explicit knowledge about what was learned. (Reber, 1993, cited in Eraut, 2004)

The most pertinent example in the context of bilingual paraprofessionals is their implicit learning of language and cultural knowledge that they bring as part of their resources to monolingual provision. Language knowledge is often referred to in cognitive models as part of implicit memory (e.g. de Bott, 1992). Implicit learning lays down implicit memories of previous experience that affects current behaviour without any conscious awareness of the previous experience. Linguistic and cultural knowledge that bilingual co-workers share with bilingual client communities is implicit, and cannot readily be discussed as explicit cultural and linguistic knowledge.

(3) There is a relationship between making explicit that which is implicit and tacit. A specific focus of learning between bilingual paraprofessionals and monolingual professionals is to transform tacit and implicit knowledge of language and culture of the bilingual co-worker so as to make it explicit and accessible to co-workers and others. This can take place in the principle learning relationship (see Figure 9.1) in dyads, when knowledgeable Others, such as experienced bilingual co-workers or monolingual therapists, work with new co-workers or therapists to develop language and cultural awareness. Specialist language professionals draw on their explicit knowledge of language in working with bilingual colleagues for this learning. The

important Other helps to transform co-workers' *implicit* knowledge to explicit knowing and scientific concepts as useable conceptual and practice tools by the co-worker in work with monolingual professionals. Here is an example in which a bilingual therapist reports on her work with a new bilingual co-worker:

> she's Asian but she's aware that she doesn't know too much about other communities, such as Muslim, and the majority of the client caseload she works with are Mirpuri speakers ... so we've had to look at the fact that her vocabulary is different from theirs ... This is the type of vocabulary you need to look out for, the verb ending ... (Martin, 2005: 149)

The important Other is a bilingual therapist from a neighbouring district. She reports how she engages the new Asian co-worker to interrogate the stereotypical assumption that 'Asians' are a homogeneous group, across religion and regional language variation. She uses differentiated language and terms: *Muslim, Mirpuri speakers, client caseload, vocabulary, verb ending*. She reports that she has mediated the co-worker's implicit linguistic and cultural knowledge to an explicit knowing of conceptual knowledge that the co-worker can use with monolingual professionals. The bilingual therapist has drawn the new recruit's attention to conceptual distinctions about language and culture. The co-worker speaks an Indian variety of Panjabi and the client community speak a similar but different language variation, Mirpuri Punjabi. The client community, Pakistani Mirpuri, is a geographical neighbour to her own Indian Panjabi community and the two are different culturally and religiously. It is a good example of explicit, deliberative learning.

The extent to which interpretation (spoken) and translation (written) remain implicit knowledge is for exploration between professionals and co-workers. Bilingual co-workers and community interpreters usually receive no formal training in interpreting and translating practices or in the scientific knowledge of the professional. Nevertheless, there is the expectation that they transform scientific and professional knowledge into their community language and cultural understanding in a way that can be accessible to children, families and other professionals. For example, in translating advice for culturally and linguistically diverse parents about language interaction in play, co-workers are required to go beyond linguistic interpreting. They need to locate this new knowledge in cultural frames of reference of child rearing for parents and families in order to make it meaningful for them, that is, to 'sell' them the idea and for them to 'buy' into it, and to follow the advice.

Experienced practitioners working with novice bilingual co-workers attend to the relationship between implicit and explicit knowing by making the event of interpreting and translating a shared object of learning in order to transform it through explicit learning to usable knowledge. Co-workers can draw on explicit knowledge along two axes – language for interpretation as well as specialist knowledge about aspects of language disability – as conceptual tools for future work. Co-worker learning is supported by discussion with professionals and with other co-workers who share zones of proximal development across both axes in this learning task. Evaluation of success and efficacy of this kind of learning challenges methods of data collection. Reportage is unsatisfactory, although guided reflection *after* the action in discussion with knowledgeable practitioners may offer insights (Eraut, 2004). Linguistic ethnography may be a fruitful approach to capture the complexity of the multilayered and multivoiced nature of this learning.

How is knowledge being learned?

The response to this question shifts the focus of learning from individual relationships of novice and expert practitioners, to the organisational activity systems that they work in. From a Vygotskian perspective of learning, participants effect change on others and are themselves changed and transformed in the process of learning. Departments and organisations that operate with coordination knowledge tend to be driven by procedure; professionals and co-workers are role focused, with professional learning mainly through formalised training. At strategic levels where organisation is through coordination, indicators of effective services to bilingual clients include coordinators of provision to bilingual clients, coordinators for the bilingual co-workers and professional development about knowledge of CLD (Mennen & Stansfield, 2006). Professionals and co-workers develop effective paired working relationships with high levels of expertise (vertical knowledge) for work with culturally and linguistically diverse children with SLCN. Expertise remains highly bounded and there is little widespread effect of distributing expertise of working bilingually and biculturally across monolingual assistants, professionals and departments (Martin, 2005).

Provisions which organise through processes of cooperation, in contrast with coordination, encourage more collective learning across professional/role boundaries, so-called horizontal learning. The focus of concern is less on developing professional and coworker expertise to meet CLD needs, and more towards meeting joint needs of provision for culturally and linguistically diverse learners with SLCN. There is an emphasis on working with other practitioner groups to develop a shared object of learning. Provisions that organise through cooperative learning have a determination to respond to dilemmas, paradoxes and tensions through negotiation and joint problem solving in their work with culturally and linguistically diverse families. Yet, they continue to adhere to organising within professional roles and boundaries (e.g. Stow & Dodd, 2003).

Organising collaboration through communicative processes is characterised by building a reflective working environment, which encourages fluid and flexible work practices to dilemmas and problem solving. Communicative collaboration addresses the threat of co-workers being a 'bolt-on' facility to monolingual provision. Reflective communication with other provisions seeks to develop horizontal learning across traditional professional, linguistic and cultural boundaried domains. Discussion, planning and implementing solutions to systemic difficulties contributes to distributing expertise across practitioner boundaries for therapists, co-workers, teachers and others, and building collective understanding and new shared knowledge. For example, those involved in problem-solving distribution of work could decide that trained bilingual co-workers are better placed to discuss with culturally and linguistically diverse parents about choice of language for intervention for the child's SLCN, than professionals who do not share the parents' language or cultural practices. Bilingual co-workers may contribute equally to resolving problems as other participants. Strategic managers of provisions can prioritise developing conceptual and skill resources of monolingual practitioners for working with bilingual personnel.

Factors that orientate level and direction of learning

Factors that orientate the level and direction of learning can be interpreted according to perspectives taken by the communities of activity. The core organising processes in activity networks operate in the relationship between key elements of one community of activity, and other elements with which it interacts, as well as the shared object of their endeavours. Activity communities in agencies for educating and supporting language disabilities in culturally and linguistically diverse families can be orientated by developing perspectives in three ways

(Blacker *et al.*, 2000). *Perspective making* refers to contributions to innovating practice from each community of activity across provisions and clients. *Perspective taking* refers to relations between different communities of activity, both horizontally and vertically within an agency's or provider's hierarchy. These perspectives include assumptions that disrupt relations, such as power asymmetries and racism that can be widespread in working across CLD and with untrained colleagues.

Power asymmetries exist between professionals and co-workers for reasons such as professional status, education, gender and possibly racism (Martin-Jones & Saxena, 1996). Similar asymmetries may emerge between parents and co-workers due to gender, age, class, education, religion, standard of spoken and written minority language (Isaac, 2002). Professionals and co-workers maintain discreet roles, although they are often renegotiated in expansive learning cycles, particularly as co-workers become more knowledgeable, reflective and confident in their work with families and bilingual children with language-related disabilities.

Perspective shaping refers to strategic views of the level and direction of learning within and across organisations for multiagency working for culturally and linguistically diverse children with language disabilities. Shaping learning perspectives involves identifying shared priorities and future developments across professional boundaries in contexts of educational and social inclusion and increasing CLD.

Conclusion

Two frames of analysis have been presented in this chapter in response to strong policy drives to find more effective ways of learning to work with culturally and linguistically diverse children with language disabilities and their families. They aim to avoid fragmentation, over/underlapping, inefficiency and confusion among the various services involved. Both approaches are orientated by a Vygotskian perspective on learning in the community in order to change unsatisfactory practice. One frame of analysis examines learning for organisational collaboration and the other frame of analysis examines individual learning in dyadic work focused on collaborating across CLD in provision settings.

One approach analyses practice as activity in provisions across three levels of organising process. Practitioners collaborate across professional disciplines around shared understandings of their roles and responsibilities towards the child's needs, represented in coordination of role-focused work or cooperation through negotiation and problem solving. Less frequently, practitioners share a conceptualisation of their work as reflective communication of distributed expertise across professional roles and boundaries. These processes are applied to provisions for language disabilities for culturally and linguistically diverse communities to analyse the relationship between the nature of collaboration across professionals and bilingual co-workers and its influence in shaping and transforming current and future provision.

Ideas about explicit and implicit learning inform the second approach, which analyses developing shared knowledge between practitioners working across languages and cultures for language-related disabilities. It draws on Vygotsky's basic learning relationship to analyse intraprofessional learning between professionals and bilingual co-workers. A focused example of specialist professionals and bilingual co-workers learning to work together illustrates the complexity of the multilayered and multivoiced learning involved. Examining perspectives of people and elements involved in the communities of activity informs strategic planning towards developing a collective mind for agencies involved in meeting language-related additional needs of culturally and linguistically diverse children and their families. There are implications for all practitioner groups who work in multidisciplinary settings, with a range of stakeholders and parents and families, as well as for those who work in CLD contexts.

Chapter 10
Parents, Families and Children Working with Professionals

Case Study

Some Asian parents views on the disclosure process

C20: I think it's not just me cos a lot of other Asian people and a lot of Black people tend to think when you've got these English doctors they're not bothered 'Oh no, it's an Asian. Never mind I'll see to one of our own'.

C16: Sometimes I feel that English people are more concerned and more caring than our own people.

C24: What's going to happen. Nobody told me that. I've been really upset about that. I mean is [child with disabilities] going to be like that or is she going to get better. What is exactly wrong with her. I tried [to find out] a lot of times. That's what I said 'What's causing the troubles?' They just use the word 'She's mentally handicapped'... I like to be prepared ... Everybody was upset and disappointed. No other members of the family have had a child like that or with disabilities ... They didn't say anything to me about she's not going to talk and she's not going to be normal.

C1: It was explained that with this child we'll have to train him this way ... I was told about his feeding and his play. I was given a lot of information about his care that he needs more support and attention ... he is a special child. I believe that nobody could have informed me better than she [health visitor] did ... she told me very calmly and explained the whole future too ... she helped me a lot to accept my child was disabled. (From Hatton *et al.*, 2003: 177)

Introduction

This chapter, like the previous one, follows the theme of collaboration: *learning to work together* and *working to learn together*, with a focus on collaboration between providers and clients who are culturally and linguistically diverse families and their children with substantial communication needs. With reference to the literature, the chapter argues that approaches adopted by providers to work with this client group need to adapt to meet the needs of culturally and linguistically diverse families. It makes a case that models of collaborative *learning to work together* evidenced in the literature are more responsive to culturally and linguistically diverse families with children with disabilities, and more effective at changing provision.

Steinstra (2002) found that the studies she reviewed on culturally and linguistically diverse parents and families with children with disability tended to take one of two perspectives. Much research takes a 'provider' perspective, where studies focus on aspects of service delivery and professional behaviour with a view to improving access to and take-up of provision by these families. The relationship between minority language parents of children with special needs and majority language professionals is constructed through differentials and inequalities of power, privilege, voice and access. Critical theory has been drawn on to explicate these relationships (Baca & Cervantes, 1998: 363). Fewer research studies take the 'client' perspective, that of culturally and linguistically diverse parents', families' and children's experience of provision for language disabilities. This body of research examines parents' experiences of racism, language barriers and parenting. The quotations that open the chapter illustrate this perspective, where client families' reported experiences can clearly inform service delivery. Beyond Steinstra's review, there is a third emerging body of research literature that provides evidence and models of collaborative learning to work/working to learn together with culturally and linguistically diverse families with children with disabilities.

In this chapter, discussions are framed by theoretical perspectives already set out in earlier chapters to interpret the literature on current research and practice with culturally and linguistically diverse families with children who have a disability. I use the first section to critically engage with Cunningham's and Davis' (1985) model of provider-led services for culturally and linguistically diverse parents and families with children with language disability. In the second section, I explore an ecosystemic approach (Bronfenbrenner, 1979), which supports much research in this aspect of the field, and offer a critical perspective on the insights and constraints of this approach for provision to culturally and linguistically diverse families. In the third section, I draw on the metaphor of social capital (Bourdieu, 1993) to explain structural and institutional racism, language discrimination and barriers to access and exclusion from services for culturally and linguistically diverse families. I use the fourth section to examine literature that researches provision and practice through a sociocultural teaching/learning approach, focusing on learning to work/working to learn together. This approach offers perspectives on how capability theory may offer a way to build on a family's beliefs, values and 'capabilities' of working to include children with additional needs into families. Finally, I draw some conclusions.

Professionals' Perspectives: Service Needs-led Approaches

Professional perspectives traditionally privilege individuated and specialist provision. The dominant approach is for professionals to work with individuals – the child, the parent (usually the mother) – and less frequently families. A main disadvantage of paradigms that are individual-focused is that extended patterns of collective, social learning and behaviour may remain unnoticed. This oversight is particularly important for professionals when interrogating practice with culturally and linguistically diverse parents and families. Over the last 20 years and more, Cunningham's and Davis' (1985) model has been widely used as an analysis of professional approaches to work, by teachers and parents of children with special educational needs (SEN). Their model is based on the management of specialist knowledge by practitioners with parents and families, particularly knowledge of the child's difficulties and needs, and knowledge of the systems that can meet those needs.

Cunningham and Davis' three-pronged model is described here with a critical reflection in relation to bilingual and culturally diverse parents:

- expert model;
- transplant model;
- consumer model.

An expert model: Critical perspectives

In an expert model, professionals and parents across cultural back-grounds perceive and acknowledge that professionals are repositories of expert knowledge. Impairment is understood through a medical para-digm and professional roles and relationships are constructed around diagnosis and identification of services and provisions. Professionals draw on a similar psychological model when working with parents to cope with feelings of grief, loss, shock and denial concerning their children's disability (McCool, 1999). However, parents' response to their children's disability seems to vary along a continuum (Carpenter, 1997). Professional roles and involvement may not always be understood by parents. For example, Roberts and Gibbs (1989) note that, where there is limited shared language between practitioners and minority ethnic parents, it may be difficult to explain/understand that assessing and supporting feeding and swallowing difficulties are part of speech and language therapists' (SLT) professional role, such as for a perinatal baby with cleft palate or supporting a youngster with swallowing difficulties resulting from brain damage in a road traffic accident.

An advantage of the expert model is that it 'carries with it the imperative for the professional to deliver well' (McCool, 1999: 152). The expert model is a service-led model for 'mass production' of provisions and services that is not necessarily honed to client need. A critique of this model is that parents' role in the implementation of provision is sidelined and there is no engagement with mutual learning between parents and professionals, or reflection on parents' understanding of the information that has been given to them about their child's difficulties and needs. Parents are treated as a homogeneous entity despite, as studies show, parents are diverse across class, gender, race, ethnicity and language and personal identity. Where services are not 'delivered well', professionals and services feel threatened and often blame the client. Consequently, differences in language, attendance and punctuality, parenting practices with clients are constructed as barriers to delivering services well.

There is a mandatory requirement in many countries for parents to be included in the official identification and individual educational planning for their children's SEN. The legal processes include the allocation of special educational resources, development and implementation of Individual Educational Plans (IEPs) and annual reviews of these procedures. Studies in the USA, reviewed by Baca and Cervantes (1998; citing Smith, 1990) through a lens of critical theory, indicate that parents and mainstream teachers are minimally included in these planning procedures. Baca and Cervantes (1998: 358) attribute this marginalisation of parents and teachers to the dominance in special education of a medical model for understanding impairment. This model privileges knowledge in expert professionals such as medics, psychologists, SLTs and SEN specialist teaching staff. Research consistently reports that differences between parental and professional evaluations of children's abilities are the result of parents overestimating their children's capabilities. Research rarely reports that differences stem from professionals underestimating children's abilities (Crais, 1992).

A 'within-child' perspective on disability assumes that there is a relatively stable, context-free set of capabilities and performances in the child. It does not allow for other explanations of variations in children's performance, such as context-generated variations and multiple realities. Specialist professionals holding this view usually disregard as unsound and inaccurate, discrepancies and differences in reported performances of children by parents and mainstream teachers because they lack specialist professional training. Consequently, the nonspecialist voice rarely effects educational management decisions for their children (Mehan, 1983). Mehan noted that there were distinct characteristics between parent and professional presentations of knowledge about the child with SEN. Professional reports were presented as context-free, scientific/technical and objective, while parental reports were presented as common sense, with little technical knowledge and context bound. He argues that it is most likely the discursive practices of the presentation of knowledge about the child that imbues the reports with status and authority. This analysis resonates with the metaphor of linguistic capital, that particular ways of talking and writing are more privileged than others (Bourdieu, 1993).

Legislation in the field of special needs encourages parents to be passive and professionals to be agentive (Harry, 1992). Harry's research with minority families showed that professionals inform parents of their children's SEN and educational management, rather than parents initiating, being involved and included in the process of educational assessment and management of their children's special needs. Harry (1992) points out that the less social and cultural capital is attributed to parents, such as (im)migrant, minority ethnic and linguistic minority parents, the more likely they are to be passive in the mandatory educational process of managing their children's SEN. She suggests that teachers and other professionals are likely to be more directive with this group of parents. Participation of linguistic and ethnic minority parents in the educational and legal processes of SEN is under-researched and under-reported.

A transplant model

In a transplant model, professionals acknowledge the role of parents in the intervention process, although it is usually they who define the parents' role in the partnership. Professionals 'transplant' aspects of their scientific knowledge to parents so that they can support and implement intervention with their child. The perceived advantages of this approach by service needs-led provision is that professionals spread the workload of intervention, encouraging parents to adapt programmes of work to their child's needs and preferences. A systematic review of literature in the field of speech, language and communication needs (SLCN) (Law *et al.*, 1998) concludes that practitioners' indirect work with children, that is, work with their parents, is effective. Programmes in the transplant model are, for example, the Hanen programme (Watson, 1995) for children with SLCN, sign language such as American (ASL) and British Sign Languages (BSL), and Makaton (Walker, 1996).

Few programmes have been adapted for use with culturally and linguistically diverse parents, and professionals often have to reinvent the wheel each time they 'transplant' their skills with bilingual parents and their children. There are examples in the literature (Ara & Thompson, 1989) and very few which have been evaluated. The Portage Project established in the early 1970s in Portage, WI, USA, for children with severe disabilities has developed beyond a 'transplant' model and has evolved ecologically to be a relationship-based intervention approach with parents (Copa *et al.*, 1999), as well as developing work with culturally and linguistically diverse families through Spanish. Portage is further discussed later in the chapter.

One criticism levelled at the transplant approach is that it is not sensitive to the diverse needs of parents. Parents are not a homogenous entity; they respond uniquely to inclusion in their child's intervention. Some parents may welcome and understand what is required, and accept the shared responsibility of their child's intervention. On the other hand, some may not understand what is expected of them, while others still may resist the responsibility, believing that intervention is the professional's role and job. Studies have shown that social class is an important indicator of taking up this responsibility. White, middle-class parents who are higher educated, with positive experiences of school are more likely to work with white professionals in general mainstream education (Vincent & Martin, 2005). It is highly probable that this group will be more positive to supporting the intervention of their children's special needs. In the USA, studies show that parents from white working-class and black and minority ethnic groups find it most difficult to be in a relationship with their schools where they support their children's learning needs (Lareau & Horvat, 1999). There is a need to research more extensively the approaches which bilingual and bicultural parents bring to sharing responsibility for their children's intervention, which may challenge professionals' constructs and practice.

A further criticism of the transplant model is that professionals must take on roles as educators when working to 'transplant' knowledge and skills to parents. Some professionals may resist this as part of their role and for others it may become the major strand of their work. All professionals themselves require training in taking on this new role, in order to understand the process of teaching and learning, building on parenting skills and knowledge that already exist in the family (Harry *et al.*, 1999) and to avoid didactic, directive approaches which are largely ineffective (Vincent & Martin, 2005).

A consumer model

Cunningham's and Davis' (1985) third model constructs parents as informed consumers of the services and provision offered to their children. Parents have power over their own role and level of participation and the role of the professionals is to listen, counsel and advise on the options available to parents for their child's needs. It is argued (e.g. Hornby, 1995) that in this model, parents are likely to feel more empowered, knowledgeable and more satisfied with the provision their child receives. This is most probably the case for higher educated parents. Some parents may resist this approach, as they perceive that professionals are abandoning their responsibilities; they may fear taking on decision making responsibilities. Furthermore, they may be critical of the level of provision offered to them, which may drive them to seek better services. This response may result in competition or conflict between service providers rather than improved options for the child.

A consumer model approach towards bilingual parents is advocated in Genesee *et al.* (2004). They recommend that practitioners assess bilingual children's speech and language needs carefully and then inform the parents fully, taking account of context and language and learning demands. Well-informed parents make the decisions about language choice and language intervention for their child. Ortiz (2001, 2004) supports collaborative school–community relationships. She argues, like Cummins (1994), that parents learning English must be viewed as capable advocates for their children and as valuable resources in school improvement efforts. By being involved with the families and communities of English learners, educators come to understand the social, linguistic and cultural contexts in which the children are being raised (Ortiz, 1997). Thus, educators learn to respect cultural differences in child-rearing practices and in how parents choose to be involved in their children's education (Garcia & Dominguez, 1997). Research in the area of deafness with parents from English, Hispanic and Deaf backgrounds (Allen, 2002) showed that working in groups with parents opens up opportunities for empowerment, through the social processes of group discussion. Hispanic parents became increasingly aware of the barriers they faced to accessing resources and support, and they found ways around these barriers, such as recruiting a trilingual Spanish/English/ASL tutor to teach them ASL.

In Cunningham's and Davis' models, the voice of the child is not readily heard. The relationship is constructed either as a dyad between professionals and parents, or as a slightly more expanded network between health professionals (e.g. the SLT), educationists (class teacher, special needs teacher, bilingual/English support teacher) and parents. In some cases, certain knowledge will not be privileged at all, such as that of children. Maitra and Miller (2002) note the passivity and silence surrounding children with disabilities in their own intervention pro-grammes, which is accentuated for children from diverse cultural heritages;

> Children themselves frequently have little power in directly influen-cing the course or nature of therapeutic interventions. Referred by adults (parents, teachers or other professionals) and taken to therapy by adults, the child's feelings and wishes are often overlaid by adult fears and hopes. For the ethnic minority family the relationship with western/white systems is yet more complex, and the child's "voice" may be drowned out completely. (Maitra & Miller, 2002: 109)

Ali and colleagues' (2001) review of the literature found that 'Indeed, the voices of black and Asian children in disability research have been almost silent' (Ali *et al.*, 2001: 949). They reviewed the less than 20 studies in the last two decades that were concerned with disability, ethnicity and childhood. They conclude that black and Asian disabled children have a unique and different experience from white disabled children, attributed to discriminatory experiences of disability, race and language.

Barriers that are regularly identified in the literature are differences from professionals in language, literacy, and cultural beliefs and values about disability (Allen, 2002; Steinberg *et al.*, 2003; Powers *et al.*, 1998). The pattern of marginalisation through language and cultural diversity can be understood through sociological theories. Theorising evidence allows feelings of personal blame and incompetence to be reinterpreted in terms of social and systemic processes, which shape and are shaped by individual behaviour. It also gives perspective on the size and nature of the challenge facing providers and researchers in efforts to change the current situation for minority families of children with difficulties.

Ecosystems

The idea of ecosystems is used as a metaphor to explain development and change in society. In order for social groups to function and survive, ecosystems must have basic prerequisite abilities. The most well known are: to *adapt* to the external environment, formulate and attain *goals*, achieve internal *integration* through group rules and norms, and to reproduce the group's *latent* dispositions and resources, such as cultural patterns and language (Crossley, 2005: 321; Parsons, 1966). Bronfenbrenner took the idea of an ecosystem and modified it as a model to interpret psychological and social-emotional development of children in their 'lifeworld' of the family, school, community and state/country. His ideas of social functioning as an ecosystem are widely cited as a way of interpreting community and family functioning within society. He posits that there are four main levels or subsystems of social organisation around the child, that she/he learns to engage with through the functional prerequisites which impact on the child's development: a microlevel of organisation with parents and siblings interacting with the child; a mesolevel, such as wider family and teacher and classroom; an exosystem, that is community, school, special needs and disability services; and ultimately a macrolevel, such as legislation on migration and discrimination, national government education policies, and for minority communities, the diaspora (see Chapter 7).

Bronfenbrenner's model is also used to interpret ethnic socialisation in minority families (Rodriguez *et al.*, 2002) and for understanding interventions for refugee families (Hamilton & Moore, 2004). Where there are distinct 'lifeworlds', such as majority and minority ethnic, cultural and linguistic ecosystems, we can construct an analysis where minority parents and families must move between two ecosystems, where cohesion and coherence across the systems are dependent on meaningful interactions that protect both systems. Successful cohesion relies on the relationship across systems and subsystems based on the individual's ability to use accessible resources to achieve goals that meet needs. According to Bronfenbrenner, the idea and practices of 'culture' function within the different levels of social organisation, where culture and community are independent variables, which define and distinguish settings. So, for Bronfenbrenner, 'context' is the setting that surrounds individuals, although socioculturalists understand context differently, and define 'context as that which weaves together the individuals' (Cole, 1996) (see discussion in Chapter 1). There are implications for practitioners depending on the perspective they take. Practitioners who understand context as something created between individuals would work differently from those who understand context as something that separates or is shared by parent/child/family and the professional.

Family as a system

A family is usually considered to be a group of related people living together, along with the wider circle of other related significant people who are frequently involved in the lives of the group. Families, like individuals, have life cycles with events that have significance for them. The notion of a family life cycle allows analysis of the stage or process that the family is at and the issues that are relevant to them. The family life cycle reflects how a family adjusts and develops as it collectively copes with the changes occurring to each member of the group as she/he passes through developmental life stages.

Some life events may disrupt the family unit to such an extent that the family draws on external agencies. For example, marriages, deaths and births are important family life cycle events. Disadvantaged minority families in the UK have high infant mortality rates. Infant death is traumatic for the whole family, and is often spoken about by young siblings (Duncan, 1989a). The birth of a child with disability impacts on the whole family (Carpenter, 1997; Shah, 1992). For many families, particularly minority families, children starting school and entering the majority community is a 'life event'. For refugees and asylum seekers, migration histories tell of particularly important, disruptive family events.

A systemic analysis views individual members as part of the family system rather than a collection of separate entities. Systems are interrelated and interacting with interdependent elements that form a collective entity. Within the collective of the family there are boundaries that are across generations and may also be across gender. Language and cultural practices are often boundary markers between generations and gender, where older family members and females maintain the home language more than the younger or male family members. Language and culture may be boundary markers between culturally and linguistically diverse families and external agencies using the majority language. The introduction of an 'outside' language into the home and family may be viewed positively as a tool for engaging across the minority and majority social ecosystems. Alternatively, it may be constructed by some family members as damaging to the cohesion of the family. Such views are expressed by parents and grandparents in studies of Asian deaf youngsters, when BSL and English are introduced in the home (Ahmad *et al.*, 2002; Atkin *et al.*, 2002). English speakers and signers can no longer communicate with other family members or read important cultural and religious texts.

Each family system is unique with its own beliefs and value systems, which to greater or lesser extents will be influenced by the values of the wider community. Belief systems can be explicit, such as religious, or they may be implicit and nonverbalised, such as child-rearing practices. Evidence suggests that practitioners and researchers need to be aware of the extent to which parents and families are able to articulate the belief systems which inform their interactions, as well as being aware of their own cultural positioning (Harry *et al.*, 1999).

Families develop their own communication practices. Some families have communication practices that are damaging to their members, and may result in communication difficulties, such as stammering or language delay. Minority linguistic families may use more than one language in communication practices, and codeswitch between them, which is usually unproblematic (Myers-Scotton, 2006). Some studies suggest that codeswitching may be a site for identifying speech and language difficulties; difficulties codeswitching may indicate vulnerability in language development (Pert & Letts, 2003). Some monolingual professionals mistakenly inform parents and families that bilingualism causes language impairment and advise that there should be one language only in the child's repertoire, the dominant language. Not only is there no linguistic evidence to support this advice, it is clear that the family's communicative dynamic will be changed, creating tensions with negative impact on the social communication of the child with difficulties (see Chapter 8 for discussion).

Systems seek stability and are more easily modified than they are changed. Families differ in their flexibility to accommodate new events and ideas. Those that show resilience maintain stability by accommodating new ideas, beliefs and behaviours. Resilience is a crucial resource for families with children with difficulties, in order to regain stability and continue to develop and function in the face of major life changes. Families at particular risk are likely to be those experiencing several major life events, such as migration, unemployment and financial difficulties, housing difficulties (Anderson, 2004a, 2004b). Families with few support systems are also more at risk (Ghate & Hazel, 2002). While minority families may live in established, transplanted communities with substantial cultural support systems, other (im)migrant families may not, with few extended family members, and live relatively isolated lives (Harris, 2003). Individual children can show resilience to 'overcome adversity to achieve good developmental outcomes' (Masten & Coatesworth, 1998: 205, in Hamilton & Moore, 2004: 6).

Parenting

For many bilingual and minority ethnic parents, parenting is concerned with bringing their children up as members of their community: religious, linguistic, family and the diasporic community (Harding & Riley, 1998; Harding-Esch & Riley, 2003). Parents contribute to ethnic/ linguistic socialisation and developing identity in their children that will harmonise with the community, howsoever that community is defined. In Bourdieu's terms, they are inculcated into the 'habitus' – the way of living – of the community (Martin, 2003). Encouraging parents to change their parenting practices is an enterprise with profound implications (Dwivedi, 2002; Ghate & Hazel, 2002).

Social Capital and Symbolic Power: Access and Barriers

The literature shows that 'disability' is a site of great social injustice. Injustice for disabled people and their families is further accentuated by their social class, level of education, race, ethnicity and lack of English, or the dominant language. Ecosystem models are unable to explain this kind of structural discrimination. I draw on a sociology theory to interpret and explain how these injustices are constructed through actual and perceived social connections.

Social capital and symbolic power

In his theory of social capital, 'Bourdieu draws on all that is useful from a functionalist concept of systems' (Crossley, 2005: 49). Bourdieu (1983, 1986) interpreted the function of social systems was to produce and reproduce social capital, where social capital was the benefits accruing to individuals or families by virtue of their ties with others (Smyth, 2004: 20). Bourdieu draws attention to the central relationship between social capital, superiority and privilege, in his terms, symbolic power. He focuses on structural constraints and unequal access to institutional resources based on class, gender and race. Institutional resources are the combined actual and potential resources that are linked to membership of a resilient and stable network of essentially institutionalised relationships of shared acquaintance and recognition. According to Bourdieu, dominant positions in society are maintained by people consciously developing and maintaining social networks realised through official institutions, such as education and health. Negotiated and continuous institutionalised association over time secures a mutual relationship between these dominant social groups and the institutions. The opposite also seems to hold. The circularity of the system preserves its existence.

There are structural features and mutual recognition between the institutions and dominant groups, and their members. Economically and socially advantaged groups have educational and social experiences that empower them to network so that they 'know who' and 'know how' to access and negotiate with the institutions for resources. Dominant groups use their social capital, that is, knowledge and social ties of their group, to access resources and maintain their position. Individuals and families in these groups are also recognised by the institutions and are allowed access to pathways through the system to secure potential and actual resources. Symbolic power, that is superiority and privilege, is reproduced by social negotiation and collusion between the advantaged and the institutions for actual and potential resources. An important difference between this approach and an ecosystem approach is the circularity, production/reproduction and negotiation between people and institutions.

Applying a theory of social capital and symbolic power to the field of disability can make sense of the process of acquiring the 'right' labels that access limited resources for disabled children. Parental pushing for appropriate provision for their children is well known in practice and summed up by the adage 'squeaky wheels get the most oil', where parents who know how to work the system obtain resources. Daniels notes that entry into more socially acceptable SEN categories such as learning difficulties (LD) in the USA (dyslexia in the UK) is more difficult to achieve than entry into the category of mental retardation in the USA (learning difficulties in the UK). So it is likely to be the educationally informed middle-class who are active to ensure the LD/dyslexia label for their children, especially their sons (Daniels *et al.*, 2000b: 50, citing Carrier, 1983).

Access and barriers

Little recognition, negotiation or attribution of social capital and symbolic power between institutions and CLD groups ensures the circularity of the exclusion of many culturally and linguistically diverse families with members with disabilities. Barriers are created that prevent access for culturally and linguistically diverse families to provision for their disabled children, such as lack of recognition by the providers of the families' linguistic and cultural resources, no shared language between provider and client, stereotypical views by providers attributed to culturally and linguistically diverse families, and financial disadvantage among culturally and linguistically diverse families.

In the case of accessing support and resources from institutions such as health and specialist education services, simply knowing of the existence of resources is not enough. To be able to access them, minority ethnic, CLD and disadvantaged families not only need to know the pathways through, but at the same time be recognised as legitimate by the institutions and professionals, by having the material and symbolic *requirements*, such as appropriate language and literacy proficiency and appropriate cultural behaviour. For example, a culturally and linguistically diverse family needs to speak and be literate in English and be punctual for their appointment. Ironically, the characteristics of diversity such as language, culture and education are perceived as *barriers* to accessing services. The metaphor of symbolic power attributed to social, cultural and linguistic resources is one of the explanations for institutionalised racism.

The circularity of low social capital and symbolic power awarded by institutions and professionals to minority ethnic and linguistic parents and families with disabled children ensures low access to provision. Minority ethnic parents with severely disabled children in the UK tend to be poorer compared to the general population and consistently face greater adversity, which suggests that their minority ethnic status is important in explaining their greater poverty, lack of service provision and access to benefits (Ahmad, 2000: 5; Chamba *et al.*, 1999). Low quality of maternity services for minority ethnic and linguistic mothers is one of the causes of high infant mortality and impairment rates in this group, yet low take-up of these services is widely attributed to language and cultural barriers (Ahmad, 1993).

Attributing stereotypical beliefs to culturally and linguistically diverse families can deny access to provision. Providers are reported to attribute stereotypical views of 'Asian' parents' attitudes and behaviour towards impairment and disability, such as religious-based explanations and shame, that lead parents to have low expectations of their children's future. Reportedly, these attributed stereotypical views differ from those attributed to the majority white population (Beresford *et al.*, 1996) and are taken to explain why service uptake amongst minority ethnic families is lower than that of white families. Yet, such explanations can be interpreted as classic cases of 'blaming the victim', deflecting attention from institutional discrimination (Ahmad, 1993). Further research reports that religious-based beliefs concerning disability and impairment are held by parents and families from majority and minority ethnic groups and co-exist with medical explanations (Bywaters *et al.*, 2003). Bywaters *et al.*'s (2003) study showed that low up-take of services, such as respite care and advocacy service by Pakistani and Bangladeshi parents of disabled children, was due to lack of information and linguistically, culturally and socially created barriers by providers.

Low/no take up of financial resources is due to providers' stereotyped beliefs that South Asian extended families offer social resources among themselves. These stereotyped beliefs create barriers against culturally and linguistically diverse families accessing information from the services (Fazil *et al.*, 2002). Yet, there is substantial existing UK research that has consistently found contrary to these common stereotypes that informal and formal support received by families is not sufficient to meet the needs of disabled children, and that South Asian families receive less family and community support than their white counterparts (Beresford, 1995; Chamba *et al.*, 1999; Hatton *et al.*, 2002; Atkin & Rollings, 1996).

Some social groups may lack social capital – the 'know how', the strategic, empowering educational and social experiences to allow them to become part of the more powerful social collective. In addition, linguistic minority ethnic groups may not know of the resources available, they may be unfamiliar with the networking pathways to the resources they need and unable to negotiate for them. South Asian families, already living in disadvantaged circumstances, suffer additional material disadvantage due to lack of access to financial resources, as well as related mental health problems (Fazil *et al.*, 2002). Fazil *et al.* suggest that families were unaware of the resources because they did not understand the process due to language. 'Neither the health or education systems offered a clear gateway to information about and access to the range of services that may be available to disabled families (Fazil *et al.*, 2002: 251). Research with refugee families with adults and children who are disabled either in their country of origin or in the UK encounter 'insurmountable' barriers to welfare services and benefits in the UK (Harris, 2003). A pertinent example from the USA is the high number of middle-class, educated families that secure cochlear implants for their deaf children in comparison with the low or no numbers of minority ethnic and linguistic families (Geers & Brenner, 2003; Steinberg *et al.*, 2003). Steinberg *et al.*'s research indicates that professionals might not even inform minority families of cochlear implants.

Research with South Asian parents of the disclosure process of their child's disability, shows variable experiences, as the chapter's opening case study extracts reveal. For some parents in Hatton *et al.*'s study, the process is in the wrong language for them and most parents reported little postdisclosure support. Poor postdisclosure support and access to support services outside the hospital environment are also experienced by majority, middle-class parents and families with disabilities (Carpenter, 1997). The study also showed good practice with prompt disclosure in the appropriate language, often English, with both parents present where possible, with emotional support as part of the process, with clear practical information and linked to postdisclosure support from a key worker (Hatton *et al.*, 2003: 177). Good disclosure processes are associated with good parental understanding of their child's difficulties. Minority ethnic and linguistic parents are more likely to understand their children's difficulties the more obvious and familiar the disabilities are, such as sensory and physical difficulties. Parents have considerably more difficulty understanding disabilities which are less obvious and emerge later in development, such as autism spectrum difficulties (Warner, 1999).

Research with minority ethnic groups shows that while their social capital is drawn on unevenly by institutions because of structural inequities such as social class, ethnicity and gender, there is differentiated inclusion due to group and individual agency. In the USA, broadly speaking, Asian immigrants tend to adapt (that is, they acquire the material and symbolic requirements to develop social capital and access resources) more successfully than Black Americans (Ogbu, 1995). Moreover, while middle-class black families still benefit from their class position (and interact with schools in different ways from their less privileged counterparts), they still face an institutional setting that implicitly and invisibly privileges white families (Lareau & Horvat, 1999). Resilience and coping mechanisms were noted in minority ethnic families with severely disabled children indicating strong ecosystems, and individual relationships in the face of adversity and stressors (Fazil *et al.*, 2002).

Resistance to change

The slow response by institutions, such as education, health and professional bodies, to the challenges of disabled people and their families with cultural and linguistic diversity (CLD) could be interpreted as further evidence of social capital and symbolic power. There is overwhelming research evidence that institutions have barely changed their policies, protocols or staffing to recognise and legitimise diverse forms of social capital and negotiation. Inequities in service provision continue. Fazil and colleagues note that while limited skills in English in culturally and linguistically diverse families are a major barrier to accessing services, it is not the only one.

> Over three decades after the main contemporary period of immigration from the South Asian sub-continent, service providers still had not got effective means of offering services to non-English speakers or to those who are not familiar with the basic structures of the British welfare system. (Fazil *et al.*, 2002: 251)

For example, inaccessibility to quality genetic counselling in the home language can have serious consequences. Only 4 of the 27 UK regional genetic centres had staff trained in genetic counselling for people from minority ethnic populations (Darr, 1999). A survey (Anionwu, 1996) showed that there were 34 haemoglobinopathy counsellors in post in the UK, and only four were of Asian background with appropriate linguistic skills. For EAL pupils with SLCN in the UK, Law *et al.* (2000b) showed that SLT provision was generally absent. A study documenting the difficulties in providing equity in SLT services to linguistic minority groups in a region in the UK (Stow & Dodd, 2003) revisits many of the issues examined earlier by Winter (1999, 2001) and Miller (1984). Low numbers of linguistic minority ethnic professionals mean that services rely on interpreters, linkworkers and teaching assistants who may not be specifically trained in working with a culturally and linguistically diverse client group. In SLT services in the UK, bilingual assistants/co-workers are not required to have training, although most do (Martin, 2005). Professionals are unlikely to have had training in helping families deal with spiritual beliefs, stigma and shame (Bywaters *et al.*, 2003). Information in accessible formats is a difficulty faced by many disabled people regardless of ethnicity (Harris & Bamford, 2001).

Reflections on research procedures

The qualitative research studies with minority linguistic parents and their disabled children address some of the shortcomings of large quantitative written postal surveys, which are unable to explore in detail the key issues behind the statistical data (Fazil *et al.*, 2002). Qualitative studies research relatively small numbers through interviews and produce rich descriptions and analyses of the interface between minority linguistic parents and families with disabled children and institutions, services and professionals. They are very moving accounts of personal suffering which the researchers are sensitive to. This body of research would drive anyone who reads it to consider ways in which services that are led by provider needs and resources can be moved to become client needs-led services.

What do parents want from support?

A large national research project in the UK with families living in poor environments examined issues of stress, support and coping with parenting from the perspectives of parents themselves (Ghate & Hazel, 2002). Eleven percent of the families were from minority ethnic and linguistic groups, which reflect the UK's demographic distribution. The authors note that minority ethnic parents were among the three priority groups considered for enhanced support for parenting. The study did not have a disability dimension, although many of the families had sick children (e.g. cancer) and parental health was a feature. The study found that there was an association between families with ineffective strategies for managing a child with challenging behaviour and parental poor mental health. While the study does not directly focus on minority families with disabilities, the key findings identify some general issues about what parents want from support services, and sets the scene for discussing how providers might meet these needs with minority ethnic and linguistic parents.

Key findings by Ghate and Hazel (2002) indicated that different forms of support fulfil different functions for parents; what may work well for one service does not work well for another. Parents expect and receive different things from informal, semiformal and formal support. Parents take up informal support (e.g. parent and toddler groups, parent support groups) to broaden their social networks for coping purposes. Minority ethnic families were found to have significantly smaller social networks and had significantly lower use of informal and semiformal support which seemed to be due to parents being unaware of this kind of support or being self-sufficient and coping without them. The authors note that services could respond to this need by improving their marketing. Services' reluctance/resistance to this recommendation, often voiced as a fear of being unable to meet the subsequent high demand from minority families, is another form of institutional racism.

The neediest parents were often the ones least likely to take up informal services. They were anxious about loss of privacy, confidentiality, reciprocity and indebtedness (Ghate & Hazel, 2002: 257). This may have been enhanced for some minority families by cultural issues of 'stigma' of disability (Hatton *et al.*, 2003). Minority linguistic families may have also encountered language access problems. Some reported simply not knowing anyone in the neighbourhood they had moved to, which must be an important characteristic for many minority families, including refugees and asylum seekers. Despite/because of living in poverty, parents were resourceful and learnt from experience – parents of older children reported coping better than parents with younger children. The authors suggest that finding ways to involve these two groups might be a powerful way of boosting families' naturally occurring social support networks. On the other hand, parents reported that formal support is taken up for instrumental reasons to get professional advice and help for specific problems that required special services. While many had positive experiences, many found that their experience of receiving help was often brusque, businesslike and directive, and parents most feared 'losing control' of their parenting role.

This study has implications for providers working with poor minority ethnic families. This group is likely to be a priority, to be relatively isolated and not have ready access to support, and to be unaware of informal support and possibly unaware of formal expert services. What parents want are responsive services that give them information, advice and help relevant to them for their child's needs while allowing them to remain 'in charge'

Passing on information

The study found a large information gap in parents' perceived knowledge about key aspects of parenting and child rearing. The information parents wanted varied according to the age of their children. Thirty percent of parents with children under 11 years wanted information about children's behaviour and how to deal with behaviour problems, 20% wanted information about schooling, and 10% of parents with preschool children wanted to know about typical child development (Ghate & Hazel, 2002: 248). Over half of the parents wanted information in written form, such as leaflets or booklets, rather than audio or videotapes. The advantages of 'take home' information are that parents can manage the information themselves, confidentially and revisit it as often as required.

This finding needs to be read with reference to adult literacy research. A quarter of the US population and a fifth of the UK population has poor reading skills. The average reading age among adults is between 9 and

13 years in the UK (Pumphrey, 1991) and similarly in the USA at Grades 5–8 level (Weiss *et al.*, 1995). Limited literacy skills seem to be more prevalent in the elderly, poor, members of minority groups or (im)migrants (Weiss & Coyne, 1997). The implications are that most adults and parents taking up services for the 'at risk' will not understand the majority of educational handouts, consent forms, questionnaires and official papers they receive.

Research studies in health contexts find that typical handouts from professional organisations, used to educate clients, are written at the 10th-grade (15-year-old level) or higher. Consent forms to request permission, compliance and explain risks or research studies are typically written at the higher education level (Davis *et al.*, 1994). Services need to take on board and possibly enlist the skills of literacy specialists in drawing up information about provision and child development for parents. As Darr (1999: 13) notes, there is little evidence of efficacy from evaluation research, although videos have been documented as a cost-effective tool in genetic counselling (Fisher *et al.*, 1981). Videos as an information resource in the home may be particularly relevant for Asian families; in the mid-1980s in the UK, for reasons related to the entertainment industry, over 60% of Asian households had videos in their homes (Husband, 1994). Husband noted that this number was likely to increase as VCR continued to be an important resource for accessing entertainment in Asian homes. Videos have since been replaced by DVDs, and cable TV and the internet offer further electronic tools and resources to service providers and voluntary agencies for knowledge transfer about disabilities across languages. A role for providers is to open up pathways of negotiation with and for minority families. This is beginning to be adopted by professionals, paraprofessionals and advocates from minority ethnic and linguistic communities (Allen, 2002; Steinberg *et al.*, 2003; Jones *et al.*, 2001; Barnett, 1989) in education, social services and aspects of the health service.

Sociocultural Approaches to Working with Parents and Families

I use this section to examine, with reference to relevant literature, sociocultural perspectives as developed in earlier chapters to working with culturally and linguistically diverse parents and families.

A 'posture of cultural reciprocity' helps professionals in their work with parents to view discrepant beliefs through multiple multicultural lenses (Harry *et al.*, 1999). That is, practitioners not only need to be aware of the extent to which parents and families are able to articulate their belief systems, they also need to be able to articulate their own. Kalyanpur and Harry (1997, 1999) propose that an effective starting point for cross-cultural collaboration is for professionals to engage in a self-reflective and dialogic process toward identifying both their own and the families' cultural norms. Decisions about goals for service provision need to be informed by two principles: cultural reciprocity where professionals work in a collaborative manner with parents and families, and with a sociocultural view of learning and development which targets social, collective processes rather than individual ones (Harry *et al.*, 1999).

Collaborative work with parents that is informed by sociocultural theory emphasises social learning by participants across personal, interpersonal and community planes. Models of work across providers, parents and children with needs often describe a triangular network of communication. By contrast, a Vygotskian model of learning (first generation see p. 207) describes the three agents together in one part of the learning activity system, drawing on shared tools in order to work on a shared focus of learning – such as developing targets for development that are of value to all three agents. Hence, the focus for the professional, that is the target of intervention, is not on changing the child (although this may happen), but rather working towards setting goals for the individual through a process of social mediation with the family in their zone of proximal development. The professional is the important Other, who guides and is guided by the learning and development of the parents and families. Two examples are given of client needs-led provision. They are orientated by sociocultural approaches to learning and by capability approaches to building on families' resources to develop an inclusive environment rather than 'a fixing the child' approach.

The work of the Portage Project, referred to earlier, uses an ecological approach to frame the relationship between the legislation, which requires that services be provided in the child's natural environment and the real lives of children with language disabilities in culturally and linguistically diverse families. In addition, the Portage Project works within a sociocultural paradigm focused on learning at several levels. As a learning organisation, practitioners learn through experiences with families, other organisations and research. At a client level, studies on intervention show that the learning relationship between child and caregiver affords significant building blocks for development. Work with early intervention programmes has shown the importance of provider's reflection on work with families as key to providing family-centred/client-led services.

For example, recognising and negotiating disjuncture in beliefs and values within families and between families and practitioners; also developing materials in Spanish for culturally and linguistically diverse families. As providers learn more about relationship-based intervention, they shape training and technical assistance to incorporate concepts of negotiated learning (Copa *et al.*, 1999).

Other provision is more explicit about its sociocultural orientation and collaborative learning. In a four-year action research project, practitioners worked with seven culturally and linguistically diverse families with children with disabilities (Harry *et al.*, 1999; Kalyanpur & Harry, 1997; Kalyanpur, 1998). The aim was twofold: the goals for the lives of people with disabilities had to resemble those that would be socially valued by both them and their families and the services. Practitioners provided assistance in a family's zone of proximal development to develop targets generated with them, rather than targeting goals that were normative for 'mainstream' families but not for culturally and linguistically diverse families. The project focused on cultural reflection and learning of cultural discrepancies between professionals and families. It reported on one aspect, the families' cultural response/resistance to future planning for the young person, and the need to access disability benefits. A key site for negotiation for language disability in bilingual families is language choice and its interface with future planning and the language of care and carers around the individual. This issue was not directly addressed in Harry *et al.*'s study, other than noting that one of the young people with cerebral palsy was fluent in Spanish and English, and choice was not an issue.

Harry *et al.* (1999) identified four key findings that demonstrate the changes that service providers must engage with in work with culturally and linguistically diverse families. Practitioners need to learn to take a culturally reciprocal stance that recognises a cultural, rather than a universal, base of beliefs; so that they do not so much give up their beliefs, but rather 'cultivate a habit of learning to understand and respect others'. Practitioners need to have professional development/personal preparation to develop the skills and habits of self-reflection and flexibility to understand and practice cultural reciprocity. The preparation needs to interface with professional practice to enable practitioners to gather, in a respectful manner, necessary information regarding the 'ecocultural niche' of the family. In order to understand the ecocultural niche of each family, practitioners need to become appraised of the cultural, historical and linguistic information about the minority groups they work with. Not doing so, leaves service providers open to individual racism and perpetuating institutional racism.

From early on, parents are concerned for the future of their children with SLI and SLCN (Pratt *et al.*, 2006). In the UK, there is growing interest in researching the long-term expectations of young people and adults with SLCN and SLI, and in particular on the transition from compulsory education to adult life. Studies show that this group of young people are usually involved in basic skills and vocational education where provision is aimed more at the needs of learners with learning disabilities (Stothard *et al.*, 1998). Young people with SLCN/SLI can be deeply disappointed with the restricted training/employment opportunities available to them, when they do not match their expectations and aspirations (Haynes & Naidoo, 1991). In addition, approximately 40% of the young people followed in the studies were experiencing social difficulties, particularly with regard to social isolation. Many continue to live with their parents, few have close friends or permanent jobs, and ratings of social inter-action indicate anomalies in a number of different areas (Howlin *et al.*, 2000; Haynes & Naidoo, 1991). These studies are of monolingual English speakers and suggest a possible bias in research orientation towards excluding culturally and linguistically diverse young people with SLCN.

Approaches to research and intervention, like Harry's and colleagues, go some way to addressing the expectations and aspirations of the future lives of bilingual/EAL young people with substantial language and communication needs and their families. A cultural reciprocity approach by providers and clients that engages with the systems of families and communities building on language, values and belief systems is likely to address the issues identified in the UK studies: further training and education, employment and social inclusion of young people and adults with SLCN. Moreover, a sociocultural frame for provision has a long term, developmental perspective, and aims to be sensitive to the needs of both client and provider in an iterative cycle of reflection and accommodation of needs and resources. This approach seeks to address the life-long communication needs of young people with SLCN and SLI, their families and communities.

Conclusion

The role of providers to mediate less powerful minority ethnic and linguistic families through the social structures and processes of institutions and prepare them to mediate for themselves is not even hinted at in traditional models such as Cunningham and Davies (1985).

Indeed, the model implicitly promotes service-led needs and hierarchies of social capital and symbolic power. Research and practice with minority ethnic and linguistic families with disability forces providers, practitioners and researchers to think outside the usual boxes we work within. We need to draw on powerful sociological theories to understand and interpret the full nature of the challenge facing these children and their families and the role of practitioners and researchers working with them.

A sociocultural approach is fundamentally different from 'transplant' and 'consumer' models discussed at the beginning of the chapter, which are didactic in their approach to parents and centred on child-fixing skills and processes. A socioculural approach shifts away from potentially patronising 'parent empowering' approaches towards a more democratic collaborative and mutual learning approach. Kalyanpur advocates that special education professionals, when dealing with culturally diverse families, need to be aware of the challenge of cultural blindness and acknowledge the cultural assumptions embedded in the services they offer which can contribute to the (dis)empowerment of minority families (Kalyanpur, 1998).

An approach based on cultural reciprocity fits more easily with notions of social capital and symbolic power. Providers and professionals with cultural reciprocity are able to reflect on and recognise the social capital and cultural and linguistic resources that minority ethnic and linguistic families bring to their engagement with service provision. They can both position themselves accordingly to best develop social mediation of shared goals, and scaffold learning. Evidence suggests that when providers and parents and families work in mutual learning relationships, relationships are more sustainable and better able to meet the long-term needs of children and young people with substantial communication needs and their families in culturally and linguistically diverse contexts.

References

Adams, C., Baxendale, J., Lloyd, J. and Aldred, C. (2005) Pragmatic language impairment: Case studies of social and pragmatic language therapy. *Child Language Teaching and Therapy* 21 (3), 227–250.

Adams, C., Byers Brown, B. and Edwards, M. (1997) *Developmental Disorders of Language* (2nd edn). San Diego, CA: Singular Pub. Group.

Ahmad, W.I.U. (1993) *'Race' and Health in Contemporary Britain*. Buckingham: Open University Press.

Ahmad, W.I.U. (ed.) (2000) *Ethnicity, Disability and Chronic Illness*. Buckingham: Open University Press.

Ahmad, W., Aitkin, K. and Chamba, R. (2000a) 'Causing havoc among their children': Parental and professional perspectives on consanguinity and childhood disability. In W.I.U. Ahmad (ed.) *Ethnicity, Disability and Chronic Illness* (pp. 28–44). Buckingham: Open University Press.

Ahmad, W.I.U., Darr, A., Jones, L. *et al.* (1998) *Deafness and Ethnicity Services, Policy and Politics*. Bristol: Policy Press.

Ahmad, W., Atkin, K. and Jones, L. (2002) Being deaf and being other things: Young Asian people negotiating identities. *Social Science and Medicine* 55 (10), 1757–1769.

Ahmad, W., Darr, A. and Jones, L. (2000b) 'I send my child to school and he comes back an Englishman': Minority ethnic deaf people, Identity politics and services. In W. Ahmad (ed.) *Ethnicity, Disability and Chronic Illness* (pp. 67–84). Buckingham: Open University Press.

Al Sheik Abdullah, Sarimah (2005) Constructing understanding around text: Investigating EFL reading as a social practice. Unpublished PhD thesis, School of Education, University of Birmingham, UK.

Alexander, R. (2004) Still no pedagogy? Principle, pragmatism and compliance in primary education. *Cambridge Journal of Education* 34 (1), 7–33.

Alexander-Passe, N. (2006) How dyslexic teenagers cope: An investigation of self-esteem, coping and depression. *Dyslexia* 12 (4), 256–275.

Ali, Z., Fazil, Q., Bywaters, P., Wallace, L. and Singh, G. (2001) Disability, ethnicity and childhood: A critical review of research. *Disability and Society* 16 (7), 949–968.

Allen, B. (2002) ASL-English bilingual classroom: The families' perspectives. *Bilingual Research Journal* 26 (1), 149–168.

American College of Physicians (2004) Racial and ethnic disparities in health care: A position paper of the American College of Physicians. *Annals of Internal Medicine* 141 (3), 226–232.

American Speech-Language-Hearing Association(ASHA) (2008) *No Child Left Behind(NCLB)*: Executive Summary http://www.asha.org/about/legislation-advocacy/federal/nclb/exec-summary.htm (accessed January 2009).

Anderson, A. (2004a) Issues of migration. In R. Hamilton and D. Moore (eds) *Educational Interventions for Refugee Children: Theoretical Perspectives and Implementing Best Practice* (pp. 64–82). London: RoutledgeFalmer.

Anderson, A. (2004b) Resilience. In R. Hamilton and D. Moore (eds) *Educational Interventions for Refugee Children: Theoretical Perspectives and Implementing Best Practice* (pp. 53–63). London: RoutledgeFalmer.

Anderson, R. (2002) Practical assessment strategies with Hispanic students. In A. Brice (ed.) *The Hispanic Child: Speech, Language, Culture, and Education* (pp. 143–184). Boston, MA: Allyn & Bacon.

Anionwu, E.N. (1996) Ethnic origin of sickle and thalassaemia counsellors – does it matter? In D. Kelleher and S. Hillier (eds) *Researching Cultural Differences in Healthcare* (pp. 160–189). London: Routledge.

Ara, F. and Thompson, (1989) Intervention with bilingual pre-school children. In D. Duncan (ed.) *Working with Bilingual Language Disability* (pp. 132–153). London: Paul Chapman.

Armstrong, F., Armstrong, D. and Barton, L. (eds) (2000) *Inclusive Education: Policy, Contexts and Comparative Perspectives.* London: David Fulton.

Arnot, M. and Pinson, H. (2005) *The Education of Asylum-seeker and Refugee Children.* Faculty of Education, University of Cambridge, Cambridge, UK.

Aspinall, P.J. (2005) Why the next census needs to ask about language, Editorial. *British Medical Journal* 33 (1), 363–364.

Association of Directors of Social Services (ADSS), British Deaf Association (BDA), Local Government Association (LGA), National Children's Bureau (NCB), National Deaf Children's Society (NCDS), Royal National Institute of the Deaf (RNID) (2002) *Deaf Children: Positive Practice Standards in Social Services.* London. On WWW at http://www.deaf-friendly.org.uk/SIGN_Executive_Briefing.pdf. Accessed January 2008.

Atkin, K. (2003) Ethnicity and the politics of the new genetics: Principles and engagement. *Ethnicity and Health* 8 (2), 91–109.

Atkin, K., Ahmad, W.I.U. and Jones, L. (2002) Young South Asian deaf people and their families: Negotiating relationships and identities. *Sociology of Health and Illness* 24 (1), 21–45.

Atkin, K. and Rollings, J. (1996) Looking after their own? Family care giving Asian and Afro-Caribbean communities In W.I.U. Ahmad and K. Atkin (eds) *'Race' and Community Care.* Buckingham: Open University Press.

Au, K.H. (1979) Using the experience-text relationship method with minority children. *Reading Teacher* 32 (6), 677–679.

Australian Bureau of Statistics (ABS) (2001) *Australian Social Trends* (4102.0). Canberra: AGPS.

Baca, L. and Cervantes, H.T. (eds) (1998) *The Bilingual Special Education Interface* (3rd edn). New York: Prentice Hall.

Baca, L. and Cervantes, H.T. (eds) (2003) *The Bilingual Special Education Interface* (4th edn). New York: Prentice Hall.

Baddeley, A.D. (1990) *Human Memory. Theory and Practice.* London: Lawrence Erlbaum Associates.

Baetens-Beardsmore, H. (1986) *Bilingualism: Basic Principles.* Clevedon, UK: Multilingual Matters.

Bagga-Gupta, S. and Domfors, L-A. (2003) Pedagogical issues in Swedish Deaf Education. In L. Monaghan, K. Nakamura, C. Schmaling and G. Turner (eds)

Many Ways to be Deaf: International Variation in Deaf Communities (pp. 67–88). Washington, DC: Gallaudet University Press.

Baker, C. (1992) *Attitudes and Languages*. Clevedon: Multilingual Matters.

Baker, C. (2001) *Foundations of Bilingual Education and Bilingualism*. Clevedon: Multilingual Matters.

Balarajan, R. and Soni Raleigh, V. (1995) *Ethnicity and Health in England*. London: HMSO.

Ball, M., Müller, N. and Munro, S. (2006) Phonological development and disorder of bilingual children acquiring Welsh and English. In H. Zhu and B. Dodd (eds) *Phonological Development and Disorders in Children: A Multilingual Perspective* (pp. 346–382). Clevedon: Multilingual Matters.

Barnes, C. and Mercer, G. (eds) (1996) *Exploring the Divide: Illness and Disability*. Leeds: The Disability Press.

Barnett, S. (1989) Working with interpreters. In D. Duncan (ed.) *Working with Bilingual Language Disability* (pp. 91–112). London: Paul Chapman.

Barton, D. and Hamilton, M. (1998) *Local Literacies: Reading and Writing in One Community*. London: Routledge.

Bates, E. and McWhinney, B. (1987) Competition, variation and language learning. In B. McWhinney (ed.) *Mechanisms of Language Acquisition* (pp. 157–193). Hillsdale, NJ: Erlbaum.

Battle, D. (ed.) (2002) *Communication Disorders in Multicultural Populations* (3rd edn). Stoneham, MA: Andover Medical.

Baugh, J. (1999) *Out of the Mouths of Slaves: African American Language and Educational Malpractice*. Austin: University of Texas Press.

Baxter, C., Poonia, K. and Nadirshaw, Z. (1990) *Double Discrimination*. London: King's Fund.

Bayton, D. (1996) *Forbidden Signs: American Culture and the Campaign Against Sign Language*. Chicago, IL: University of Chicago Press.

Bedore, L. and Leonard, L. (2002) Grammatical morphology deficits in Spanish-speaking children with specific language impairment *Journal of Speech, Language and Hearing Research* 44, 905–924 45.

Belsky, J. (1996) Parent, infant and social-contextual antecedents of father-son attachment security. *Developmental Psychology* 32, 905–913.

Belsky, J., Rosenberger, K. and Crnic, K. (1995) The origins of attachment security: Classical and contextual determinants. In S. Goldberg, R. Muir and J. Kerr (eds) *Attachment Theory, Social, Developmental and Clinical Perspectives* (pp. 153–184). London: The Analytic Press.

Benjamin, S. (2002) *The Micropolitics of Inclusive Education: An Ethnography*. Buckingham: Open University Press.

Beresford, B., Sloper, P. and Baldwin, S. (1996) *What Works in Services for Families with a Disabled Child?* London: Barnardos.

Berg, F.S., Blair, J.C. and Benson, P.V. (1996) Classroom acoustics: The problem, impact, and solution. *Language, Speech and Hearing Services in Schools* 27, 16–22.

Bernstein, B. (1999) Vertical and horizontal discourse: An essay. *British Journal of Sociology of Education* 20 (2), 157–173.

Bhatt, R. (1994) Word order and case in Kashmiri. PhD dissertation, University of Illinois.

Bialystok, E. (2001) *Bilingualism in Development: Language, Literacy and Cognition*. New York: Cambridge University Press.

Bishop, D. (1992) The underlying nature of specific language impairment. *Journal of Child Psychology and Psychiatry* 33 (1), 3–66.

Bishop, D. and Mogford, K. (eds) (1993) *Language Development in Exceptional Circumstances*. Lawrence Erlbaum.

Bishop, D.V.M. (1986) Is otitis media a major cause of specific developmental language disorders? *First Language* 6 (18), 225–266.

Bishop, D.V.M. (2006) What causes specific language impairment in children? *Current Directions in Psychological Science* 15, 217–221. On WWW at http://www.blackwell-synergy.com.

Bishop, D.V.M., Adams, C.V. and Rosen, S. (2006) Resistance of grammatical impairment to computerized comprehension training in children with specific and non-specific language impairments. *International Journal of Language & Communication Disorders* 41 (1), 19–40.

Bishop, D.V.M. and Baird, G. (2001) Parent and Teacher report of pragmatic aspects of communication: Use of the Children's Communication Checklist in a clinical setting. *Developmental Medicine and Child Neurology* 43, 809–818. (Erratum on p. 817, items 22–23 belong with scale D not scale C.).

Bishop, D.V.M. and Leonard, L.B. (eds) (2000) *Speech and Language Impairments in Children: Causes, Characteristics, Intervention and Outcome*. New York: Psychology Press.

Bishop, D.V.M., North, T. and Donlan, C. (1996) Nonword repetition as a behavioural marker for inherited language impairment: Evidence from a twin study, *Journal of Child Psychology and Psychiatry* 37, 4, 391–403.

Blacker, F., Crump, N. and McDonald, S. (2000) Organizing processes in complex activity networks. *Organization* 7 (2), 277–300.

Blackledge, A. (ed.) (1994) *Teaching Bilingual Children*. Stoke: Trentham Books.

Blackledge, A. (2000) *Literacy, Power and Social Justice*. Stoke: Trentham Books.

Blair, M. and Bourne, J. with Coffin, C., Creese, A. and Kenner, C. (1998) *Making the Difference: Teaching and Learning Strategies in Successful Multi-ethnic Schools*. Research Brief No 59. London: DfEE.

Blum, L.A. (2002) *I'm Not a Racist, But..: The Moral Quandary of Race*. London: Cornell University Press.

Bonnett, A. and Carrington, B. (2000) Fitting into categories or falling between them? Rethinking ethnic classification. *British Journal of Sociology of Education* 21 (4), 487–500.

Bortolini, U., Arfé, B., Caselli, M.C., Degasperi, L., Deevy, P. and Leonard, L. (2006) Clinical markers for specific language impairment in Italian: The contribution of clitics and nonword repetition. *International Journal of Language and Communication Disorders* 41 (6), 695–712.

Bortolini, U., Caselli, M.C., Deevey, P. and Leonard, L. (2002) Specific impairment in Italian: The first steps in the search for a clinical marker. *International Journal of Language and Communication Disorders* 37 (2), 77–93.

Bortolini, U. and Leonard, L. (1991) The speech of phonologically-disordered children acquiring Italian. *Clinical Linguistics and Phonetics* 5, 1–12.

Bortolini, U., Leonard, L. and Caselli, M.C. (1998) Specific language impairment in Italian and English: Evaluating alternative accounts of grammatical deficits. *Language and Cognitive Processes* 13, 1–20.

Bosch, L. and Sebastián-Gallés, N. (1997) Native-language recognition abilities in 4-month-old infants from monolingual and bilingual environments. *Cognition* 65 (1), 33–69.

Botting N. and Conti-Ramsden, G. (2000) Social and behavioural difficulties in children with language impairment. *Child Language Teaching and Therapy* 16 (2), 105–120.

Botting, N. and Conti-Ramsden, G. (2001) Non-word repetition and language development in children with specific language impairment (SLI). *International Journal of Language & Communication Disorders* 36 (4), 421–432.

Bourdieu, P. (1977) *Outline of a Theory of Practice* (R. Nice trans.). Cambridge: Cambridge University Press.

Bourdieu, P. (1983, 1986) The forms of capital. In J.G. Richardson (ed.) *Handbook of Theory and Research for the Sociology of Education* (pp. 241–258). New York: Greenwood Press (in French, 1983).

Bourdieu, P. (1993) *Sociology in Question*. London: Sage (Chapter 10, The Linguistic Market, pp. 78–89) (originally published in French as *Questions de Sociologie* by Les Editions de Minuit, Paris, 1984).

Bourne, J. (1997) The continuing revolution: Teaching as learning in the mainstream multilingual classroom. In C. Leung and C. Cable (eds) *English as an Additional Language* (pp. 77–88). York: NALDIC Publications.

Bourne, J. and McPake, J. (1991) *Partnership Teaching: Co-operative Teaching Strategies for Language Support in Multilingual Classrooms*. London: HMSO.

Bowd, A.D. (2002) *Otitis Media: Its Health, Social and Educational Consequences Particularly for Canadian Inuit, Métis, and First Nations Children and Adolescents*. Thunder Bay, Ontario: Centre of Excellence for Children and Adolescents with Special Needs, Lakehead University.

Bowd, A.D. (2005) Otitis media: Health and social consequences for aboriginal youth in Canada's north. *International Journal of Circumpolar Health* 64 (1), 5–15.

Bowd, A.D. (2008) *Otitis Media: Education and Prevention, a Follow-up Investigation*. Thunder Bay, Ontario: Centre of Excellence for Children and Adolescents with Special Needs, Lakehead University.

Bradley, L. and Bryant, P.E. (1983) Categorizing sounds and learning to read: A causal connection. *Nature* 30, 419–421.

Bradley, L. and Bryant, P.E. (1985) *Rhyme and Reason in Reading and Spelling*. Ann Arbor, MI: University of Michigan Press.

British Association for Applied Linguistics (BAAL) (2004) *Guidelines for the Use of Language Analysis in Relation to Questions of National Origin in Refugee Cases*. British Association for Applied Linguistics. On WWW at http://www.baal.org.uk/sitemap.htm.

Bronfenbrenner, U. (1970) *Two Worlds of Childhood: US and USSR*. New York: Sage.

Bronfenbrenner, U. (1979) *The Ecology of Human Development*. Cambridge, MA: Harvard University Press.

Brown, R. (1973) *A First Language: The Early Stages*. Cambridge, MA: Harvard University Press.

Bruck, M. (1984) The suitability of immersion education for children with special needs. In C. Rivera (ed.) *Communicative Competence Approaches to Language proficiency Assessment: Research and Application* (pp. 123–131). Clevedon: Multilingual Matters.

Bruck, M. and Genesee, F. (1995) Phonological awareness in young second language learners. *Journal of Child Language* 22, 307–324.

Bruner, J. (1978) The role of dialogue in language acquisition. In A. Sinclair, R.J. Jarvella and W.J. Levelt (eds) *The Child's Conception of Language* (pp. 241–256). New York: Springer-Verlag.

Bruner, J. (1986) *Actual Minds, Possible Worlds*. London: Harvard University Press.

Bullock, C. and Khalid, F.N. (1995) Health issues related to customary consanguineous marriage among British Pakistanis. *Health Promotion International* 10 (3), 209–217.

Burch, S. (2000) In a different voice: Sign language preservation in America's Deaf Community. *Bilingual Research Journal* 24 (4), 443–464.

Bury, M. (1996) Defining and researching disability: Challenges and responses. In C. Barnes and G. Mercer (eds) *Exploring the Divide: Illness and Disability* (pp. 17–38). Leeds: The Disability Press.

Bywaters, P., Ali, Z., Fazil, Q., Wallace, L. and Singh, G. (2003) Attitudes towards disability amongst Pakistani and Bangladeshi parents of disabled children in the UK: Considerations for service providers and the disability movement. *Health and Social Care in the Community* 11 (6), 502–509.

Cameron, L. (2003) *Metaphor in Educational Discourse*. London: Continuum.

Campbell, C. and McLean, C. (2001) Representations of ethnicity in people's accounts of local community participation in a multi-ethnic community in England. *Journal of Community and Applied Social Psychology* 12 (1), 13–29.

Campbell, R. and Sais, E. (1995) Accelerated metalinguistic (phonological) awareness in bilingual children. *British Journal of Developmental Psychology* 13, 61–68.

Campbell, T., Dollaghan, C., Needleman, H. and Janosky, J. (1997) Reducing bias in language assessment: Processing-dependent measures. *Journal of Speech, Language, and Hearing Research* 40, 519–525.

Canagarajah, A.S. (1999) *Resisting Linguistic Imperialism in English Teaching*. Oxford; Oxford University Press.

Carpenter, B. (ed.) (1997) *Families in Context: Emerging Trends in Family Support and Early Intervention*. London: David Fulton.

Carr, M. (2002) Emerging learning narratives: A perspective from early childhood education. In G. Wells and G. Claxton (eds) *Learning for Life in the 21st Century* (pp. 99–111). Oxford: Blackwell.

Carr-Hill, R., Passingham, S., Wolf, A. and Kent, N. (1996) *Lost Opportunities: The Language Skills of Linguistic Minorities in England and Wales*. London: Basic Skills Agency.

Carrier, J.G. (1983) Explaining educability: An investigation of political support for children with learning disabilities. *British Journal of Sociology of Education* 4 (2), 28.

Carter, J.A., Lees, J.A., Murira, G.M., Gona J., Neville, B. and Newton, C. (2005) Issues in the development of cross-cultural assessments of speech and language for children. *International Journal of Language and Communication Disorders* 40 (4), 385–401.

Cashman, J., Linehan, P. and Rosser, M. (2007) *Communities of Practice: A New Approach to Solving Complex Educational Problems*. Alexandria, VA: National Association of State Directors of Special Education. On WWW at www.ideapartnership.org.

Castles, A. and Coltheart, M. (1993) Varieties of developmental dyslexia, *Cognition* 47, 149–180.

Castro, A., Nunes, T. and Strecht-Ribeiro, O. (2004) Relacao entre consciencia grammatical na linguagem maternal e progresso na apredizagem de uma lingua estrangeira. *Da Investigacao as practicas. Estudos de Natureza Educacional* 5, 51–66.

Catts, H.W., Adlof, S.M., Hogan, T.P. and Ellis Weismer, S. (2005) Are specific language impairment and dyslexia distinct disorders? *Journal of Speech, Language, and Hearing Research* 48, 1378–1396.

Caulfield, M.B., Fischel, J.E., DeBaryshe, B.D. and Whitehurst, G.J. (1989) Behavioural correlates of developmental expressive language disorder. *Journal of Abnormal Child Psychology* 19, 187–201.

Centeno, J., Anderson, R. and Obler, L. (eds) (2007) *Communication Disorders in Spanish Speakers.* Clevedon: Multilingual Matters.

Chamba, R., Ahmad, W., Hirst, M., Lawton, D. and Beresford, D. (1999) *On the Edge: Minority Ethnic Families Caring for a Severely Disabled Child.* Bristol: Policy Press.

Chen, X., Rubin, K.H. and Sun, Y. (1992) Social reputation and peer relationships in Chinese and Canadian children: A cross-cultural study. *Child Development* 63, 1336–1343.

Cheng, L., Battle, D., Murdoch, B. and Martin, D. (2001) Educating speech-language pathologists for a multicultural world. *Folia Phoniatrica et Logopaedica* 53, 121–127.

Chiat, S. (2000) *Understanding Children with Language Problems.* Cambridge: Cambridge University Press

Christie, F. and Martin, J.R. (eds) (2007) *Knowledge and Pedagogy: Functional Linguistic and Sociological Perspectives.* London: Continuum.

Clark, E.V. (1993) *The Lexicon in Acquisition.* Cambridge: Cambridge University Press.

Clark, M., Owen, D.W., Szcepura, A. and Johnson, M.R.D. (1998) *Assessment of the Costs to the NHS Arising from the Need for Interpreter, Advocacy and Translation (IAT) Services.* Report prepared for the Department of Health Technical Advisory Group. Warwick: Centre for Health Services Studies and Centre for Research in Ethnic Relations, University of Warwick.

Claxton, G. (2002) Educating for the learning age: A sociocultral approach to learning to learn. In G. Wells and G. Claxton (eds) *Learning for Life in the 21ˢᵗ Century: Sociocultural Perspectives on the Future of Education* (pp. 21–33). Oxford: Blackwell.

Clegg, J., Hollis, C., Mawhood, L. and Rutter, M. (2005) Developmental language disorders – a follow-up in later adult life. Cognitive, language and psycho-social outcomes. *Journal of Child Psychology and Psychiatry* 46 (2), 128–149.

Cline, T. (1997) Educating for bilingualism in different contexts: Teaching the deaf and teaching children with English as an additional language. *Educational Review* 49 (2), 151–158.

Cline, T. (2000) Multilingualism and dyslexia: Challenges for research and practice. *Dyslexia* Special Issue: *Multilingualism and Dyslexia (Part One)* 6 (1), 3–12.

Cline, T., de Abreu, G., Fihosy, C., Gray, H., Lambert, H. and Neale, J. (2002) *Minority Ethnic Pupils in Mainly White Schools*. London: Department for Education and Skills.

Cline, T. and Frederickson, N. (1999) Identification and assessment of dyslexia in bi/multilingual children. *International Journal of Bilingual Education and Bilingualism* 2, 81–93.

Cline, T., Ganschow, L. and Reason, R. (eds) (2000) Multilingualism and dyslexia: Including the teaching of modern foreign languages. *Dyslexia*, Special Issue: *Multilingualism and Dyslexia (Part One)* 6 (1), 1–84 (Editorial 1–2).

Cline, T. and Reason, R. (1993) Specific learning difficulties (dyslexia): Equal opportunities issues. *British Journal of Special Education* 20 (1), 30–34.

Cline, T. and Shamsi, T. (2000) *Language Needs or Special Needs? The Assessment of Learning Difficulties in Literacy Among Children Learning English as an Additional Language: A Literature Review*. Research Report 184. London: Department for Education and Employment.

Cloud, N. (1994) Special education needs of second language students. In F. Genesee (ed.) *Educating Second Language Children: The Whole Child, the Whole Curriculum, The Whole Community* (pp. 243–277). New York: Cambridge University Press.

Clough, P. and Barton, L. (eds) (1995) *Making Difficulties – Research and the Construction of SEN*. London: Paul Chapman.

Coard, B. (1971) *How the West Indian Child is Made Educationally Subnormal in the British School System: The Scandal of the Black Child in Schools in Britain*. First published by the Caribbean Education and Community Workers' Association: New Beacon Books Ltd.

Coard, B. (2005) *How the West Indian Child is Made Educationally Subnormal in the British School System: The Scandal of the Black Child in Schools in Britain*. Republished in B. Richardson (ed.) *Tell It How It Is: How our Schools Fail Black Children* (pp. 27–59). Bookmarks Publication, Trentham Books.

Cobo-Lewis, A.B., Eilers, R.E., Pearson, B.Z. and Umbel, V.C. (2002) Interdependence of Spanish and English knowledge in language and literacy among bilingual children. In D.K. Oller and R.E. Eilers (eds) *Language and Literacy in Bilingual Children* (pp. 118–134). Clevedon: Multilingual Matters.

Cole, M. (1996) *Cultural Psychology: A Once and Future Discipline*. Cambridge, MA: The Bellknap Press of Harvard University Press.

Cole, P. and Taylor, O.L. (1990) Performance of working class African American children on three tests of articulation. *Language, Speech and Hearing Services in Schools* 21 (3), 171–176.

Coleman, J.S. (1990) *Foundations of Social Theory*. Cambridge, MA: Harvard University Press.

Commission for Racial Equality (CRE) (1992) *Ethnic Monitoring in Education*. London: CRE.

Commission for Racial Equality (CRE) (1996) *Special Educational Needs Assessment in Strathclyde: Report of a Formal Investigation*. London: CRE.

Conrad, R. (1979) *The Deaf Schoolchild: Language and Cognitive Function*. London: Harper & Row.

Constable, A. (1993) Investigating word-finding difficulties in children. Unpublished MSc thesis, College of Speech Sciences, University College London.

Constable, A. (2001) A psycholinguistic approach to word-finding difficulties. In J. Stackhouse and B. Wells (eds) *Children's Speech and Language Difficulties 2* (pp. 330–365). London: Whurr.

Conti-Ramsden, G. and Botting, N. (1999) Characteristics of children attending language units in England: A national study of 7-year-olds. *International Journal of Language and Communication Disorders* 34, 359–366.

Conti-Ramsden, G. and Botting, N. (2004) Social difficulties and victimization in children with SLI at 11 years of age. *Journal of Speech, Language, and Hearing Research* 47 145–161.

Cooper, P., Drummond, M., Hart, S., Lovey, J. and McLaughlin, C. (2000) *Positive Alternatives to Exclusion*. London: Routledge Falmer.

Cooper, P. (2006) Supporting minority ethnic children adolescents with social, emotional, and behavioural difficulties in the United Kingdom. *Preventing School Failure* 50 (2), 21–28.

Copa, A., Loraine Lucinski, B., Olsen, E. and Wollenburg, K. (1999) Promoting Professional and Organizational Development: A Reflective Practice Model, *ZERO TO THREE: National Center for Infants Toddlers and Families, (Aug/Sept Issue)* Portage, WI: The Portage Project. On WWW at http://www.zeroto three.org.

Corbett, J. (1996) *The Language of Special Needs*. London: Falmer Press.

Craig, H.K. and Washington, J.A. (1993) Access behaviors of children with specific language impairment. *Journal of Speech and Hearing Research* 36, 322–337.

Craig, H.K. and Washington, J.A. (2002) Oral language expectations for African American preschoolers and kindergartners. *American Journal of Speech-Language Pathology* 11, 59–70.

Craig, H.K. and Washington, J.A. (2004) Grade-related changes in the production of African American English. *Journal of Speech, Language, and Hearing Research* 47, 450–463.

Craig, H.K. Thompson, C.A., Washington, J.A. and Potter, S.L. (2003) Phonological features of child African American English. *Journal of Speech, Language, and Hearing Research* 46, 623–635.

Craig, J., Huber, J. and Lownsbrough, H. (2004) *Schools Out: Extended schools*. HayGroup: Demos. On WWW at http://www.demos.co.uk.

Crais, E.R. (1992) "Best practices" with preschoolers: Assessing within the context of a family centered approach. *Best Practices in School Speech-Language Pathology* 2, 33–42.

Creese, A. (2002) The discursive construction of power in teacher partnerships: Language and subject specialists in mainstream schools. *TESOL Quarterly* 36 (4), 597–616.

Creese, A. (2005) *Teacher Collaboration and Talk in Multilingual Classrooms*. Clevedon: Multilingual Matters.

Creese, A., Bhatt, A., Bhojani, N. and Martin, P. (2006) Multicultural heritage and learner identities in complementary schools. *Language and Education* 20, 23–43.

Creese, A., Daniels, H. and Norwich, B. (1997) *Teacher Support Teams in Secondary Schools*. London: David Fulton.

Creese, A., Norwich, B. and Daniels, H. (2000) Evaluating teacher support teams in secondary schools: Supporting teachers for SEN and other needs. *Research Papers in Education* 15 (3), 307–324.

Croll, P. and Moses, D. (2000) Continuity and change in special school provision; some perspectives on local education authority policy-making. *British Educational Research Journal* 26 (2), 177–190.

Crosbie, S., Holm, A. and Dodd, B. (2005) Intervention for children with severe speech disorder: A comparison of two approaches. *International Journal of Language Communication Disorders* 40, 467–491.

Crossley, N. (2005) *Critical Social Theory*. London: Sage.

Crutchley, A. (1999) Professional attitudes and experience in relation to bilingual children attending language units. *British Educational Research Journal* 25 (3), 371–388.

Crystal, D. (1987) Towards a bucket theory of language disability: Taking account of interaction between linguistic levels. *Clinical Linguistics and Phonetics* 1, 7–22.

Cummins, J. (1977) Cognitive factors associated with the attainment of intermediate levels of bilingual skills. *Modern Language Journal* 61, 3–12.

Cummins, J. (1981) *Bilingualism and Language Minority Children*. Ontario: Ontario Institute for Studies in Education.

Cummins, J. (1984) *Bilingualism and Special Education: Issues in Assessment and Pedagogy*. Clevedon: Multilingual Matters (Co-published in USA by College-Hill Press).

Cummins, J. (1994). Knowledge, power and identity in teaching English as a second language. In F. Genesee (ed.) *Educating Second Language Children: The Whole Child, the Whole Curriculum, the Whole Community* (pp. 33–58). Cambridge: Cambridge University Press.

Cummins, J. (2000) *Language, Power and Pedagogy: Bilingual Children in the Crossfire*. Clevedon: Multilingual Matters.

Cunningham, C. and Davis, H. (1985) *Working with Parents: Frameworks for Collaboration*. Open University Press.

Cunningham-Andersson, U. and Andersson, S. (1999) *Growing Up with Two Languages: A Practical Guide*. London: Routledge.

Dale, P., Simonoff, E., Bishop, D., Eley, T., Oliver, B., Price, T., Purcell, S., Stevenson, J. and Plomin R. (1998) Genetic influence on language delay in two-year-old children. *Nature Neuroscience* 1, 324–328.

D'Anglejan, A. and Renaud, C. (1985) Learner characteristics and second language acquisition: A multivariate study of adult immigrants and some thoughts on methodology. *Language Learning* 35, 1–19.

Daniels, H. (2001) *Vygotsky and Pedagogy*. London: RoutledgeFalmer.

Daniels, H. and Anghileri, J. (1995) *Secondary School Mathematics and Special Educational Needs*. London: Cassell.

Daniels, H., Creese, A., Fielding, S., Hey, V., Leonard, D. and Smith, M. (2001a) The gendering of social practices in special needs education. In M. Hedegaard (ed.) *Learning in Classrooms: A Cultural-historical Approach* (pp. 39–58). Aarhus: Aarhus University Press.

Daniels, H., Creese, A., Hey, V., Leonard, D. and Smith, M. (2001b) Gender and learning: Equity, equality and pedagogy. *Support for Learning* 16 (3), 112–116.

Daniels, H., Creese, A. and Norwich, B. (2000a) Supporting collaborative problem-solving in schools. In H. Daniels (ed.) *Special Education Re-formed. Beyond Rhetoric?* (pp. 173–186). London: Falmer Press.

Daniels, H., Hey, V. Leonard, D. and Smith, M. (2000b) Issues of equity in special needs education as seen from the perspective of gender. In H. Daniels (ed.) *Special Education Reformed: Beyond Rhetoric?* (pp. 47–66). London: Falmer Press.

Darr, A. (1999) *Access to Genetic Services by Minority Ethnic Populations: A Pilot Study.* London: Genetic Interest Group. On WWW at www.gig.org.uk.

Datta, M. (ed.) (2007) *Bilingualism and Biliteracy: Principles and Practice.* London: Continuum.

Davis, R. (1997) *The Gift of Dyslexia* (rev. edn). New York: Perigee.

Davis, P. and Florian, L. (2004) *Teaching Strategies and Approaches for Children with Special Educational Needs. A scoping study.* Research Report 516. London: Department of Education and Skills.

Davis, T.C., Mayeaux, E.J., Fredrickson D., Bocchini, J.A. Jr., Jackson, R.H. and Murphy, P.W. (1994) Reading ability of parents compared with reading level of pediatric patient education materials. *Pediatrics* 93, 460–468 [Abstract].

de Bot, K. (1992) A bilingual production model: Levelt's 'speaking' model adapted. *Applied Linguistics* 13, 1–24.

de Houwer, A. (1990) *The Acquisition of Two Languages from Birth: A Case Study.* Cambridge, MA: Cambridge University Press.

de la Mata, M. and Santamaria, A. (2001) Teacher–student interaction, text comprehension and memory: A semiotic analysis of instructional actions. In M. Hedegaard (ed.) *Learning in Classrooms: A Cultural-historical Approach* (pp. 258–279). Aarhus: Aarhus University Press.

Del Giudice, E., Luigi Trojano, L., Fragassi. N., Posteraro, S., Crisanti, A., Tanzarella, P., Marino, A. and Grossi, D. (2000) Spatial cognition in children. II. Visuospatial and constructional skills in developmental reading disability. *Brain and Development* 22 (6), 368–372.

Delgado-Gaitan, C. (1991) Involving parents in the schools: A process of empowerment. *American Journal of Education* 100 (1), 20–46.

Demie, F. (2001) Ethnic and gender differences in educational achievement and implications for school improvement strategies. *Educational Research* 43 (1), 91–106.

Department for Education and Science (DES) (1985) *Education for All* (Report of Committee of Enquiry into the education of children from ethnic minorities: The Swan Report). London: HMSO.

Department for Education (DfE) (1994) *Code of Practice on the Identification and Assessment of Special Educational Needs.* London: HMSO.

Department for Education and Employment (DfEE) (1997) *Excellence for All Children: Meeting Special Educational Needs.* London: DfEE.

Department for Education and Employment (DfEE) (1999) Ethnic Minority Pupils and Pupils for whom english is an Additional Language: England 1996/97. Statistical Bulletin No. 3/99. London: HMSO.

Department for Education and Employment (DfEE) (2000) *Provision of Speech and Language Therapy Services to Children with Special Educational Needs (England): Report of the Working Group.* London: DfEE.

Department for Education and Employment (DfEE) (2001a) *Code of Practice on the Identification and Assessment of Special Educational Needs, and SEN Thresholds: Good Practice Guidance on Identification and Provision for Pupils with Special Educational Needs.* London: HMSO.

Department for Education and Employment (DfEE) (2001b) *Permanent Exclusions from Schools, England, 1999/2000.* London: DfE.

Department for Education and Skills (2003) *Every Child Matters.* Green Paper. London: HMSO

Department of Health (2005) *A Practical Guide to Ethnic Monitoring in the NHS and Social Care.* London: HMSO.

Deponio, P., Landon J., Mullin, K. and Reid G. (2000) An audit of the processes involved in identifying and assessing bilingual learners suspected of being dyslexic: A Scottish study. *Dyslexia* 6 (1), 29–41.

Diniz, F.A. (1999) Race and special educational needs in the 1990s. *British Journal of Special Education* 26 (4), 213–217.

Diniz, F.A. and Usmani, K. (2001) Changing the discourse on 'race' in special educational needs. *Multicultural Teaching* 20 (1), 25–28.

Dockrell, J. and Lindsay, G. (1998) The ways in which speech and language difficulties impact on children's access to the curriculum. *Child Language Teaching and Therapy* 14 (2), 117–133.

Dockrell, J. and McShane, J. (1993) *Children's Learning Difficulties.* Oxford: Blackwell.

Dodd, B. (ed.) (1995) *The Differential Diagnosis and Treatment of Children with Speech Disorder.* London: Whurr.

Dodd, B., Crosbie, S., MacIntosh, B., Teitzel, T. and Ozanne, A., (2000) *Primary and Preschool Battery of Phonological Awareness (PIPA).* London: Psychological Corporation.

Dodd, B. and McCormack, P. (1995) A model of speech processing of phonological disorders. In B. Dodd (ed.) *The Differential Diagnosis and Treatment of Children with Speech Disorder* (pp. 65–89). San Diego, CA: Singular Publishing Group.

Dollaghan, C. and Campbell, T.F. (1998) Nonword repetition and child language impairment. *Journal of Speech, Language, and Hearing Research* 41, 1136–1146.

Donato, R. (2000) Sociocultural contributions to understanding the foreign and second language classroom. In J. Lantolf (ed.) *Sociocultural Theory and Second Language Learning* (pp. 27–50). Oxford: Oxford University Press.

Dowling, E. and Osborne, E. (1994) *The Family and the School: A Joint Systems Approach to Problems with Children* (2nd edn). London: Routledge.

Dromi, E., Leonard, L.B., Adam, G. and Zadunaisky-Ehrlich, S. (1999) Verb agreement morphology in Hebrew-speaking children with specific language impairment. *Journal of Speech, Language and Hearing Research* 42 (6), 1414–1431.

Duchan, J.F. and Kovarsky, D. (eds) (2005) *Diagnosis as Cultural Practice.* New York: Mouton de Gruyter.

Dulay, H. and Burt, M. (1974) Natural sequences in child second language acquisition. *Language Learning* 24 (1), 37–53.

Duncan*, D. (1989a) Semantic relations and Vocabulary in L2 English. Unpublished PhD thesis. CNAA

Duncan*, D. (ed.) (1989) *Working with Bilingual Language Disability.* London: Paul Chapman.

* D. Duncan previous name of D. Martin.

Duncan*, D. and Gibbs, D. (1987) Acquisition of syntax in Panjabi and English. *The British Journal of Disorders of Communication* 22 (2), 129–144.

Dunn, L.M. and Dunn, L.M. (1981) *Peabody Picture Vocabulary Test-III*. Circle Pines, MN: American Guidance Service.

Dunn, L.M. and Dunn, L.M. (1997) *Peabody Picture Vocabulary Test-III*. Circle Pines, MN: American Guidance Service.

Durgunoglu, A., Nagy, W. and Hancin-Bhatt, B. (1993) Cross-language transfer of phonological awareness. *Journal of Educational Psychology* 85, 453–465.

Durgunoglu, A.Y. and Verhoeven, L. (1998) Epilogue: Multilingualism and literacy development across different cultures. In A.Y. Durgunoglu and L. Verhoeven (eds) *Literacy Development in a Multilingual Context: Cross-cultural Perspectives* (pp. 289–298). Mahwah, NJ: Lawrence Erlbaum Associates.

Dwivedi, K.N. (ed.) (2002) *Meeting the Needs of Ethnic Minority Children: A Handbook for Professionals* (2nd edn). London: Jessica Kingsley.

Eadie, P. (2004a) The evidence base for the management of late talkers. In S. Reilly, J. Douglas and J. Oates (eds) *Evidence Based Practice in Speech Pathology* (pp. 206–218). London: Whurr.

Eadie, P. (2004b) The evidence base for the diagnosis of developmental language disorders: Research to clinical practice. In S. Reilly, J. Douglas and J. Oates (eds) *Evidence Based Practice in Speech Pathology* (pp. 185–205). London: Whurr.

Ebbels, S.H. (2007) Teaching grammar to school-aged children with specific language impairment using shape coding. *Child Language Teaching and Therapy* 23 (1), 67–93.

Ebbels, S. and van der Lely, H.K.J. (2001) Meta-syntactic therapy for children with severe persistent SLI using visual coding. *International Journal of Language and Communication Disorders* 36 (supplement), 345–350.

The Education Act (1981) London: Houses of Parliament, UK.

Ellis Weismar, S., Evans, J. and Hesketh, L.J. (1999) An examination of verbal working memory capacity in children with specific language impairment. *Journal of speech, Language and Hearing Research* 42, 1249–1260.

Ellis Weismer, S. and Hesketh, L. (1996) Lexical learning by children with specific language impairment: Effects of linguistic input presented at varying speaking rates. *Journal of Speech and Hearing Research* 39, 177–190.

Ellis Weismer, S., Tomblin, B., Zhang, X., Buckwalter, P., Chynoweth, J. and Jones, M. (2000) Nonword repetition performance in school-age children with and without language impairment. *Journal of Speech, Language, and Hearing Research* 43, 865–878.

Enderby, P. and Emerson, J. (1995) *Does speech and language therapy work?* London: Whurr.

Engeström, Y. (1987) *Learning by Expanding: An Activity-Theoretical Approach to Development Research*. Helsinki, Orienta-Konsultit.

Engeström, Y. (1995) Voice as communicative action. *Mind, Culture and Activity* 2, 192–214.

Engeström, Y. (1999) Innovative learning in work teams: Analyzing cycles of knowledge creation in practice. In Y. Engeström, R. Miettinen and R-L. Punamki (eds) *Perspectives on Activity Theory*. New York: Cambridge University Press.

Engeström, Y. (2007) Putting Vygotsky to work: The Change Laboratory as an application of double stimulation. In H. Daniels, M. Cole and J. Wertsch (eds)

The Cambridge Companion to Vygotsky (pp. 363–382). New York: Cambridge University Press.

Engeström, Y., Brown, K., Christopher, L.C. and Gregory, J. (1997) Coordination, co-operation and communication in the courts: Expansive transitions in legal work. In M. Cole, Y. Engeström and O. Vasquez (eds) *Mind, Culture and Activity.* Cambridge: Cambridge University Press.

Eraut, M. (1995) Schon Shock: A case for reframing reflection-in-action? Teachers and Teaching 1 (1), 9–22.

Eraut, M. (2000) Non-formal learning, implicit learning and tacit knowledge in professional work. *British Journal of Educational Psychology* 70, 113–136.

Eraut, M. (2002) Conceptual analysis and research questions: Do the concepts 'learning community' and 'community of practice' provide added value? Paper presented at American Education Research Association (AERA) conference, New Orleans, LA, April 2002.

Eraut, M. (2004) Informal learning in the workplace. *Studies in Continuing Education* 26 (2), 247–273.

Evans, P. (1995) *Intergrating Students with Special Needs into Mainstream Schools.* Paris, OECD.

Evans, P. (2000) Evidence-based practice: How will we know what works? An international perspective. In H. Daniels (ed.) *Special Education Reformed: Beyond Rhetoric?* (pp. 69–84). London: Falmer Press.

Every Child Matters (2003) Green Paper. London: HMSO.

Fagundes, D., Haynes, W., Haak, N. and Moran, M. (1998) Task variability effects on the language test performance of southern lower socioeconomic class African American and Caucasian five year olds. *Language, Speech and Hearing Services in Schools* 29, 148–157.

Fantini, A.E. (1985) *Language Acquisition of a Bilingual Child.* Clevedon: Multilingual Matters.

Fathman, A. (1975) The relationship between age and second language productive ability. *Language Learning* 25 (2), 245–253.

Fawcett, A. and Lynch, L. (2000) Systematic identification and intervention for reading difficulty: Case studies of children with EAL. *Dyslexia* 6 (1), 57–71.

Fazil, Q., Bywaters, P., Ali, Z., Wallace, L. and Singh, G. (2002) Disadvantage and discrimination compounded: The experience of Pakistani and Bangladeshi parents of disabled children in the UK. *Disability and Society* 17 (3), 237–253.

Feliciano, C. (2001) The benefits of biculturalism: exposure to immigrant culture and dropping out of school among Asian and Latino youths, *Social Science Quarterly* 82 (4), 865–879.

Fey, M.E., Long, S.H. and Finestack, L.H. (2003) Ten principles of grammatical intervention for children with specific language impairments. *American Journal of Speech-Language Pathology* 12, 3–15.

Fisher, C., Hall, D.G., Rakowitz, S. and Gleitman, L. (1994) When it is better to receive than to give: Syntactic and conceptual constraints on vocabulary growth. *Lingua* 92, 333–375.

Fisher, L., Rowley, P.T. and Lipkin, M.R. Jr. (1981) Genetic counseling for beta-thalasseamia trait following health screening in a health maintenance organisation: Comparison of programmed and conventional counseling. *American Journal of Human Genetics* 33 (6), 987–994.

Fitzgerald, T., Duva, S., Ostrer, H., Pass, K., Oddoux, C., Ruben, R. and Caggana, M. (2004) The frequency of GJB2 and GJB6 mutations in the New York State newborn population: Feasibility of genetic screening for hearing defects. *Clinical Genetics* 65, 338–342.

Fitzpatrick, F. (1987) *The Open Door: The Bradford Bilingual Project*. Clevedon: Multilingual Matters.

Fletcher, P. and Hall, D. (eds) (1992) *Specific Speech and Language Disorders in Children*. London: Whurr.

Fletcher-Campbell, F. (2001) Issues of exclusion: Evidence from three recent research studies. *Emotional and Behavioural Difficulties* 6 (2), 69–89.

Fodor, J. (1983) *The Modularity of Mind*. Cambridge, Mass: MIT Press.

Foster-Galasso, M.L. (2005) Diagnosis as an aid and a curse in dealing with others. In J.F. Duchan and D. Kovarsky (eds) *Diagnosis as Cultural Practice* (pp. 17–32). New York: Mouton de Gruyter.

Fox, A. (2006) Evidence from German speaking children. In H. Zhu and B. Dodd (eds) *Phonological Development and Disorders in Children: A Multilingual Perspective* (pp. 56–80). Clevedon: Multilingual Matters.

Fox, A. and Dodd, B. (2001). Phonological disorders in German-speaking children. *American Journal of Speech and Language-Pathology* 10, 291–307.

Fredrickson, N. and Cline, T. (eds) (1990) *Curriculum Related Assessment with Bilingual Children*. London: Educational Psychology Publishing.

Fredrickson, N. and Cline, T. (2002) *Special Educational Needs, Inclusion and Diversity: A Textbook*. Buckingham: Open University Press.

Frederickson, N.L. and Frith, U. (1998) Identifying dyslexia in bilingual children: A phonological approach with Inner London Sylheti speakers. *Dyslexia* 4, 119–131.

Frederickson, N.L., Frith, U. and Reason, R. (1997) *The Phonological Assessment Battery (PhAB), Standardisation Edition*. Windsor: NFER-Nelson.

Fujiura, G.T. and Yamaki, K. (2000) Trends in demography of childhood poverty and disability. *Exceptional Children* 66 (2), 187–199.

Gadesmann, M. and Miller, N. (2008) Reliability of speech diadochokinetic test measurement. *International Journal of Language and Communication Disorders* 43 (1), 41–54.

Gallagher, A. M. (1997) Educational Achievement and Gender: a review of research evidence of the apparent underachievement of boys. Dept. of Education, Northern Ireland, Research Report No. 6.

Gallaudet Research Institute (1996) *Stanford Achievement Test, 9th Edition, Form S, Norms Booklet for Deaf and Hard of Hearing Students*. Washington, DC: Gallaudet University. On WWW at http://gri.gallaudet.edu/Literacy.

Galton, M., Simon, B. and Croll, P. (1980) *Inside the Primary Classroom* (The ORACLE Report). London: Routledge and Kegan Paul.

Ganschow, L. and Sparks, R. (1993) Foreign language and learning disabilities: Issues, research and teaching implications. In S.A. Vogel and P.B. Adelman (eds) *Success for College Students with Learning Disabilities* (pp. 283–322). New York: Springer-Verlag.

Garcia, S.B. and Dominguez, L. (1997) Cultural contexts that influence learning and academic performance. In L.B. Silver (ed.) *Child and Adolescent Psychiatric Clinic of North America: Academic Difficulties* (pp. 621–655). Philadelphia, PA: Saunders Co.

Gathercole, S. and Baddeley, A. (1996) *The Children's Test of Non-Word Repetition.* London: Psychological Corporation.

Gaulin, C. and Campbell, T. (1994) Procedure for assessing verbal working memory in normal school-age children: Some preliminary data. *Perceptual and Motor Skills* 79, 55–64.

Gee, J.P. (2005) *An Introduction to Discourse Analysis: Theory and Method* (2nd edn). London: Routledge.

Geers, A. and Brenner, C. (2003) Background and educational characteristics of prelingually deaf children implanted by five years of age. *Ear and Hearing* 24 (1), 2S–14S.

Genesee, F. (1989) Early bilingual development: One language or two. *Journal of Child Language* 6, 161–179.

Genesee, F., Paradis, J. and Crago, M. (2004) *Dual Language Development and Disorders: A Handbook on Bilingualism and Second Language Learning.* Baltimore, MD: Paul Brookes.

Gersten, R. and Woodward, J. (1994) The language-minority student and special education: Issues, trends, and paradoxes. *Exceptional Children* 60 (4), 310–322.

Ghate, D. and Hazel, N. (2002) *Parenting in Poor Environments: Stress, Support and Coping.* London: Jessica Kingsley.

Gibbons, P. (2002) *Scaffolding Language, Scaffolding Learning: Teaching Second Language Learners in the Mainstream Classroom.* Westport, CT: Heinemann.

Gibbons, P. (1993) *Learning to Learn in a Second Language.* Westport, CT: Heinemann.

Gibbs, J.T. and Huang, L.N. (1989) A conceptual framework for assessing and treating minority youth. In J.T. Gibbs and L.N. Huang (eds) *Children of Color: Psychological Interventions with Minority Youth* (pp. 1–29). San Francisco, CA: Jossey-Bass.

Giddens, A. (1992) *The Transformation of Intimacy: Sexuality, Love and Eroticism in Modern Societies.* Cambridge: Polity.

Gillborn, D. (1997) Racism and reform: New ethnicities/old inequalities? *British Educational Research Journal* 23 (3), 345–360.

Gillborn, D. and Gipps, C. (1996) *Recent Research on the Achievements of Ethnic Minority Pupils.* London: OFSTED.

Gillborn, D. and Mirza, H.S. (2000) *Educational Inequality: Mapping Race, Class and Gender: A Synthesis of Research Evidence.* London: OFSTED.

Gillborn, D. and Youdell, D. (2000) *Rationing Education: Policy, Practice, Reform and Equity.* Buckingham: Open University Press.

Gindis, B. (2003) Remediation through education: Sociocultural theory and children with special needs. In A. Kozulin, B. Gindis, V.S. Ageyev and S. Miller (eds) *Vygotsky's Educational Theory in Cultural Context* (pp. 200–221). Cambridge: Cambridge University Press.

Girbau, D. and Schwartz, R.G. (2007) Non-word repetition in Spanish-speaking children with specific language impairment (SLI). *International Journal of Language and Communication Disorders* 42 (1), 59–75.

Glisson, C. and Hemmelgarn, A. (1998) The effects of organizational climate and interorganizational coordination on the quality and outcomes of children's service systems. *Child Abuse and Neglect* 22 (5), 401–421.

Goldfus, C. (2001) Reading comprehension and EFL adolescents with difficulties: A cognitive processing model. Unpublished doctoral thesis, University of Birmingham.

Goldstein, B. (2005) Substitutions in the phonology of Spanish-speaking children. *Journal of Multilingual Communication Disorders* 3, 56–63.

Gopnik, M. and Crago, M.B. (1991) Familial aggregation of a developmental language disorder. *Cognition* 39 (1), 1–50.

Goswami, U. (1992) Annotation: Phonological factors in spelling development. *Journal of Child Psychology and Psychiatry* 33 (6), 967–975.

Goswami, U. (2004) Neuroscience and education. *British Journal of Educational Psychology* 74 (1), 1–14.

Graf Estes, K., Evans, J.L. and Else-Quest, N.M. (2007) Differences in the nonword repetition performance of children with and without specific language impairment: A meta-analysis. *Journal of Speech, Language, and Hearing Research* 50, 177–195.

Gregory, E. (1996) Learning from the community: A family project with Bangladeshi origin children in London. In S. Wolfendale and K. Topping (eds) *Family Involvement in Literacy. Effective Partnerships in Education*. London. Cassell.

Gregory, E. (ed.) (1997) *One Child: Many Worlds*. London: David Fulton.

Gregory, E. (1998) Siblings as mediators of literacy in linguistic minority communities. *Language and Education* 12 (1), 33–54.

Gregory, E. and Biarnes, J. (1994) Tony and Jean-Francois looking for sense in the strangeness of school. In H. Dombey and M. Meek Spencer (eds) *First Steps Together*. Stoke: Trentham Books.

Grundy, K. (1989) *Linguistics in Clinical Practice*. London: Whurr.

Grunwell, P. (1987) *Clinical Phonology* (2nd edn). London: Croom Helm.

Gupta, A. (2004) Reading difficulties of Hindi-speaking children with developmental dyslexia. *Reading and Writing: An Interdisciplinary Journal* 17, 79–99.

Gutierrez, K. and Rogoff, B. (2003) Cultural ways of learning: Individual traits or repertoires of practice. *Educational Researcher* 32 (5), 19–25.

Gutierrez-Clellen, V.F. (1999) Language choice in interventions with bilingual children. *American Journal of Speech Language Pathology* 6, 291–302.

Gutiérrez-Clellen, V.F. (2002) Narratives in two languages: Assessing performance of bilingual children. *Linguistics and Education* 13 (2), 175–197.

Gutierrez-Clellen, V., Calderon, J. and Ellis Weismer, S. (2004) Verbal working memory in bilingual children. *Journal of Speech, Language, and Hearing Research* 47, 863–876.

Gutiérrez-Clellen, V.F. and Peña, E. (2001) Dynamic assessment of diverse children, a tutorial. *Language, Speech, and Hearing Services in Schools* 32, 212–224.

Gutiérrez-Clellen, V.F. and Quinn, R. (1993) Assessing narratives in diverse cultural/linguistic populations: Clinical implications. *Language, Speech, and Hearing Services in Schools* 24, 2–9.

Hager, P. (2004) Lifelong learning in the workplace? Challenges and issues. *Journal of Workplace Learning* 16 (1/2), 22–32.

Håkansson, G. (2001) Tense morphology and verb-second in Swedish L1 children, L2 children and children with SLI. *Bilingualism, Language and Cognition* 4, 85–99.

Håkanssson, G. (2005) Similarities and differences in L1 and L2 development: Opening up the perspective: Including SLI. In M. Pienemann (ed.) *Cross-linguistic Aspects of Processability Theory* (pp. 179–197). Amsterdam: John Benjamins.

Håkansson, G. and Nettelbladt, U. (1996) Similarities between SLI and L2 children: Evidence from the acquisition of Swedish word order. In C. Johnson and J. Gilbert (eds) *Children's Language, 9* (pp. 135–151). Hillsdale, NJ: Lawrence Erlbaum.

Håkansson, G., Salameh, E.K. and Nettelbladt, U. (2003) Measuring language development in bilingual children: Swedish-Arabic children with and without language impairment. *Linguistics* 41 (2), 255–288.

Hale, S.B. (2007) *Community Interpreting*. Basingstoke: Palgrave Macmillan.

Hall, D., Griffiths, D., Haslam, L. and Wilkin, Y. (2001) *Assessing the Needs of Bilingual Pupils: Living in Two Languages*. London: David Fulton.

Hallam, S., Rogers, L. and Shaw, J. (2006) Improving children's behaviour and attendance through the use of parenting programmes: An examination of practice in five case study local authorities. *British Journal of Special Education* 33 (3), 107–113.

Halliday, M.A.K. (1975) *Learning How to Mean: Explorations in the Development of Language*. London: Edward Arnold.

Halliday, M.A.K. (1979/1980) Three aspects of children's language development: Learning language, learning through language, learning about language. In Y. Goodman, M. Hausser and D. Strickland (eds) *Oral and Written Language Development: Impact on Schools. Proceedings from the 1979 and 1980 IMPACT Conferences*. Urbana, IL: International Reading Association and National Council of Teachers of English.

Halliday, M.A.K. (1993) Towards a language-based theory of learning. *Linguistics and Education* 5 (2), 93–116.

Halliday, M.A.K. and Hasan, R. (1985) *Language, Context and Text: A Social Semiotic Perspective*. Geelong, Vic.: Deakin University Press.

Hamblin, L. and Kitson, N. (1992) Springfield supra-regional deaf unit: A retrospective case note survey. *Abstracts, Royal College of Psychiatrists Annual Meeting, London, UK* (p. 73).

Hamilton, R. and Moore, D. (eds) (2004) *Educational Interventions for Refugee Children: Theoretical Perspectives and Implementing Best Practice*. London: RoutledgeFalmer.

Hannon, P. (1995) *Literacy, Home and School: Research and Practice in Teaching Literacy with Parents*. London: Falmer Press.

Hanson, M., Gutierrez, S., Morgan, M., Brennan, E. and Zerecher, C. (1997) Language, culture and disability: Interacting influences on preschool inclusion. *Topics in Early Childhood Special Education* 17, 307–336.

Hanson, M., Wolfberg, P., Zerecher, C., Morgan, M., Gutierrez, S., Barnwell, D. and Beckman, P. (1998) The culture of inclusion: Recognising diversity at multiple levels. *Early Childhood Research Quarterly* 13, 185–210.

Harding, E. and Riley, P. (1998) *The Bilingual Family: A Handbook for Parents*. New York: Cambridge University Press.

Harding-Esch, E. and Riley, P. (2003) *The Bilingual Family: A Handbook for Parents* (2nd edn). New York: Cambridge University Press.

Harris, J. (2003) 'All doors are closed to us': A social model analysis of the experiences of disabled refugees and asylum seekers in Britain. *Disability and Society* 18 (4), 395–410.

Harris, J. and Bamford, C. (2001) The uphill struggle: Services for Deaf and hard of hearing people – issues of equality, participation and access. *Disability & Society* 16 (7), 969–980.

Harry, B. (1992) *Cultural Diversity, Families, and the Special Education System: Communication and Empowerment.* New York: Teachers College Press.

Harry, B., Rueda, R. and Kalyanpur, M. (1999) Cultural reciprocity in sociocultural perspective: Adapting the normalisation principle for family collaboration. *Exceptional Children* 66 (1), 123–136.

Hatton, C., Akram, Y., Robertson, J., Shah, R. and Emerson, E. (2002) *Supporting South Asian Families with a Child with Severe Intellectual Disabilities.* A report to the Department of Health, Institute of Health Research, Lancaster University, Lancaster.

Hatton, C., Akram, Y., Robertson, J., Shah, R. and Emerson, E. (2003) The disclosure process and its impact on South Asian families with a child with severe intellectual disabilities. *Journal of Applied Research in Intellectual Disabilities* 16 (3), 177–188.

Hatton, C., Azmi, S., Emerson, E. and Caine, A. (1997) Researching the needs of South Asian people with learning difficulties and their families. *Mental Health Care* 1 (3), 91–94.

Haynes, C. and Naidoo, S. (1991) *Children with Specific Speech and Language Impairments.* Oxford: Blackwell.

Hayward, H.C. and Tzuriel, D. (2002) Applications and challenges in dynamic assessment. *Peabody Journal of Education* 77 (?), 40–63.

Health Advisory Service (1995) *Child and Adolescent Mental Health Services: Together We Stand.* London: HMSO.

Hedegaard, M., Chaiklin, S. and Pedraza, P. (2001) Culturally sensitive teaching within a Vygotskian perspective. In M. Hedegaard (ed.) *Learning in Classrooms: A Cultural-historical Approach* (pp. 121–143). Aarhus: Aarhus University Press.

Hernandez, A.E. and Kohnert, K.J. (1999) Aging and language switching in bilinguals. *Aging Neuropsychology and Cognition* 6, 69–83.

Hill, M. (1994) 'They are not our brothers': The disability movement and the black disability movement. In N. Begum, M. Hill and A. Stevens (eds) *Reflections: The Views of Black Disabled People on Their Lives and Community Care.* London: Central Council for Education and Training in Social Work.

Hirschman, C., Alba, R. and Farley, R. (2000) The meaning and measurement of race in the U.S. Census: Glimpses into the future. *Demography* 37 (3), 381–393.

Holm, A. and Dodd, B. (1997) An intervention case study of a bilingual child with phonological disorder. *Child Language Teaching and Therapy* 15 (2), 139–158.

Holm, A. and Dodd, B. (1999) Differential diagnosis of phonological disorder in two bilingual children acquiring Italian and English. *Clinical Linguistics and Phonetics* 13, 113–129.

Holm, A., Ozanne, A. and Dodd, B. (1997) Efficacy of intervention for a bilingual child making articulation and phonological errors. *International Journal of Bilingualism* 1 (1), 55–69.

Holt, J.A. (1993) Stanford Achievement Test – 8th edition [Reading Comprehension Subgroup Results]. *American Annals of the Deaf* 128, 172–175.

Home Office RDS Directorate (2004) *Asylum Statistics, United Kingdom. Home Office Statistical Bulletin 11/04*. London: Home Office RDS Directorate.

Hornberger, N.H. (1989) Continua of Biliteracy. *Review of Educational Research* 59 (3), 271–296.

Hornberger, N.H. and Skilton-Sylvester, E. (2000) Revisiting the continua of biliteracy: International and critical perspectives. *Language and Education* 14 (2), 96–122.

Hornby, G. (1995) *Working with Parents of Children with Special Needs*. New York: Cassell.

Howell, J. and Dean, E. (1991) *Treating Phonological Disorders in Children: Metaphon – Theory to Practice*. San Diego, CA: Singular.

Howlin, P., Mawhood, L. and Rutter, M. (2000) Autism and developmental receptive language disorder – A follow-up comparison in early adult life. II: Social, behavioural, and psychiatric outcomes. *Journal of Child Psychology and Psychiatry* 41 (5), 561–578.

Hsiau, A-chin (1997) Language ideology in Taiwan: The KMT's language policy, the Tai-yu language movement, and ethnic politics. *Journal of Multilingual and Multicultural Development* 18 (4), 302–315.

Hughes, D., McGillivray, L. and Schmidek, M. (1997) *Guide to Narrative Language*. Eau Claire, WI: Thinking Publications.

The Human Rights Act (1998) Ministry of Justice UK; www.humanrights.gov.uk

Husband, C. (1994) *A Richer Vision: The British Experience*. Perth, W.A.: Paradigm Books.

Hymes, D. (1972) Models of interaction of language and social life. In J.J. Gumperz and D. Hymes (eds) *Directions in Sociolinguistics: The Ethnography of Communication*. New York: Holt, Rinehart and Winston.

Ingram, D. (1989) *Phonological Disability in Children* (2nd edn). London: Whurr.

Isaac, K. (2002) *Speech Pathology in Cultural and Linguistic Diversity*. London: Whurr.

Ivanič, R. (2006) Language, learning and identification. In R. Kiely, P. Rae-Dickins, H. Woodfield and G. Clibbon (eds) *Language, Culture and Identity in Applied Linguistics* (pp. 7–29). London: British Association for Applied Linguistics in association with Equinox.

James, M. and Woll, B. (2004) Black Deaf or Deaf Black? In A. Blackledge and A. Pavlenko (eds) *Negotiation of Identities in Multilingual Contexts* (pp. 125–160). Clevedon: Multilingual Matters.

Jenner, A.R., Rosen, G.D. and Galaburda, A.M. (1999) Neuronal asymmetries in primary visual cortex of dyslexic and nondyslexic brains. *Annals of Neurology* 46 (2), 189–196.

John-Steiner, V. and Meehan, T. (2000) Creative collaboration in knowledge construction. In C. Lee and P. Smagorinsky (eds) *Vygotskian Perspectives on Literacy Research: Constructing Meaning Through Collaborative Inquiry* (pp. 31–48). Cambridge: Cambridge University Press.

Jones, L., Atkin, K. and Ahmad, W. (2001) Supporting Asian Deaf young people and their families: The role of professionals and services. *Disability and Society* 16 (1), 51–70.

Jun Yamada (1998) Script makes a difference: The induction of deep dyslexic errors in logograph reading. *Dyslexia* 4 (4), 197–211.

Kalantzis, M. and Cope, B. (1999) Multicultural education: Transforming the mainstream. In S. May (ed.) *Critical Multiculturalism: Rethinking Multicultural and Antiracist Education* (pp. 245–276). London: Falmer Press.

Kalyanpur, M. (1998) The challenge of cultural blindness: Implications for family-focused service delivery. *Journal of Child and Family Studies* 7 (3), 317–332.

Kalyanpur, M. and Harry, B. (1997) A posture of reciprocity: A practical approach to collaboration between professionals and parents of culturally diverse backgrounds. *Journal of Child and Family Studies* 6 (4), 487–509.

Kalyanpur, M. and Harry, B. (1999) *Culture in Special Education: Building Reciprocal Family-Professional Relationships*. Baltimore, MD: Paul Brookes.

Kamhi, A. (1998) Trying to make sense of developmental language disorders. *Language, Speech and Hearing Services in Schools* 29, 35–44.

Karanth, P. (1992) Developmental dyslexia in bilingual-biliterates. *Reading and Writing* 4 (3), 297–306.

Kasen, S., Ouellette, R. and Cohen, P. (1990) Mainstreaming and postsecondary educational and employment status of a rubella cohort. *American Annals of the Deaf* 135 (1), 22–26.

Kayser, H. (ed.) (1995) *Bilingual Speech-Language Pathology: An Hispanic Focus*. San Diego, CA: Singular.

Keith, R.W. (2000a) Development and standardization of SCAN-C test for auditory processing disorders in children. *Journal of American Academic Audiology* 11, 438–445.

Keith R.W. (ed.) (2000b) *SCAN-C Test for Auditory Processing Disorders in Children-Revised*. San Antonio, CA: Psychological Corporation.

Kenner, C. (1997) A child writes from her everyday world: Using home texts to develop biliteracy at school. In E. Gregory (ed.) *One Child: Many Worlds* (pp. 75–86). London: David Fulton.

Kenner, C. (2000) *Home Pages: Literacy Links for Bilingual Children*. Stoke: Trentham Books.

Kirk, R. (2004) *Skills Audit of Refugees*. Home Office Online Report 37/04. London: Home Office. On WWW at http://www.homeoffice.gov.uk/rds/pdfs04/rdsolr3704.pdf. Accessed January 2008.

Knox, E. and Conti-Ramsden, G. (2003) Bullying risks of 11-year-old children with specific language impairment (SLI): Does school placement matter? *International Journal of Language and Communication Disorders* 38 (1), 1–12.

Kohnert, K. (2002) Picture naming in early sequential bilinguals. A 1-year follow up. *Journal of Speech, Language and Hearing Research* 45, 759–771.

Kohnert, K. (2007) *Language Disorders in Bilingual Children and Adults*. San Diego, CA: Plural.

Kohnert, K., Bates, E. and Hernandez, A. (1999) Balancing bilinguals: Lexical-semantic production and cognitive processing in children learning Spanish and English. *Journal of Speech, Language, and Hearing Research* 42, 1400–1413.

Kohnert, K. and Derr, A. (2004) Language intervention with bilingual children. In B. Goldstein (ed.) *Bilingual Language Development and Disorders in Spanish-English Speakers* (pp. 315–343). Baltimore, MD: Brookes.

Kohnert, K., Kennedy, M., Glaze, L., Kan, P. and Carney, E. (2003) Breadth and depth of diversity in Minnesota: Challenges to clinical competency. *American Journal of Speech-Language Pathology* 12, 259–272.

Kohnert, K., Windsor, J. and Yim, D. (2006) Do language-based processing tasks separate children with language impairment form typical bilinguals? *Learning Disabilities Research and Practice* 21 (1) 19–29.

Kovarsky, D., Duchan, J. and Maxwell, M. (eds) (1999) *Constructing (In) Competence: Disabling Evaluations in Clinical and Social Interaction.* Mahwah, NJ: Lawrence Erlbaum.

Kozulin, A. (1999) Cognitive learning in younger and older immigrant students. *School Psychology International* 20 (2), 177–190.

Kramsch, C. (1998) *Language and Culture.* Oxford: Oxford University Press.

Krashen, S., Long, M. and Scarcella, R. (1979) Age, rate and eventual attainment in second language acquisition. *TESOL Quarterly* 13 (4), 573–582.

Krausneker, V. (2003) Has something changed? Sign languages in Europe: The case for minorised minority languages. *Deaf Worlds: International Journal of Deaf Studies* 19 (2), 33–46.

Kress, G. and van Leeuwen, T. (1996) *Reading Images: Grammar of Visual Design.* London: Routledge.

Krezmien, M.P., Leone, P.E. and Achilles, G.M. (2006) Suspension, race, and disability: Analysis of statewide practices and reporting. *Journal of Emotional and Behavioral Disorders* 14 (4), 217–226.

Labov, W. (1994) *Principles of Linguistic Change.* Oxford: Blackwell.

Lacey, P. (2000) Multidisciplinary work: Challenges and possibilities. In H. Daniels (ed.) *Special Education Re-formed. Beyond Rhetoric* (pp. 157–172). London: Falmer Press.

Lacey, P. (2001) Support Partnerships: Collaboration in Action. London: David Fulton.

Laing, S. and Kamhi, A. (2003) Alternative assessment of language and literacy in culturally and linguistically diverse populations. *Language Speech and Hearing Services in Schools* 34, 44–55.

Lane, H. (2002) Do deaf people have a disability? *Sign Language Studies* 2 (4), 356–379.

Lane, H. (2005) Ethnicity, ethics, and the Deaf-world. *The Journal of Deaf Studies and Deaf Education* 10 (3), 291–310.

Langdon, H. (1992) Language communication and sociocultural patterns in Hispanic families. In H. Langdon and L.L. Cheng (eds) *Hispanic Children and Adults with Communication Disorders: Assessment and Intervention* (pp. 99–131) Gaithersburg, MD: Aspen Publishers.

Lantolf, J. (ed.) (2000) *Sociocultural Theory and Second Language Learning.* Oxford: Oxford University Press.

Lantolf, J. and Poehner, M. (eds) (2008) *Sociocultural Theory and the Teaching of Second Languages.* London: Equinox.

Lareau, A. and Horvat, E.M. (1999) Moments of social inclusion and exclusion: Race, class and cultural capital in family–school relationships. *Sociology of Education* 72 (1), 37–53.

Lave, J. and Wenger, E. (1991) *Situated Learning: Legitimate Peripheral Participation.* Cambridge: Cambridge University Press.

Law, J., Boyle, J., Harris, F., Harkness, A. and Nye, C. (1998) *Screening for Speech and Language Delay: A Systematic Review of the Literature.* Health Technology Assessment, NHS R&D HTA Programme, Southampton: The National Co-ordinating Centre for Health Technology Assessment.

References 277

Law, J., Boyle, J., Harris, F., Harkness, A. and Nye, C. (2000a) Prevalence and natural history of primary speech and language delay: Findings from a systemic review of the literature. *International Journal of Language and Communication Disorders* 35, 165–188.

Law, J., Lindsay, G., Peacey, N., Gascoigne, M., Soloff, N., Radford, J., Band, S. and Fitzgerald, L. (2000b) *Provision for Children with Speech and Language Needs in England and Wales.* Research Report RR239. London: DfEE.

Lawn, J.E., Reef, S., Baffoe-Bonnie, B., Adadevoh, S., Caul, E.O. and Griffin, G.E. (2000) Unseen blindness, unheard deafness, and unrecorded death and disability: Congenital rubella in Kumasi, Ghana. *American Journal of Public Health* 90, 1555–1561.

Lee, D.J., Gomez-Marin, O. and Lee, H.M. (1998) Prevalence of unilateral hearing loss in children: The National Health and Nutrition Examination Survey II and the Hispanic Health and Nutrition Examination Survey. *Ear and Hearing* 19 (4), 329–332.

Lemke, J. (1988) Genres, semantics, and classroom education. *Linguistics and Education* 1, 81–99.

Leonard, L. (1985) Unusual and subtle phonological behavior in the speech of phonologically-disordered children. *Journal of Speech and Hearing Disorders* 50, 4–13.

Leonard, L. (1998) *Children with Specific Language Impairment.* Cambridge, MA: MIT Press.

Leonard, L. and Bortolini, U. (1998) Grammatical morphology and the role of weak syllables in the speech of Italian-speaking children with specific language impairment. *Journal of Speech, Language, and Hearing Research* 41, 1363–1374.

Leont'ev A.N. (1978) *Activity, Consciousness and Personality.* Englewood Cliffs, NJ: Prentice Hall.

Leont'ev A.N. (1981) The problem of activity in psychology. In J. Wertsch (ed.) *The Concept of Activity in Soviet Psychology.* Armonk, NY: M.E. Sharpe.

Levelt, W.J.M. (1989) *Speaking: From Intention to Articulation.* Cambridge, MA: MIT Press.

Levinson, M. (2003) The language of race. *Theory and Research in Education* 1 (3), 267–281.

Lewis, A. and Norwich, B. (2000) *Mapping a special educational needs pedagogy.* Exeter: University of Exeter and University of Warwick.

Lewis, A. and Norwich, B. (eds) (2005) *Special Teaching for Special Children? Pedagogies for Inclusion.* Maidenhead: Open University Press.

Lewis, B.A., Freebairn, L.A., Hansen, A., Gerry Taylor, H., Iyengar, S. and Shriberg, L.D. (2004) Family pedigrees of children with suspected childhood apraxia of speech. *Journal of Communication Disorders* 37, 157–175.

Li, G. (2007) Home environment and second-language acquisition: The importance of family capital. *British Journal of Sociology of Education* 28 (3), 285–299.

Li Wei (ed.) (2000) *The Bilingualism Reader.* London: Routledge.

Lidz, C. and Pena, E. (1996) Dynamic assessment: The model, its relevance as a nonbiased approach and its implications to Latino American preschool children. *Language, Speech and Hearing Services in Schools* 27, 367–384.

Lindsay, G. and Dockrell, J.E. (2004) Whose job is it? Parents' concerns about the needs of their children with language problems. *Journal of Special Education* 37, 225–235.

Lindsay, G., Dockrell, J., Mackie, C. and Letchford, B. (2005) The roles of specialist provision for children with specific speech and language difficulties in England and Wales: A model for inclusion? *Journal of Research in Special Educational Needs* 5 (3), 88–96.

Lindsay, G., Pather, S. and Strand, S. (2006) *Special Educational Needs and Ethnicity: Issues of Over-and Under-representation*. London: Department for Education and Skills.

Linguistic Minorities Project (LMP) (1985) *The Other Languages of England*. London: Routledge and Kegan Paul.

Linton, S. (1998) *Claiming Disability*. New York: New York University Press.

Locke, J. (1993) *The Child's Path to Spoken Language*. Cambridge: Cambridge University Press.

Locke, J. (1994) Gradual emergence of developmental language disorders. *Journal of Speech and Hearing Disorders* 37, 608–616.

Lock, R.H. and Layton, C.A. (2002) Isolating intrinsic processing disorders from second language acquisition. *Bilingual Research Journal* 26, 213–224.

Lopez, L.M. and Greenfield, D.B. (2004) The cross-language transfer of phonological skills of Hispanic Head Start children. *Bilingual Research Journal* 28, 1–18.

Lozano-Rodriguez, J.R. and Castellano, J.A. (1999) *Assessing LEP Migrant Students for Special Education Services. ERIC Digest*. Charleston, WV: ERIC Clearinghouse on Rural Education and Small Schools.

Luria, AR. (1973) *The Working Brain. An Introduction to Neuropsychology*. Newyork: Bazic Books.

Luria, AR. (1979) (1997) *The Making of Mind. A Personal Account of Personal Psychology*. Cambridge, MA: Harvard University Press.

Luria, AR. (1981) *Language Cognition*. New York: Wiley.

MacPherson of Cluny, W. (1999) *The Stephen Lawrence Enquiry*, CM 4262-1. London: HMSO.

MacSwan, J. and Rolstad, K. (2003) Linguistic diversity, schooling, and social class: Rethinking our conception of language proficiency in language minority education. In C.B. Paulston and R. Tucker (eds) *Sociolinguistics: The Essential Readings* (pp. 329–340). Oxford: Blackwell.

MacSwan, J., Rolstad, K. and Glass, G.V. (2002) Do some school-age children have no language? Some problems of construct validity in the pre-LAS Español. *Bilingual Research Journal* 26 (2), 213–238.

Mahon, M. (2007) Early Communication: Language learning with deaf children in the early years. *BATOD Magazine* November, 8–9.

Mahon, M., Crutchley, A. and Quinn, C. (2003) Editorial: New directions in the assessment of bilingual children (special issue). *Child Language Teaching and Therapy* 19 (3), 237–244.

Maitra, B. and Miller, A. (2002) Children, families and therapists: Clinical considerations and ethnic minority cultures. In K.N. Dwivedi (ed.) *Meeting the Needs of Ethnic Minority Children: A Handbook for Professionals* (2nd edn, pp. 108–129). London: Jessica Kingsley.

Maratsos, M. (1982) The child's construction of grammatical categories. In L.R. Gleitman and E. Wanner (eds) *Language Acquisition: The State of the Art* (pp. 240–266). New York: Cambridge University Press.

Marbley, A.F., Bonner, F.A., McKisick, S., Henfield, M. and Watts, L.M. (2007) interfacing culture specific pedagogy with counseling: A proposed diversity training model for preparing preservice teachers for diverse learners. *Multicultural Education* 14 (3), 8–16.

Marquardt, T.P., Sussman, H.M., Snow, T. and Jacks, A. (2002) The integrity of the syllable in developmental apraxia of speech. *Journal of Communication Disorders* 35, 31–49.

Martin, D. (1999) Bilingualism and literacies in primary school: Implications for professional development. *Educational Review* 51 (1), 67–79.

Martin, D. (2003) Constructing discursive practices in school and community: Bilingualism, gender and power. *International Journal of Bilingual Education and Bilingualism* 6, Special issue 3&4, 237–252.

Martin, D. (2003) Constructing discursive practices in school and community: Bilingualism, gender and power. In A Creese and P. Martin (eds) *Multilingual Classroom Ecologies: Inter-relationships, interactions and ideologies* (pp. 77–92). Clevedon: Multilingual Matters.

Martin, D. (2005) Communities of practice and learning communities: Do bilingual co-workers learn in community? In D. Barton and K. Tusting (eds) *Beyond Communities of Practice: Language, Power and Social Context* (pp. 139–157). Cambridge: Cambridge University Press.

Martin, D. (2008) A New paradigm to inform inter-professional learning for integrating speech and language provision into secondary Schools. A sociocultural activity theory approach. *Child Language Teaching and Therapy* 24 (2), 173–192.

Martin, D., Colesby, C. and Jhamat, K. (1997) Phonological awareness in Panjabi/English children with phonological difficulties. *Child Language Teaching and Therapy* 13 (1), 59–72.

Martin, D., Krishnamurthy, R., Bhardwaj, M. and Charles, R. (2003) Language change in young Panjabi/English children: Implications for bilingual language assessment. *Child Language Teaching and Therapy* 19 (3), 245–265.

Martin-Jones, M. (1993) Code switching in the classroom: Two decades of research. In L. Milroy and P. Muysken (eds) *One Speaker, Two Languages: Cross-disciplinary Perspectives on Code-switching* (pp. 90–111). Cambridge: Cambridge University Press.

Martin-Jones, M. and Romaine, S. (1986) Semilingualism: A half-baked theory of communicative competence. *Applied Linguistics* 7 (1), 26–38.

Martin-Jones, M. and Saxena, M. (1996) Turn-taking, power asymmetries, and the positioning of bilingual participants in classroom discourse. *Linguistics and Education* 8 (1), 105–123.

Marton, K., Schwartz, R.G., Farkas, L. and Katsnelson, V. (2006) The effect of sentence length and complexity on working memory performance in Hungarian children with specific language impairment (SLI): A cross-linguistic comparison. *International Journal of Language and Communication Disorders* 41 (6), 653–673.

Masten, A.S. and Coatesworth, J.D. (1998) The development of competence in favourable and unfavourable environments. Lessons from research on successful children. *American Psychologist* 53, 205–220.

Mattes, L.J. and Omark, D.R. (1984) *Speech and Language Assessment for the Bilingual Handicapped.* San Diego, CA: College-Hill Press.

Mayer, C., Akmatsu, C.T. and Stewart, D. (2002) A model for effective practice: A dialogic inquiry with students who are deaf. *Exceptional Children* 68 (4), 485–502.

McCartney, E. (ed.) (1999) *Speech/Language Therapists and Teachers Working Together: A systems approach to collaboration.* London: Whurr.

McConachie, H. (2002) Appropriate research design in evaluating interventions for children with disabilities. *Child: Care, Health and Development* 28, 195–197.

McCool, S. (1999) Collaboration with parents. In E. McCartney (ed.) *Speech/ Language Therapists and Teachers Working Together: A systems approach to collaboration* (pp. 150–161). London: Whurr.

McCormick, L. (1997) Ecological assessment and planning. In L. McCormick, D.F. Loeb and R.L Schiefelbusch (eds) *Supporting Children with Communication Difficulties in Inclusive Settings: School-based Language Intervention* (pp. 223–256). Boston, MA: Allyn & Bacon.

McGuinness, C. (1999) *From Thinking Skills to Thinking Classrooms: A Review and Evaluation of Approaches for Developing Pupils' Thinking.* Research Report RR115. London: Department for Education and Employment.

McPherson, B. and Swart, S.M. (1997) Childhood hearing loss in sub-Saharan Africa: A review and recommendations. *International Journal of Pediatric Otorhinolaryngology* 40 (1), 1–18.

McSwan, D. (2001) *A Whole Community Approach to Otitis Media – Reducing Its Incidence and Effects: Abstract.* Report from Rural Education, Research and Development Centre, James Cook University of North Queensland, Townsville. Australia. On WWW at eric.ed.gov.

McWilliam, N. (1998) *What's in a Word? Vocabulary Development in Multilingual Classrooms.* Stoke: Trentham Books.

Mead, G.H. (1967) *Mind, Self and Society,* London: Chicago University Press.

Mehan, H. (1983) The role of language and the language of role in institutional decision making. *Language in Society* 12, 187–211.

Meisel, J.M. (1989) Early differentiation of languages in bilingual children. In K. Hyltenstam and L.K. Obler (eds) *Bilingualism Across the Lifespan: Aspects of Acquisition, Maturity and Loss* (pp. 13–40). Cambridge: Cambridge University Press.

Mennen, I. and Stansfield, J. (2006) Speech and language therapy service delivery for bilingual children: A survey of three cities in Great Britain. *International Journal of Language and Communication Disorders* 41 (6), 635–652.

Mercer, N. (2000) *Words and Minds: How We Use Language to Think Together.* London: Routledge.

Middleton, D. and Brown, S. (2005) *The Social Psychology of Experience.* London: sage.

Miller, C. (1996) Relationships between teachers and speech-language therapists: Influencing practice by distance education, *Child Language Teaching and Therapy* 12 (1), 29–38.

Miller, N. (ed.) (1984) *Bilingualism and Language Disability: Assessment and Remediation*. San Diego, CA: College Hill Press.

Mills, J. (1994) Finding a voice: Bilingual classroom assistants and their role in primary school. In A. Blackledge (ed.) *Teaching Bilingual Children* (pp. 131–142). Stoke: Trentham.

Mir, G., Nocon, A., Ahmad, W. and Jones, T. (2001) *Learning Difficulties and Ethnicity*. London: Department of Health.

Mirza, M. (1998) 'Same voices, same lives?': Revisiting black feminist standpoint epistemology. In P. Connolly and B. Troyna (eds) *Researching Racism in Education: Politics, Theory and Practice* (pp. 79–94). Buckingham: Open University Press.

Mitchell, D. and Scott, L. (1994) Professional and institutional perspectives on interagency collaboration. In *The Politics of Linking Schools and Social Services: The 1993 Yearbook of the Politics of Education Association*. London: Falmer.

Modood, T. (2005) *Multicultural Politics: Racism, Ethnicity, and Muslims in Britain*. Minneapolis, MN: University of Minnesota Press.

Modood, T., Berthoud, R., Lakey, J., Nazroo, J. Smith, P., Virdee, S. and Beishon, S. (1997) *Ethnic Minorities in Britain: Diversity and Disadvantage*. London: Policy Studies Institute.

Moll, L. (1992) Bilingual classroom studies and community analysis. *Educational Researcher* 21 (2), 20–24.

Moll, L.C. (2000) Inspired by Vygotsky: Ethnographic experiments in education. In C. Lee and P. Smagorinsky (eds) *Vygotskian Perspectives on Literacy Research: Constructing Meaning Through Collaborative Inquiry* (pp. 256–268). Cambridge: Cambridge University Press.

Moll, L. and Gonzalez, N. (2005) *Fund of Knowledge: Theorizing Practices in Households, Communities and Classrooms*. Mahwah, NJ: Erlbaum.

Montgomery, J. (2000) Relation of working memory to off-line and real-time sentence processing in children with specific language impairment. *Applied Psycholinguistics* 21, 117–148.

Montgomery, J. (2002) Examining the nature of lexical processing in children with specific language impairment: Temporal processing or processing capacity deficit? *Applied Psycholinguistics* 23 (3), 447–470.

Moriarty, B.C. and Gillon, G.T. (2006) Phonological awareness intervention for children with childhood apraxia of speech. *International Journal of Language and Communication Disorders* 41, 713–734.

Morris, B. (1991) The nature and role of educational therapy. *The Journal of Educational Therapy* 3 (3), 5–14.

Morton, N.E. (1991) Genetic epidemiology of hearing impairment. *Annals of New York Academy of Science* 630, 16–31.

Moss, C. (1999) Selection of topics and questions for the 2001 census. *Population Trends* 97, 28–36.

Muñoz-Sandoval, A., Cummins, J., Alvarado, C. and Ruef, M. (1998) *Bilingual Verbal Ability Tests* (BVAT). Itasca, IL: Riverside Publishing, Houghton Mifflin Co.

Muñoz-Baell, I.M. and Ruiz, T.M. (2000) Empowering the deaf. Let the deaf be deaf. *Journal of Epidemiological Community Health* 54, 40–44.

Murphy, V.A., Messer, D. and Dockrell, J. (2003) *Lexical Representation in Children with Word Finding Difficulties*. ESRC End of Award Full Report, Swindon, UK.

Myers-Scotton, C. (2006) *Multiple Voices: An Introduction to Bilingualism.* Oxford: Blackwell.

National Institute for Mental Health Education (NIMHE/DH) (2005) *Mental Health and Deafness. Towards Equity and Access.* London: HMSO.

National Statistics and Department for Education and Skills (2004) *Statistics of Education: Schools in England* (2004 edn). London: HMSO.

Nazroo, J. (1997) *The Health of Britain's Ethnic Minorities: Fourth National Survey of Ethnic Minorities.* London: Policy Studies Institute.

Nazroo, J.Y. (1998) Genetic, cultural or socio-economic vulnerability? Explaining ethnic inequalities in health. *Sociology of Health and Illness* 20 (5), 710–730.

Nazroo, J.Y. (2003) The structuring of ethnic inequalities in health: Economic position, racial discrimination, and racism. *American Journal of Public Health* 93 (2), 277–284.

Negueruela, E. (2008) Revolutionary pedagogies: Learning that leads (to) second language development. In J.P. Lantolf and M.E. Poehner (eds) *Sociocultural Theory and the Teaching of Second Languages* (pp. 189–227). London: Equinox.

Nelson, C. (2005) The diagnosis of the constituents of communication in everyday discourse: Some functions, enabling conditions, consequences, and remedies. In J.F. Duchan and D. Kovarsky (eds) *Diagnosis as Cultural Practice* (pp. 277–297). New York: Mouton de Gruyter.

Nelson, C.S. (2006) Listening comprehension in the primary school: A metacognitive approach to transactional listening. Unpublished MPhil thesis, School of Education, University of Birmingham.

Nelson, P., Kohnert, K., Sabur, S. and Shaw, D. (2005) Double jeopardy? Classroom noise and children learning through a second language. *Language, Speech and Hearing Services in Schools* 36, 219–229.

New London Group (1996) A pedagogy of multiliteracies: Designing social future. *Harvard Educational Review* 66 (1), 60–92.

Newton, C. and Wilson, D. (1999) *Circles of Friends.* Dunstable: Folens.

New Zealand Census of Population and Dwellings Government Statistics for Census (2006). *QuickStats about Culture and Identity.* On WWW at http://www.stats.govt.nz/census/about-2006-census/default.htm. Accessed July 2007.

Nic Craith, M. (2000) Contested identities and the quest for legitimacy. *Journal of Multilingual and Multicultural Development* 21 (5), 399–413.

Nias, J. (1993) Changing times, changing identities; grieving for a lost self. In R.G. Burgess (ed.) *Educational Research and Evaluation: For Policy and Practice* (pp. 139–156). London: Routledge.

Nieto, S. (1999) *The Light in their Eyes: Creating Multicultural Learning Communities.* New York: Teachers College Press.

Noels, K.A. and Clément, R. (1996) Communicating across cultures: Social determinants and acculturative consequences. *Canadian Journal of Behavioural Science* 28, 214–228.

Norbury, C.F. and Bishop, D.V.M. (2002) Inferential processing and story recall in children with communication problems: A comparison of specific language impairment, pragmatic language impairment and high-functioning autism. *International Journal of Language and Communication Disorders* 37 (3), 227–251.

Norwich, B. (1990) *Reappraising Special Needs Education.* London: Cassell Educational.

Nunes, T. and Bryant, P. (2006) *Improving Literacy by Teaching Morphemes.* Abingdon: Routledge.

Nunes, T., Bryant, P. and Olsson, J.M. (2003) Learning morphological and phonological spelling rules: An intervention study. *Reading and Writing 7,* 298–307.

Nuru, N. (1993) Multicultural aspects of deafness. In D. Battle (ed.) *Communication Disorders in Multicultural Populations* (pp. 287–305). Stonehaven: Andover Medical.

Nuru, N. (1998) Multicultural aspects of deafness. In D. Battle (ed.) *Communication Disorders in Multicultural Populations* (2nd edn, pp. 355–378). Boston, MA: Butterworth-Heineman.

O'Connor, T. and Colwell, J. (2002) The effectiveness and rationale of the 'nurture group' approach to helping children with emotional and behavioural difficulties remain within mainstream education. *British Journal of Special Education* 29 (2), 96–100.

Odom, S., Vitztum, J., Wolery, R., Lieber, J., Sandall, S., Hanson, M., Beckman, P. Schwartz, I. and Horn, E. (2004) Preschool inclusion in the United States: A review of research from an ecological systems perspective. *Journal of Research in Special Educational Needs* 4 (1), 17–49.

Office for Standards in Education (OFSTED) (2002) *The National Literacy Strategy: The First Four Years 1998–2002.* London: OFSTED.

Office for National Statistics (ONS) (2005) *The 2011 Census: Initial View on Content for England and Wales.* London: ONS.

Ogbu, J.U. (1995) Cultural problems in minority education: Their interpretations and consequences – Part two: Case studies. *The Urban Review* 4, 271–297.

Okamura-Bichard, F. (1985) Mother-tongue maintenance and second language learning: A case of Japanese children. *Language Learning* 35 (1), 63–69.

Oliver, M. (1990) *The Politics of Disablement.* Tavistock: Macmillan.

Oliver, M. (1992) Changing the social relations of research production. *Disability, Handicap and Society* 7 (2), 101–115.

Ortiz, A.A. (1997) Learning disabilities occurring concomitantly with linguistic differences. *Journal of Learning Disabilities* 30, 321–332.

Ortiz, A.A. (2001, 2004) *English Language Learners with Special Needs: Effective Instructional Strategies.* Washington, DC: ERIC Clearinghouse on Languages and Linguistics. Posting date on web: April 26, 2004.

Organisation for Economic Co-operation and Development (OECD) (2001) *Knowledge and Skills for Life, First Results from the OECD Programme for International Student Assessment (PISA) 2000.* Paris: OECD.

Osler, A. (1997) *Exclusion for School and Racial Equality.* London: Commission for Race Equality.

Osler, A. and Hill, J. (1999) Exclusion from school and racial equality: An examination of government proposals in the light of recent research evidence. *Cambridge Journal of Education* 29, 1–33.

Owens, R. (1995, 1999) *Language Disorders: A Functional Approach to Assessment and Intervention* (2nd and 3rd edn). Boston, MA: Allyn & Bacon.

Ozanne, A. (1995) The search for developmental verbal dyspraxia (DVD). In B. Dodd (ed.) *The Differential Diagnosis and Treatment of Children with Speech Disorder* (pp. 91–109). London: Whurr.

Painter, C. (2007) Language for learning in early childhood. In F. Christie and J.R. Martin (eds) *Knowledge and Pedagogy: Functional Linguistic and Sociological Perspectives* (pp. 131–155). London: Continuum.

Palincsar, A.S. and Brown, A.L. (1984) Reciprocal teaching of comprehension-fostering and comprehension-monitoring activities. *Cognition and Instruction* 2 (2), 117–175.

Paradis, J. (2005) Grammatical morphology in children learning English as a second language: Implications of similarities with specific language impairment. *Language, Speech, and Hearing Services in Schools* 36, 172–187.

Paradis, J., Crago, M. and Genesee, F. (2003a) Object clitics as a clinical marker of SLI in French: Evidence from French-English bilingual children. In B. Beachley *et al.* (eds) *Proceedings of the Boston University Conference on Language Development* (pp. 638–649). Sommerville, MA: Cascadilla.

Paradis, J., Crago, M., Genesee, F. and Rice, M. (2003b) Bilingual children with specific language impairment: How do they compare with their monolingual peers? *Journal of Speech, Language and Hearing Research* 46, 1–15.

Parsons, T. (1966) *Societies.* Englewood Cliffs, NJ: Prentice Hall.

Parsons, C. and Howlett, K. (1996) Permanent exclusions form school: A case where society is failing its children. *Support for Learning* 11 (3), 109–112.

Parsons, C., Godfrey, R., Annan, G., Cornwall, J., Dussart, M., Hepburn, S., Howlett, K. and Wennerstrom, V. (2004) *Minority Ethnic Exclusions and the Race Relations (Amendment) Act 2000*, DfES Research Report RR616. London: HMSO.

Pavlenko, A. (2004) The making of an American: Negotiation of identities at the turn of the twentieth century. In A. Pavlenko and A. Blackledge (eds) *Negotiation of Identities in Multilingual Contexts* (pp. 34–67). Clevedon: Multilingual Matters.

Pavlenko, A. and Blackledge, A. (eds) (2004) *Negotiation of Identities in Multilingual Contexts.* Clevedon: Multilingual Matters.

Pavlenko, A. and Lantolf, J. (2000) Second language learning as participation and the (re)construction of selves. In J. Lantolf (ed.) *Sociocultural Theory and Second Language Learning* (pp. 155–177). Oxford: Oxford University Press.

Pearl, A. (1997) Cultural and accumulated environmental deficit models. In R. Valencia (ed.) *The Evolution of Deficit Thinking: Educational Thought and Practice* (pp. 132–159). London: Falmer Press.

Peer, L. and Reid, G. (eds) (2000) *Multilingualism, Literacy and Dyslexia: A Challenge for Educators.* London: David Fulton.

Pembrey, M. (1992) Genetics and language disorder. In P. Fletcher and D. Hall (eds) *Specific Speech and Language Disorders in Children* (pp. 51–62). London: Whurr.

Peña, E., Bedore, L. and Rappazzo, C. (2003) Comparison of Spanish, English and bilingual children's performance across semantic tasks. *Language, Speech and Hearing Services in Schools* 34, 5–16.

Peña, E. and Gillam, R. (2000) Dynamic assessment of children referred for speech and language evaluations. *Dynamic Assessment: Prevailing Models and Applications* 6, 543–575.

Peña, E., Quinn, R. and Iglesias, A. (1992) The application of dynamic methods to language assessment: A non biased procedure. *Journal of Special Education* 26 (3), 269–280.

Peña, E. and Valles, L. (1995) Language assessment and instructional programming for linguistically different learners: Proactive classroom processes. In H. Kayser (ed.) *Bilingual Speech-language Pathology: An Hispanic Focus* (pp. 129–152). San Diego, CA: Singular Press.

Perani, D., Dehaene, S., Grassi, F., Cohen, L., Cappa, S.F., Dupoux, F.F. and Mehler, J. (1996) Brain processing of native and foreign languages. *NeuroReport* 7, 2439–2444.

Perera, C. (1986) Language acquisition and writing. In P. Fletcher and M. Garman (eds) *Language Acquisition* (2nd edn, pp. 494–533). Cambridge: Cambridge University Press.

Perez-Arce, P. (1999) The influence of culture on cognition. *Archives of Clinical Neuropsychology* 14, 581–592.

Perkins, D.N. (1983) Person plus: A distributed view of thinking and learning. In G. Salmon (ed.) *Distributed Cognitions* (pp. 88–110). Cambridge: Cambridge University Press.

Pert, S. and Letts, C. (2003) Developing an expressive language assessment for children in Rochdale with a Pakistani heritage background. *Child Language Teaching and Therapy* 19 (3), 267–289.

Pienemann, M. (1998) *Language Processing and Second Language Development: Processability Theory.* Amsterdam: John Benjamins.

Pienemann, M. (ed.) (2005) *Cross-linguistic Aspects of Processability Theory.* Amsterdam: John Benjamins.

Pienemann, M., Di Biase, B., Kawaguchi, S. and Håkansson, G. (2005) Processability, typological distance and L1 transfer. In M. Pienemann (ed.) *Cross-linguistic Aspects of Processability Theory* (pp. 85–116). Amsterdam: John Benjamins.

Pienneman, M. and Håkansson, G. (1999) A unified approach towards the development of Swedish as L2: A processability account. *Studies in Second Language Acquisition* 10, 217–224.

Pinker, S. (1989) *Learnability and Cognition: The Acquisition of Argument Structure.* Cambridge, MA: MIT Press.

Pinker, S. (1994) *The Language Instinct.* New York: William Morrow.

Plante, E. (1998) Criteria for SLI: The Stark and Tallal legacy and beyond. *Journal of Speech, Language and Hearing Research* 41, 951–957.

Pöchhacker, F. and Kadric, M. (1999) The hospital cleaner as healthcare interpreter: A case study. *The Translator* 5 (2), 161–178.

Polich, L. (2005) The diagnosis of deafness in Nicaragua. In J.F. Duchan and D. Kovarsky (eds) *Diagnosis as Cultural Practice* (pp. 223–237). New York: Mouton de Gruyter.

Portage Project. Cooperative Educational Service Agency. On WWW at http://www.portageproject.org.

Portes, A and Hao, L. (2002) The price of uniformity: Language, family and personality adjustment in the immigrant second generation. *Ethnic and Racial Studies* 25 (6) 1, 889–912.

Potter, J. (1996) *Representing Reality: Discourse, Rhetoric and Social Construction.* London: Sage.

Powers, S. (1998) Deaf pupils' achievements in ordinary schools. *Journal of the British Association of Teachers of the Deaf* 20 (4), 111–123.

Powers, S. (2002) The educational achievements of deaf school leavers. On WWW at www.deafnessatbirth.org.uk.
Powers, S., Gregory, S. and Thoutenhoofd, E.D. (1998) *The Educational Achievements of Deaf Children*, DfEE Research Report RR65. London: Department for Education and Employment.
Prathanee, B., Thanaviratananich, S. and Pongjanyakul, A. (2003) Oral diadochokinetic rates for Thai children. *International Journal of Language and Communication Disorders* 38 (4), 417–428.
Pratt, C., Botting, N. and Conti-Ramsden, G. (2006) The characteristics and concerns of mothers of adolescents with a history of SLI. *Child Language Teaching and Therapy* 22, 177–196.
Pray, L. (2005) How well do commonly used language instruments measure English oral-language proficiency? *Bilingual Research Journal* 29, 387–409.
Pumphrey, P. (1991) *Improving Children's Reading in the Junior School: Challenges and Responses*. New York: Cassell.
Rampton, B. (1995) *Crossing: Language and Ethnicity Among Adolescents*. London: Longman.
Rassool, N. (2000) Uncommon languages: The challenge and possibilities of minority language rights. *Journal of Multilingual and Multicultural Development* 21 (5), 386–398.
Rassool, N. (2002) Literacy: In search of a paradigm. In J. Soler, J. Wearmouth and G. Reid (eds) *Contextualising Difficulties in Literacy Development* (pp. 17–46). London: RoutledgeFalmer, Open University, University of Edinburgh.
Rawls, J. (1999) *A Theory of Justice* (rev. edn). Oxford: Oxford University Press.
Reid, G. and Peer, L. (eds) (2000) *Dyslexia: A Complete Guide for Parents*. London: David Fulton.
Reilly, S. (2004) What constitutes evidence? In S. Reilly, J. Douglas and J. Oates (eds) *Evidence Based Practice in Speech Pathology* (pp. 18–34). London: Whurr.
Reis, P. (1994) Prevalence and characteristics of persons with hearing trouble: United States 1990–91. *Vital and Health Statistics* 10, 188.
Rescorla, L. and Alley, A. (2001) Validation of the Language Development Survey (LDS): A parent report tool for identifying language delay in toddlers. *Journal of Speech, Language and Hearing Research* 44 (2), 434–445.
Rescorla, L., Roberts, J. and Dahlsgaard, K. (1997) Late talkers at 2 outcome at age 3. *Journal of Speech, Language and Hearing Research* 40, 556–566.
Restrepo, M.A., Schwanenflugel, P., Blake, J., Neuharth-Pritchett, S., Cramer, S. and Ruston, H. (2006) Applicability of the measured with African American and European American preschool children. *Language, Speech and Hearing Services in Schools* 37, 17–27.
Rice, M. (1994) Grammatical categories of children with specific language impairment. In R. Watkins and M. Rice (eds) *Specific Language Impairment in Children* (pp. 69–89). Baltimore, MD: Brookes.
Rice, M. and Wexler, K. (1996) Toward tense as a clinical marker of specific language impairment. *Journal of Speech, Language and Hearing Research* 39, 1236–1257.
Riddick, B., Sterling, C., Farmer M. and Morgan S. (1999) Self-esteem and anxiety in the educational histories of adult dyslexic students. *Dyslexia* 5 (4), 227–248.
Rinaldi, W. (1992a) *Working with Children with Moderate Learning Difficulties*. London: ICAN.

Rinaldi, W. (1992b) *The Social Use of Language Programme*. Windsor: NFER-Nelson.

Rinaldi, W. (2000) Pragmatic comprehension in secondary school-aged students with specific developmental language disorder. *International Journal of Language & Communication Disorders* 35 (1), 1–29.

Roaf, C. (2002) *Coordinating Services for Included Children. Joined Up Action.* Buckingham: Open University Press.

Roberts, A. and Gibbs, D. (1989) The bilingual child with special educational needs. In D. Duncan (ed.) *Working with Bilingual Language Disability* (pp. 154–175). London: Chapman and Hall.

Robinson, R.M., Anning, A., Cottrell, D. Frost, N. and Green, J.M. (2004) *New Forms of Professional Knowledge in Multi-agency Delivery of Services for Children.* End of Award report to the Economic and Social Research Council, UK.

Rodriguez, J., Cauce, A.M. and Wilson, L. (2002) A conceptual framework of identity formation in a society of multiple cultures: Applying theory to practice. In K.N. Dwivedi (ed.) *Meeting the Needs of Ethnic Minority Children: A Handbook for Professionals* (2nd edn, pp. 299–320). London: Jessica Kingsley.

Roeser, R.J. and Downs, M.P. (2004) *Auditory Disorders in School Children.* New York: Thieme Medical.

Rogers, D. and Whetton, D. (1982) *Interorganizational Coordination Theory and Implementation.* Iowa: Iowa State University.

Romaine, S. (1995) *Bilingualism* (2nd edn). Oxford: Blackwell.

Roulstone, S., Owen, R. and French, L. (2005) Speech and language therapy and the Knowles Edge Standards Fund project: An evaluation of the service provided to a cluster of primary schools. *British Journal of Special Education* 32 (2), 78–85.

Royal College of Speech and Language Therapists (RCSLT) (2006) *Communicating Quality RCSLT's guidance on best practice in service organisation are provision.* Royal College of Speed and Language Therapists, London, UK.

Royal National Institute for the Deaf (RNID) (2004) *A Simple Cure.* London: RNID and the British Medical Association (BMA).

Rumberger, R. and Larson, K. (1998) Toward explaining differences in educational achievement among Mexican American language-minority students. *Sociology of Education* 71 (1), 69–93.

Rutter, J. (1994) *Refugee Children in the Classroom.* Stoke: Trentham Books.

Rutter, J. and Jones, C. (eds) (1998) *Refugee Education: Mapping the Field.* Stoke: Trentham Books.

Ryan, J. and Thomas, F. (1980) *The Politics of Mental Handicap.* Harmondsworth: Penguin.

Saenz, T.I., Black, K.G. and Pellegrini, L. (1999) The social competence of children diagnosed with Specific Language Impairment. In D. Kovarsky, J.F. Duchan and M.M. Maxwell (eds) *Constructing (In) Competence: Disabling Evaluations in Clinical and Social Interaction* (pp. 111–124). Mahwah, NJ: Lawrence Erlbaum.

Salameh, E-K. (2003) *Language Impairment in Swedish Bilingual Children – Epidemiological and Linguistic Studies.* Sweden: Department of Logopedics and Phoniatrics, Lund University.

Salameh, E-K., Håkansson G. and Nettelbladt, U. (2004) Developmental perspectives on bilingual Swedish-Arabic children with and without language impairment: A longitudinal study. *International Journal of Language & Communication Disorders* 39 (1), 65–90.

Salend, S.J., Dorney, J.A., Mazo, M. (1997) The roles of bilingual special educators in creating inclusion classrooms. *Remedial and Special Education*, 18, 1, 54–64.

Sandel, T.L. (2003) Linguistic capital in Taiwan: The KMT's Mandarin language policy and its perceived impact on language practices of bilingual Mandarin and Tai-gi speakers. *Language in Society* 32, 523–551.

Saxena, M. (1994) Literacies among the Panjabis in Southall (Britain). In J. Maybin (ed.) *Language and Literacy in Social Practice* (pp. 96–116). Clevedon: Multilingiual Matters.

Saxton, M. (1997) The contrast theory of negative input. *Journal of Child Language* 24, 139–161.

Saxton, M. (2005) 'Recast' in a new light: Insights for practice from typical language studies. *Child Language Teaching and Therapy* 21 (1), 23–38.

Schieffelin, B.B. and Ochs, E. (1986) Language socialization. *Annual Review of Anthropology* 15, 163–191.

Schneider, E. and Crombie, M. (2003) *Dyslexia and Foreign Language Learning*. London: David Fulton.

Schneider, E. and Ganschow, L. (2000) Dynamic assessment and instructional strategies for learner who struggle to learn a foreign language. *Dyslexia* 6 (1), 72–82.

Schoenbrodt, L., Kerins, M. and Gessell, J. (2003) Using narrative language intervention as a tool to increase communicative competence in Spanish-speaking children. *Language, Culture and Curriculum* 16 (1), 48–59.

Schwartz, I.S. (2000) Standing on the shoulders of giants: Looking ahead to facilitating membership and relationships for children with disabilities. *Topics in Early Childhood Special Education* 20, 123–128.

Selinker, L. (1972) Interlanguage. *IRAL* 10 (2), 209–231.

Semel, E., Wiig, E. and Secord, W.A. (1995) *Clinical Evaluation of Language Fundamentals-3*. San Antonio, TX: The Psychological Corporation.

Semel, E., Wiig, E. and Secord, W.A. (1997) *Clinical Evaluation of Language Fundamentals-3: Spanish Edition*. San Antonio, TX: The Psychological Corporation.

Sen, A. (1992) *Inequality Re-examined*. Cambridge, MA: Harvard University Press.

Sen, A. (1999) *Development as Freedom*. New York: Alfred A. Knopf.

Serrano-Lopez, M. and Poehner, M. (2008) Materialising linguistic concepts through 3-D clay modelling: A tool-and-result approach to mediating L2 Spanish development. In J.P. Lantolf and M.E. Poehner (eds) *Sociocultural Theory and the Teaching of Second Languages* (pp. 321–346). London: Equinox.

Seymour, P.H.K. (1986) *Cognitive Analysis of Dyslexia*. London: Routledge and Kegan Paul.

Sfard, A. (1998) On two metaphors for learning and the dangers of choosing just one. *Educational Researcher* 27 (2), 4–13.

Shah, R. (1992) *The Silent Minority: Children with Disabilities in Asian Families*. London: National Children's Bureau.

Shah, R., Draycott, S., Wolpert, M., Christie, D. and Stein, S. (2004) A comparison of Pakistani and Caucasian mothers' perceptions of child health problems. *Emotional and Behavioural Difficulties* 9 (3), 181–190.

Shriberg, L.D., Tomblin, J.B. and McSweeny, J.L. (1999) Prevalence of speech delay in 6-year-old children and comorbidity with language impairment. *Journal of Speech, Language, and Hearing Research* 42, 1461–1481.

Sign and Mental Health Foundation (2006) *Executive Briefing on Mental Health Services for Deaf and Hard Hearing People*. London: Sign and Mental Health Foundation.

Silliman, E.R.., Huntley Bahr, R., Brea, M.R., Hnath-Chisolm, T. and Mahecha, N.R. (2002) Spanish and English proficiency in the linguistic encoding of mental states in narrative retellings. *Linguistics and Education* 13, 199–234.

Simmons, F. and Singleton, C. (2007) Do weak phonological representations impact on arithmetic development? A review of research into arithmetic and dyslexia. *Dyslexia online*. On WWW at http://www3.interscience.wiley.com/cgi-bin/abstract/114290906/ABSTRACT.

Skutnabb-Kangas, T. (1981) *Bilingualism or Not: The Education of Minorities*, Clevedon: Multilingual Matters.

Skutnabb-Kangas, T., Phillipson, R. and Rannut, M. (1995) *Linguistic Human Rights: Overcoming Linguistic Discrimination*. New York: de Gruyter.

Slaghuis, W.L., Lovegrove, W.J. and Davidson, J.A. (1993) Visual and language processing deficits are concurrent in dyslexia. *Cortex* 29, 601–615.

SLI Consortium (2002) A genome-wide scan identifies two novel loci involved in specific language impairment (SLI). *American Journal of Human Genetics* 70, 384–398.

SLI Consortium (2004) Highly significant linkage to SLI1 locus in an expanded sample of individuals affected by specific language impairment (SLI). *American Journal of Human Genetics* 94, 1225–1238.

Slobin, D. (1973) Cognitive prerequisites for the development of grammar. In C. Ferguson and D. Slobin (eds) *Studies of Child Language Development* (pp 485–496), New York: Holt, Rinehart, Winston.

Smith, F. (1971) *Understanding Reading*. New York: Holt, Rinehart and Winston.

Smith, S.W. (1990) Individualized educational programs (IEPs) in special education – From intent to acquiescence. *Exceptional Children* 57 (1), 6–14.

Smythe, J. (2004) Social capital and the 'socially just school'. *British Journal of Sociology of Education* 25 (1), 1–19.

Sneddon, R. (1993) Children developing bilingualism at home and at school, Unpublished MA dissertation, Department of Applied Linguistics, Birkbeck College, University of London.

Sneddon, R. (2000) Language and literacy: Children's experiences in multilingual environments. *International Journal of Bilingual Education and Bilingualism* 3 (4), 265–282.

Snow, C.E. (2002) *Reading for Understanding: Toward a R&D Program in Reading Comprehension*. Santa Monica, CA: Rand.

Snow, C.E., Burns, M.S. and Griffin, P. (eds) (1998) *Preventing Reading Difficulties in Young Children*. Committee on the Prevention of Reading Difficulties in Young Children, National Research Council, USA. Washington, DC: National Academy Press.

Snow, M.A. and Brinton, D.B. (eds) (2001) *The Content-based Classroom: Perspectives on Integrating Language and Content*. White Plains, NY: Longman.

Snowling, M. (2001) From language to reading and dyslexia. *Dyslexia* 7 (1), 37–46.

Snowling, M. and Stackhouse, J. (2006) *Dyslexia, Speech and Language: A Practitioner's Handbook*. Chichester: John Wiley & Sons.

So, L.K.H. and Dodd, B. (1994) Phonologically-disordered Cantonese-speaking children. *Clinical Linguistics and Phonetics* 8 (3), 235–255.

So, L.K.H. and Dodd, B. (1995) The acquisition of phonology by Cantonese-speaking children. *Journal of Child Language* 22 (3), 473–495.

Soler, J., Wearmouth, J. and Reid, G. (eds) (2002) *Contextualising Difficulties in Literacy Development*. London: RoutledgeFalmer, Open University, University of Edinburgh.

Spolsky, B. (1989) *Conditions for Second Language Learning*. New York: Oxford University Press.

Stackhouse, J. and Snowling, M.J. (1992a) Developmental verbal dyspraxia II: A developmental perspective on two case studies. *European Journal of Speech and Language Therapists* 27, 35–54.

Stackhouse, J. and Snowling, M.J. (1992b) Barriers to literacy development in two cases of developmental verbal dyspraxia. *Cognitive Neuropsychology* 9, 273–299.

Stackhouse, J. and Wells, B. (1997) *Children's Speech and Literacy Difficulties: A Psycholinguistic Framework*. London: Whurr.

Stackhouse, J. and Wells, B. (2001) *Children's Speech and Literacy Difficulties: Book Two: Identification and Intervention*. London: Whurr.

Stampe, D. (1979) *A Dissertation on Natural Phonology*. New York: Garland.

Stanovich, K.E. (1998) Toward a more inclusive definition of dyslexia. *Dyslexia* 2 (3), 154–166.

Stanovich, K.E. (1994) Annotation: Does dyslexia exist? *Journal of Child Psychology and Psychiatry* 35 (4), 579–595.

Stanovich, K.E. and Siegel, L. (1994) The phenotypic performance profile of reading-disabled children: A regression-based test of the phonological-core based test of the phonological-core variable difference model. *Journal of Educational Psychology* 86, 24–53.

Statistics Canada (2006) *Census of Canada 2001*. On WWW at http://www12.statcan.ca/english/census06/release/index.cfm.

Statistics South Africa (2003) *Census 2001: Census in Brief*. Report No: 03-03-03. Pretoria: Statistics South Africa. On WWW at http://www.statssa.gov.za/census01/html/CInBrief/CIB2001.pdf.

Steinberg, A., Bain, L., Yeulin Li, Delgado, G. and Ruperto, V. (2003) Decisions Hispanic families make after the identification of deafness. *Journal of Deaf Studies and Deaf Education* 8 (3), 291–314.

Steinberg, A., Davila, J., Loew, R. and Fischgrund, J. (1997) A little sign and a lot of love: Attitudes, perceptions and beliefs of Hispanic families with deaf children. *Qualitative Health Research* 7 (2), 202–222.

Steinstra, D. (2002) The intersection of disability and race/ethnicity/official language/religion. Prepared for the 'Intersections of Diversity' seminar, Canadian Centre on Disability Studies, University of Winnipeg.

Stirling, M. (1992) How many pupils are being excluded? *British Journal of Special Education* 19 (4), 128–130.

Stockman, I.J. (2000) The New Peabody Picture Vocabulary Test-III, an illusion of unbiased assessment? *Language, Speech, and Hearing Services in Schools* 31, 340–353.

Stoddart, T., Pinal, A., Latzke, M. and Canaday, D. (2002) Integrating inquiry science and language. *Journal of Research on Science Teaching* 39 (8), 664–687.

Stokes, S., Wong, A.M-Y., Fletcher, P. and Leonard, L. (2006) Nonword repetition and sentence repetition as clinical markers of SLI: The case of Cantonese. *Journal of Speech, Language, and Hearing Research* 43, 865–878.

Stoltenberg, C., Magnus, P., Lie, R.T., Daltveit, A.K. and Irgens, L.M. (1997) Birth defects and parental consanguinity in Norway. *American Journal of Epidemiology* 145 (5), 439–448.

Stoltenberg, C., Magnus, P., Lie, R.T., Daltveit, A.K. and Irgens, L.M. (1998) Risk of stillbirth and infant death in Norway, 1967–1993. *American Journal of Epidemiology* 148 (5), 452–459.

Stothart, S., Snowling, M., Bishop, D.V.M., Chipchase, C. and Kaplan C. (1998) Language impaired pre-schoolers: A follow-up into adolescence. *Journal of Speech Language and Hearing Research* 41, 407–418.

Stow, C. and Dodd, B. (2003) Providing an equitable service to bilingual children in the UK: A review. *International Journal of Language and Communication Disorders* 38, 351–377.

Stow, C. and Dodd, B. (2005) A survey of bilingual children referred for investigation of communication disorders: A comparison with monolingual children referred in one area in England. *Journal of Multilingual Communication Disorders* 3 (1), 1–23.

Stow, C. and Pert, S. (2006) Phonological acquisition in bilingual Pakistani heritage children in England. In II. Zhu and B. Dodd (eds) *Phonological Development and Disorders in Children: A Multilingual Perspective* (pp. 326–345). Clevedon: Multilingual Matters.

Strand, S. (1999) Ethnic group, sex and economic disadvantage: Associations with pupils' educational progress from baseline to the end of Key Stage 1. *British Educational Research Journal* 25 (2), 179–202.

Street, B. (1984) *Literacy in Theory and Practice*. Cambridge: Cambridge University Press.

Street, B. (1993) *Cross-cultural Approaches to Literacy*. Cambridge: Cambridge University Press.

Street, B. (1994) Cross-cultural perspectives on literacy. In L. Verhoeven (ed.) *Functional Literacy* (pp. 95–112). Amsterdam: Johns Benjamins.

Street, B. (2003) The implications of the 'New literacy Studies' for literacy education. In S Goodman, T. Lillis, J. Maybin and N. Mercer (eds) *Language, Literacy and Education: A Reader* (pp. 77–88). Stoke: Trentham Books in association with The Open University.

Stringer, R. and Stanovich, K.E. (2000) The connection between reaction time and variation in reading ability: Unravelling covariance relationships with cognitive ability and phonological sensitivity. *Scientific Studies of Reading* 4 (1), 41–53.

Stromswold, K. (2000). The cognitive neuroscience of language acquisition. In M.S. Gazzaniga (ed.) *The New Cognitive Neurosciences* (pp. 909–932). Cambridge, MA: MIT Press.

Stromswold, K. (1998) Genetics of spoken language disorders. *Human Biology* 70, 297–324.

Svanberg, P. (1998) Attachment, resilience and prevention. *Journal of Mental Health* 7 (6), 543–578.

Swanepoel, D.W., Hugo, R. and Louw, B. (2006) Infant hearing screening at immunization clinics in South Africa. *International Journal of Pediatric Otorhinolaryngology* 70 (7), 1241–1249.

Tabors, P.O. (1997) *One Child, Two Languages: A Guide for Preschool Educators of Children Learning English as a Second Language*. Baltimore, MD: Paul Brookes.

Tager-Flusberg, H. and Cooper, J. (1999) Present and future possibilities for defining a phenotype for specific language impairment. *Journal of Speech, Language, and Hearing Research* 42, 1001–1004.

Tallal, P. (2000) Experimental studies of language learning impairments: From research to remediation. In D.V.M. Bishop and L.B. Leonard (eds) (2000) *Speech and Language Impairments in Children: Causes, Characteristics, Intervention and Outcome* (pp. 131–155). New York, NY: Psychology Press.

Tallal, P., Hirsch, L., Realpe-Bonilla, T., Miller, S., Brzustowicz, L., Bartlett, C. and Flax, J. (2001) Familial aggregation in specific language impairment. *Journal of Speech, Language, and Hearing Research* 44, 1172–1182.

Terrell, S.L. and Terrell, F. (1993) *Communication Disorders in Multicultural Populations*. Boston, MA: Butterworth-Heinemann.

Terzi, L. (2005) A capability perspective on impairment, disability and special needs. *Theory and Research in Education* 3 (2), 197–223.

Tharp, R. and Gallimore, R. (1988) *Rousing Minds to New Life*. New York: Cambridge University Press. In Mayer et al. 2002.

Thomas, W. and Collier, V. (1997) *School Effectiveness for Minority Language Students*. Washington, DC: National Clearinghouse for Bilingual Education. (NCBE) Resource Collection Series, No. 9, December. On WWW at http://www.ncbe.gwuu.edu.

Thordardottir, E.T. (2005) Early lexical and syntactic development in Quebec French and English: Implications for cross-linguistic and bilingual assessment. *International Journal of Language and Communication Disorders* 40 (3), 243–278.

Thorne, S. (2000) Second language acquisition theory and the truth(s) about relativity. In J. Lantolf (ed.) *Sociocultural Theory and Second Language Learning* (pp. 219–243). Oxford: Oxford University Press.

The Children Act (2004) London: Houses of Parliament, UK.

Tizard, B. and Hughes, M. (1984) *Young Children Learning: Talking and Thinking at Home and at School*. London: Fontana.

Tizard, J., Schofield, W.N. and Hewison, J. (1982) Collaboration between teachers and parents in assisting children's reading. *British Psychological Society* 52 (1), 1–15.

Tolfree, D. (ed.) (1996) *Restoring Playfulness: Different Approaches to Assisting Children who are Psychologically Affected by War or Displacement*. Sweden: Radda Barnen, Swedish Save the Children.

Tomasello, M. and Brooks, P. (1999) Early syntactic development: A construction grammar approach. In M. Barrett (ed.) *The Development of Language* (pp. 161–190). London: Psychology Press.

Tomblin, B.J., Records, N.L., Buckwalter, P., Zhang, X., Smith, E. and O'Brien, M. (1997) Prevalence of specific language impairment in kindergarten children. *Journal of Speech, Language, and Hearing Research* 40, 1245–1260.

Tomlinson, S. (1982) *A Sociology of Special Education*. London: Routledge.

Topbas, S. and Konrot, A. (1996) Variability in phonological disorders: A search for systematicity? Evidence from Turkish speaking children. *International Clinical Phonetics and Linguistics Association 5th Annual Conference*. Munich, Germany, 16–18 September.

Topbas, S. and Yavas, M (2006) Phonological acquisition and disorders in Turkish. In H. Zhu and B. Dodd (eds) *Phonological Development and Disorders in Children: A Multilingual Perspective* (pp. 233–261). Clevedon: Multilingual Matters.

Towell, R. and Hawkins, R. (1994) *Approaches to Second Language Acquisition.* Clevedon: Multilingual Matters.

Troyna, B. (1991) Underachievers or underrated? The experiences of students of South Asian origin in a secondary school. *British Educational Research Journal* 17 (4), 361–376.

Troyna, B. and Siraj-Blatchford, I. (1993) Providing support or denying access? The experiences of students designated as 'ESL' and 'SN' in a multi-ethnic secondary school. *Educational Review* 45 (1), 3–11.

Troyna, B. and Vincent, C. (1996) The ideology of expertism: The framing of special education and racial quality policies in the local state. In C. Christensen and F. Rizvi (eds) *Disability and the Dilemmas of Education and Justice* (pp. 131–144). Buckingham: Open University Press.

Ukrainetz, T., Harpell, S., Walsh, C. and Coyle, C. (2000) A preliminary investigation of dynamic assessment with Native American kindergartners. *Language, Speech, and Hearing Services in Schools* 31, 142–154.

UNESCO (1994) *The Salamanca Statement and Framework for Action on Special Needs Education.* World Conference in Special Needs Education: Access and Quality.

United Nations High Commissioner for Refugees (UNHCR) (2007) *Statistical Yearbook 2006, Trends in Displacement, Protection and Solutions.* Geneva: UNHCR.

Unsworth, L. (ed.) (2000) *Researching Language in Schools and Communities.* London: Continuum/Cassell.

US Census Bureau (USCB) (2007) *Census 2000: Language Use.* On WWW at http://www.census.gov/population/www/socdemo/lang_use.html.

Valdes, G. and Figueroa, R. (1994) *Bilingualism and Testing: A Special Case of Bias.* Stamford, CT: Ablex.

Valencia, R. (ed.) (1997) *The Evolution of Deficit Thinking: Educational Thought and Practice.* Washington, DC: Routledge.

Van Eldik, T., Tieffers, P.D., Veerman, J.W. and Verhulst, F.C. (2004) Mental health problems of deaf Dutch children as indicated by parent's responses to the child behavior checklist. *American Annals of the Deaf* 148, 390–396.

van Lier, L. (2000) From input to affordance: Social-interactive learning from an ecological perspective. In J. Lantolf (ed.) *Sociocultural Theory and Second Language Learning* (pp. 245–259). Oxford: Oxford University Press.

van Lier, L. (2008) Agency in the classroom. In J.P. Lantolf and M.E. Poehner (eds) *Sociocultural Theory and the Teaching of Second Languages* (pp. 163–186). London: Equinox.

van Tuijl, C., Leseman, P. and Rispens, J. (2001) Efficacy of an intensive home-based educational intervention programme for 4- to 6-year-old ethnic minority children in the Netherlands. *International Journal of Behavioral Development* 25 (2), 148–159.

Verhoeven, L. (1994) Transfer in bilingual development: The linguistic interdependence hypothesis revisited. *Language Learning* 44, 381–415.

Vincent, C. and Martin, J. (2005) Parents as citizens: Making the case. In G. Crozier and D. Reay (eds) *Activating Participation: Parents and Teacher Working Towards Partnership* (pp. 113–135). Stoke: Trentham Books.

Volterra, V. and Taeschner, T. (1978) The acquisition and development of language by a bilingual child. *Journal of Child Language* 5, 311–326.

Von Hapsburg, D. and Peña, E.D. (2002) Understanding bilingualism and its impact on speech audiometry. *Journal of Speech, Language, and Hearing Research* 45, 202–213.

Vostanis, P., Hayes, M., Du Feu, M. and Warren, J. (1997) Detection of behavioural and emotional problems in deaf children and adolescents: Comparison of two rating scales. *Child: Care, Health and Development* 23 (3), 233–246.

Vygotsky, L.S. (1978) *Mind in Society: The Development of Higher Psychological Processes.* Cambridge, MA: Harvard University Press.

Vygotsky, L.S. (1987) *The Collected Works of L.S. Vygotsky. Vol 1: Problems of General Psychology,* including the volume *Thinking and Speech,* R.W. Rieber and A.S. Carton (eds) (N. Minick trans.). New York: Plenum Press.

Walker, M. (1973) An experimental evaluation of the success of a system of communication for the deaf mentally handicapped. Unpublished MSc. thesis, University of London.

Walker, M. (1996) *The Makaton Core Vocabulary (1996 Revision): SYMBOLS.* Camberley, Surrey: Makaton Vocabulary Development Project.

Walker, M. and Armfield, A. (1981) What is the Makaton vocabulary? *Special Education: Forward Trends* 8 (3), 19–20.

Warner, R. (1999) The views of Bangladeshi parents on the special school attended by their young children with severe learning difficulties. *British Journal of Special Education* 26 (6), 218–223.

Wartofsky, M. (1979) Introduction. In *Model: Representation and the Scientific Understanding,* Volume XLVIII in the *Boston Studies in the Philosophy of Science.* Dordrecht/Boston/London: D. Reidel.

Washington, J.A. (1996) Issues in assessing language skills in African American children. In A.G. Kamhi, K.E. Pollock and J.L. Harris (eds) *Communication Development and Disorders in African American Children: Research, Assessment, and Intervention* (pp. 35–54). Baltimore, MD: Brookes.

Washington, J.A. and Craig, H.K. (1999) Performances of at-risk, African American preschoolers on the Peabody Picture Vocabulary Test-III. *Language, Speech, and Hearing Services in Schools* 30, 75–82.

Watson, C. (1995) *Making Hanen Happen: Leader's Guide.* Toronto: Hanen Centre.

Wauters, L.N., Van Bon, W.H.J. and Tellings, A.E.J.M. (2006) Reading comprehension of Dutch deaf children. *Reading and Writing* 19 (1), 49–76.

Wedell, K. (2005) Dilemmas in the quest for inclusion. *British Journal of Special Education* 32 (1), 3–11.

Weiss, B.D. and Coyne, C. (1997) Communicating with patients who cannot read. *The New England Journal of Medicine* 337 (4), 272–274.

Weiss, B.D., Reed, R., Kligman, E.W. and Abyad, A. (1995) Literacy and performance on the Mini-Mental State Examination. *Journal of American Geriatric Society* 43, 807–810.

Wells, G. (1986) *The Meaning Makers.* Sevenoaks: Hodder and Stoughton.

Wells, G. (1996) Using the tool-kit of discourse in the activity of learning and teaching. *Mind, Culture and Activity* 3 (2), 74–101.

Wells, G. (1999) *Dialogic Inquiry: Towards a Sociocultural Practice and Theory of Education.* Cambridge: Cambridge University Press.

Wells, G. (2000) Dialogic enquiry in education: Building on the legacy of Vygotsky. In C. Lee and P. Smagorinsky (eds) *Vygotskian Perspectives on Literacy Research:*

Constructing Meaning Through Collaborative Inquiry (pp. 51–85). Cambridge: Cambridge University Press.

Wenger, E. (1998) *Communities of Practice: Learning, Meaning and Identity.* Cambridge: Cambridge University Press.

Wertsch, J. (2000) Vygotsky's two minds on the nature of meaning. In C. Lee and P. Smagorinsky (eds) *Vygotskian Perspectives on Literacy Research: Constructing Meaning Through Collaborative Inquiry* (pp. 19–30). Cambridge: Cambridge University Press.

West, A. and Pennell, H. (2003) *Underachievement in Schools.* London: Routledge-Falmer.

West, T.G. (1997) *In the Minds Eye.* New York: Prometheus Books.

Westby, C. (1990) Ethnographic interviewing: Asking the right questions to the right people in the right ways. *Journal of Childhood Communication Disorders* 13 (1), 101–111.

Westby, C., Moore, C., Roman, R. (2002) Reinventing the enemy's language: Developing narratives in Native American children. *Linguistics and Education* 13 (2) 235–269.

Wheldall, K., Gibbs, D., Duncan, D. and Saund, S. (1987) Assessing the receptive language development of young children from Panjabi-speaking homes: The Panjabi Bilingual Version of the Sentence Comprehension Test. *Child Language Teaching and Therapy* 3, 170–181.

Winter, K. (1999) Speech and language therapy provision for bilingual children: Aspects of the current service. *International Journal of Language and Communication Disorders* 34, 1–85.

Winter, K. (2001) Numbers of bilingual children in speech and language therapy: Theory and practice of measuring their representation. *International Journal of Bilingualism* 5 (4), 465–495.

Wong-Fillmore, L. (1982) Instructional language as linguistic input: Second language learning in classrooms. In L.C. Wilkinson (ed.) *Communicating in the Classroom* (pp. 283–296). New York: Academic Press.

Woo, E.Y.C. and Hoosain, R. (1984) Visual and auditory functions of Chinese dyslexics. *Psychologia* 27, 164–170.

Wood, D., Bruner, J. and Ross, G. (1976) The role of tutoring in problem-solving. *Journal of Child Psychology and Child Psychiatry* 17, 89–100.

Woodcock, R.W. and Muñoz-Sandoval, A.F. (2001a) *Woodcock-Muñoz Language Survey – Normative Update, English Form.* Itasca, IL: Riverside.

Woodcock, R.W. and Muñoz-Sandoval, A.F. (2001b) *Woodcock-Muñoz Language Survey – Normative Update, Spanish Form.* Itasca, IL: Riverside.

Woods, A.G., Pena, E.D. and Martin, F.N. (2004) Exploring possible sociocultural bias on the SCAN-C. *American Journal of Audiology* 13, 173–184.

World Health Organisation (2004) *Chronic Suppurative Otitis Media: Burden of Illness and Management Options.* Child and Adolescent Health and Development, Prevention of Blindness and Deafness. Geneva: WHO.

World Health Organisation (WHO) *International Classification of Impairments, Disabilities and Handicaps.* Geneva: World Health Organisation.

Wright, J. (1996) Teachers and therapists: The evolution of a partnership. *Child Language Teaching and Therapy* 12 (1), 3–14.

Wyatt, T. (1999) An Afro-centred view of communicative competence. In D. Kovarsky, J. Duchan and M. Maxwell (eds) *Constructing (In) Competence:*

Disabling evaluations in clinical and social interaction (pp. 197–221). Mahwah, NJ: Lawrence Erlbaum.

Wyatt, T.A. (2002) Assessing the communicative abilities of clients from diverse cultural and language backgrounds. In D.E. Battle (ed.) *Communication Disorders in Multicultural Populations* (3rd edn, pp. 415–59). Boston, MA: Butterworth-Heinemann.

Wydell, T.N. and Butterworth, B. (1999) A case study of an English-Japanese bilingual with monolingual dyslexia. *Cognition* 70 (3), 273–305.

Yopp, H.K. (1992) Developing phonemic awareness in young children. *The Reading Teacher* 45, 696–703.

York, R., Heron, J.M. and Wolff, S. (1972) Exclusion from school. *Journal of Child Psychology and Psychiatry* 13 (4), 259–266.

Yoshinaga-Itano, C., Sedel, A.L., Coulter, D.K. and Mehl, A.L. (1998) Language of early- and later-identified children with hearing loss. *Pediatrics* 102 (5), 1161–1171.

Yuet-Yee Yim-Ng, Varley, R. and Andrade, J. (2000) Contribution of finger tracing to the recognition of Chinese characters. *International Journal of Language and Communication Disorders* 35 (4), 561–571.

Zentella, A.C. (1997) *Growing Up Bilingual: Puerto Rican Children in New York.* Oxford: Blackwell.

Zhu, H. and Dodd, B. (eds) (2006a) *Phonological Development and Disorders in Children: A Multilingual Perspective.* Clevedon: Multilingual Matters.

Zhu, H. and Dodd, B. (2006b) Towards developmental universals. In H. Zhu and B. Dodd (eds) *Phonological Development and Disorders in Children: A Multilingual Perspective* (pp. 431–449). Clevedon: Multilingual Matters.

Index

NB. Page numbers in **bold** show a whole chapter on a subject. Abbreviations used are CLD (Cultural and Linguistic Diversity), EAL (English as an Additional Language) and SEN (Special Educational Needs).
Author's note: I am indebted to Helen Bilton for compiling the index.